Advances in
Modern Environmental Toxicology v. / 2

VOLUME XII

Mechanisms and Toxicity
of Chemical
Carcinogens and Mutagens

Editors:

W. G. FLAMM
R. J. LORENTZEN

Published by:

PRINCETON SCIENTIFIC PUBLISHING CO., INC.
Princeton, New Jersey

Printed and bound in the United States of America.

PRINCETON SCIENTIFIC PUBLISHING CO., INC.
P.O. Box 2155
Princeton, New Jersey 08540
Tel.: 609/683-4750

LIBRARY OF CONGRESS CATALOG CARD NUMBER: 85-062106
ISBN 0-911131-12-4
Cover Art: From K. Palmer, Figure 2.

TABLE OF CONTENTS

EDITORIAL BOARD

William Lijinsky, Ph.D.
National Cancer Institute

Howard Maibach, M.D.
University of California, San
  Francisco School of Medicine

Edward J. Massaro, Ph.D.
The Pennsylvania State University

Irving Mauer, Ph.D.
United States Environmental
  Protection Agency

Vel Nari, Ph.D.
University of Health Sciences,
  The Chicago Medical School

Mr. R. Parkhi, D.V.M., Ph.D.
United States Environmental
  Protection Agency

Michael A. Pereira, Ph.D.
United States Environmental
  Protection Agency

William R. Pool, Ph.D.
G.D. Searle & Co.

Leonard D. Saslaw, Ph.D.
United States Food and Drug
  Administration

B.V. Rama Sastry, D.Sc., Ph.D.
Vanderbilt University

Russell P. Sherwin, M.D.
University of Southern California

Andrew Sivak, Ph.D.
Arthur D. Little, Inc.

Edward A. Smuckler, Ph.D., M.D.
University of California

B. L. Van Duuren, Sc.D.
New York University Medical Center

Jerry R. Williams, D.Sc.
George Washington University
  Medical Center

James Withey, Ph.D.
Bureau of Chemical Safety
  Ottawa, Canada

EDITORS' INTRODUCTION

This volume provides both a status report and an indication of future directions of research on the genetic mechanisms of carcinogenesis. This introduction briefly reviews two etiological factors involved in cancer causation and shows, where possible, how various theories on the mechanism of carcinogenesis relate to what is known about the etiology of cancer. In the final section of this introduction, the experimental evidence supporting the somatic mutation theory of cancer induction is discussed briefly. No attempt is made to discount the importance of other theories of cancer causation, particularly those dealing with oncogenes and immunosurveillance, but these subjects are beyond the scope of this text.

There are several major classes of agents which are known to induce cancer. These range from viruses to asbestos fibers, representing such diversity of cause as to appear virtually unique in the field of medicine. This diversity of causal agents has resulted in a long and arduous search for a common denominator to explain how such widely different agents can be responsible for the disease complex we call cancer. However, cancer is not a single disease but many diseases with features in common, such as lack of control of tissue growth. The possibility that certain specific cancers are caused by only one or a restricted number of etiological agents cannot be excluded. This raises the possibility that in efforts to prove or disprove theories of cancer causation, we may be imposing too great a burden on the theory by expecting that any single theory be compatible with all known causes of cancer.

Nevertheless, the temptation to conceptualize cancer as resulting from some single yet fundamental mechanism is extremely compelling. At the present time, the vast bulk of experimental evidence favors the long-held notion that the genome is critically involved in at least the very earliest steps of carcinogenesis. It is also important to keep in mind that carcinogenesis is a multi-stage process which offers the possibility of modulation by different etiological agents at many of the steps or stages involved. Therefore, it seems reasonable that research on mechanisms of carcinogenesis will, in the future, attempt to integrate the major and most promising theories of carcinogenesis into a more unified view, rather than attempting to prove one theory at the expense of another by using data selectively.

CHEMICALS

The ability of chemicals to induce cancer has been known for more than 200 years. It was first observed in 1776 by a physician, Sir Percival Pott, who found that chimney sweeps developed scrotal carcinomas due to contact with soot and tars. Since cancer was preceded by skin irritation and inflammation, the generally held belief at that time and for at least another 150 years was that the induced carcinoma was a consequence of chronic irritation—not an unreasonable conclusion considering the nature of the evidence available at that time. Subsequently, it became clear that the chronic irritation theory of carcinogenesis failed to explain other observations in which exposure lasted for only a short period of time while cancer developed many years later. Some of these observations were based on dye workers exposed to aromatic amines around the turn of the last century. Such observations were partly responsible for a mushrooming of experimental work in chemical carcinogenesis. One chemical after another was found to be carcinogenic, but more disturbing was the finding that so many different chemical classes were being implicated. In addition to polycyclic aromatic hydrocarbons and polycyclic aromatic amines, inorganic metals, nitrosamines, nitrosamides, nitro-aromatics, certain types of lactones, epoxides, mustards, and other alkylating agents were demonstrated as carcinogenic.

More recently, tests conducted by the National Cancer Institute/National Toxicology Program have shown that many other classes of chemicals have carcinogenic activity. Halogenated aromatics, halogenated aliphatics, certain esters of carboxylic acids, and monocyclic aromatic amines have been shown to induce cancer in rats and/or mice. The fact that such a diverse group of chemical structures can induce cancer in either animals or humans has been a puzzling feature in the etiology of cancer, particularly since these chemicals bear no apparent relationship to one another on structural grounds. The argument could be made, however, that while there are great dissimilarities in structure, there might be some commonality in their chemical properties. However, even a cursory examination of these diverse classes would indicate that they are dissimilar in terms of chemical reactivity, as well. The finding that the metabolites of certain carcinogens are more carcinogenic than the carcinogen itself led to the speculation that the metabolite of the carcinogen is actually responsible for cancer induction, and that the question concerning similarities in the chemistry of carcinogenic chemicals should focus on the active metabolite as opposed to the carcinogenic compound, *per se*. This approach has preoccupied a large number of cancer researchers for the last two decades and it has revealed that aromatic amines, polycyclic aromatic hydrocarbons, nitrosamines, and other classes of chemical carcinogens are metabolized to electrophiles. Such metabolites are then capable of interacting with the nucleophilic centers of cellular macromolecules, i.e., proteins and nucleic acids. Indeed, these revelations can be viewed as a unification theory for the initiation of carcinogenesis, explaining why such diverse compounds with such diverse structures and chemistry can have such similar biological activity.

It should be pointed out, however, that there are other classes of chemical compounds which do not appear to belong to this general grouping. That is, they do not appear to interact with the nucleophilic centers of proteins or nucleic acids and act by some as yet unknown mechanisms. Finding either a general or specific explanation for the ability of this equally diverse class of chemicals to produce cancer is becoming the new *raison d'etre* of chemical carcinogenesis. To repeat, carcinogenesis is a multi-step process and different classes of chemical carcinogens may be acting by totally different mechanisms to effect different steps in the process. It is generally believed that those chemical carcinogens which either are or become electrophiles through metabolic transformation effect the first important steps in this multi-step process. There is substantial evidence for implicating DNA and changes in the genetic material as constituting the critical first step. Much of the basis for believing that somatic mutation or, more generally, that permanent changes in the genome is a critical and obligatory feature of carcinogenesis, derives from this concept. But the fact that such a chemical as saccharin produces bladder cancer in rats but does not appear to belong to the group of chemicals which are either electrophiles or are metabolized to electrophiles forces the conclusion that chemicals may act in a variety of ways to effect the cancer incidence found in groups of treated animals.

In the last five years, debate has raged in the scientific community and in federal regulatory circles over whether these non-electrophilic carcinogens sometimes referred to as non-genotoxic or "epigenetic" carcinogens should be regulated and controlled in the same way that electrophilic carcinogens are handled. In the final chapter of this text, there is a discussion of the contemporary means by which the risk to humans from animal carcinogens can be assessed mathematically. Even so, these methods of assessing risk are controversial and do not completely resolve the ongoing disputes.

As pointed out in this final chapter, conservative assumptions and methodology are used to assure that the risk of cancer to exposed human populations is not underestimated. One of the reasons for the controversy concerning the non-electrophilic carcinogens relates to whether they should be treated with the same degree of conservatism. The argument put forth by some is that the need for mathematical approaches which embody the concept of no threshold, ergo zero response exists only at zero dose, is appropriate and applicable only to the electrophilic carcinogens. For the non-electrophilic carcinogens, it is argued that they may be effecting any of a variety of processes for which thresholds may exist. Rather than assume that cancer incidence data in the observable range should be extrapolated through zero, zero using an appropriate mathematical model, it is argued that these compounds are amenable to the traditional toxicological approach of determining a "no-observed effect level" (NOEL) and applying to it a safety factor. Indeed, there have been recent proposals that a classification scheme should be developed for chemical carcinogens which would enable regulatory scientists to apply different approaches to determining the levels of acceptable risks from electrophilic and non-electrophilic groups of chemical carcinogens.

In the current nomenclature, genotoxic carcinogens or their metabolites are electrophilic and as such react with DNA, resulting in genetic damage. The so-called non-genotoxic carcinogens are of the saccharin type and appear to act by some as yet undiscovered mechanism. The emphasis in this text is on the former group and on the scientific methods and approaches used to characterize it. But it is also possible that such studies will eventually lead to a better understanding of the so-called epigenetic carcinogens and how they function.

Finally, it should be pointed out that dietary changes, the amount of protein or fat in the diet, can result in dramatic and reproducible changes in tumor incidence. Hormonal imbalances and other critical disturbances in homeostasis are also known to affect tumor incidence. Probably most scientists would argue that micro and macronutrients and other dietary substances which affect cancer incidence should not be regarded as carcinogens *per se*. Historically, these affectors of cancer incidence have been called modifying factors, but it should be kept in mind that the possibility exists that certain of the non-genotoxic substances found to induce cancer in experimental animals at high dosage levels may be affecting endocrine balance and other homeostatic mechanisms to produce cancer in ways similar to the way modifying factors induce cancer. The possibility that such substances may be active only at high dose and not at low dose is an important consideration with public health implications.

ONCOGENIC VIRUSES

While there is no question that chemicals can induce cancer in both humans and experimental animals, it is equally true that viruses produce cancer. The viral origin of cancer was the subject of speculation in the early 1900's, during the period of rapidly expanding knowledge about acute infectious diseases in humans. The first evidence of viral involvement in tumor formation came from the studies by Rous, who discovered that cell-free filtrates of sarcomas obtained from chickens produced tumors when injected into normal chickens.

It is clearly not the purpose of this volume to address the vast literature and body of scientific knowledge dealing with the viral origin of cancer. It is mentioned here simply to point out a few current and fundamental facts. First, while many RNA and DNA viruses are known to be the cause of certain types of cancer in a variety of experimental animal species, no conclusive evidence yet exists to prove that any human cancer is caused by a specific virus, and the laborious search for a viral etiology of human cancer has been disappointing thus far. At a basic mechanistic level, it can be argued that both chemicals and viruses have the same fundamental properties of affecting and permanently altering the genetic material of a cell. One of the major discoveries of the 1960's was the surprising finding that oncogenic RNA viruses are able to produce DNA complementary to the nucleotide sequence in their RNA, using an enzyme originally called reverse transcriptase. The synthesized DNA then incorporates itself into the DNA of the host cell and, as with oncogenic DNA viruses, carcinogenic chemicals, UV and ionizing radiation, alters the genetic material of the host cell.

There are two basic types of oncogenic viruses, those that can be transmitted horizontally as a contagious neoplastic disease and those that are transmitted vertically from one generation to the next. In some cases, oncogenic viruses are essentially harmless to the species in which the virus is ordinarily found, but when injected into a different species produces cancer. A classical example of this is the SV40 virus (simian virus) which is harbored in monkeys without causing disease, but induces sarcomas upon injection into hamsters. In fact, there are viruses of human origin, adenoviruses, known to be oncogenic to hamsters, mice and rats.

While there is no evidence that adenoviruses are causally involved in human cancer, there is evidence to implicate certain viruses as a possible cause of human cancer. Burkitt's lymphoma, discovered in 1958 in East Africa, represents one such possiblity. Clinically characterized by a swelling of facial bones with extensive metastases to internal organs, it is a highly malignant form of lymphoma.

SOMATIC MUTATION THEORY OF CARCINOGENESIS

The very fact that exposure to a chemical carcinogen may precede by decades the development of the cancer it induces implies some type of "permanent" alteration in the transformed somatic cell(s). For the exposure to be "remembered" from one cell generation to the next until neoplasia ultimately develops, the easiest and perhaps most reasonable explanation is that a somatic "mutation" is responsible. This model is examined in much greater detail in Chapter II. Actual experimental evidence is voluminous but proof is lacking and a host of questions remain concerning the subcellular events which follow initial exposure to the carcinogen.

Empirical evidence that chemical carcinogens function by altering the genetic material of a somatic cell derives from a decade of study in which known chemical carcinogens were tested for their ability to induce mutations in bacteria. Leading this effort was Bruce Ames, who developed specific histidine requiring strains of *Salmonella typhimurium*. By treating these bacteria with a large series of carcinogenic chemicals and determining whether they reverted to histidine independence, it was possible to demonstrate that many so-called classic carcinogens were indeed mutagenic in bacteria. Often, however, these chemicals required metabolic transformation to an active electrophile before their mutagenic properties could be evidenced. Such metabolic transformation was generally achieved by adding the supernatant fraction ($9000 \times G$) of a homogenate from rat liver. Despite the early success of these efforts to show with certain classes of chemical carcinogens a high degree of correlation between mutagenicity in bacteria and chemical carcinogenicity in rodents, a large and troubling number of chemicals (and classes of chemicals) remain outside the correlation.

Perhaps the most compelling evidence that many carcinogenic agents function by inducing somatic "mutation" are the studies that show that DNA repair can alter the frequency of mutations induced by carcinogens and can alter the frequency of neoplastic transformation in tissue culture. Most critical, however, is the evidence that DNA repair can alter the frequency of tumors induced in animals or humans by carcinogenic treatment. Direct evidence in humans is provided by a disease known as *Xeroderma pigmentosa*, whose sufferers lack the ability to repair damage to DNA due to exposure to the UV portion of sunlight. The consequence of this inability is the development of skin tumors, often at young age, following exposure to sunlight. There are many forms of the disease, ranging from mild to very severe. Takehe et al. have demonstrated a high degree of correlation between the deficiency to repair DNA and the frequency of skin tumors arising from exposure to sunlight. These findings, along with parallel ones in animals, strongly suggest that damage to DNA followed by "fixation" (replication of DNA prior to repair of damage) is a critical first step in the development of neoplasia.

—*W. Gary Flamm and R.J. Lorentzen*

CHAPTER I

A HISTORICAL PERSPECTIVE OF CHEMICAL CARCINOGENESIS

Philippe Shubik
Green College
Oxford University
Oxford, United Kingdom

A. SOOT, COAL TAR, CARCINOGENIC HYDROCARBONS

I. Locally Induced Tumors

A reiteration of many of the well known facts about chemical carcinogenesis often bores the author and speaker as much as the reader and audience. Everyone who has attended a series of lectures on chemical carcinogenesis is sooner or later exposed to a slide of a portrait of Percival Pott and another of either an English or Danish chimney sweep of 200 years ago. However much one tries to write a brief historical introduction to the subject that is a little more interesting, one is inevitably forced back to the chimney sweeps and their scrotal cancers.

The fact that all our present studies in chemical carcinogenesis owe their beginnings to clinical observations is, I believe, of great importance and to be remembered carefully; however, at the same time, the precise nature of those observations and their experimental confirmation require detailed evaluation. Our requirements for experimental demonstration of "facts" have changed perceptibily during the past two decades; one has an impression that newer techniques allowing for more rapid and more mechanized experiments have imposed much less stringency upon the research worker to draw general conclusions. Facts that may or may not be relevant are accumulated and eventually sorted out and correlated. In the past, far fewer experiments were, of course, undertaken; those that were done were often done laboriously and subjected to much peer criticism and were often the subject of prolonged polemical arguments.

The fact that soot was undoubtedly associated with the occurrence of skin cancers in man was well known for many years. Various attempts were made to test this material in animals, but no one successfully induced cancer because (i)

1

the experiments were not conducted long enough, and (ii) the criteria for the induction of real cancer were most rigid. Various suggestions that neoplasm had been induced chemically were dismissed since the lesions induced were not thought to be "real" cancer. In fact, it is difficult to believe that a thorough search of the literature and experimental notes of the last century would not reveal many instances in which lesions that would now satisfy certain present day scientists as "tumours" could not be found. Indeed, in some cases, the present attitude that often includes benign tumors as end points of significance seems justified. Perhaps the best example of early day conservatism is that benign bladder tumors induced in rabbits by aromatic amines were dismissed as inconsequential and it was only when unequivocal invasive malignant tumors occurred in the aromatic amine fed dog that a conclusive result was believed to have been obtained.

Early Japanese scientists (Yamagiwa and Itchikawa, 1918), can, without doubt, be credited with starting the science of chemical carcinogenesis by inducing skin cancer in rabbits' ears by painting them with coal tar for many months. Their first description of these lesions is made in great detail and merits careful reading as the first dynamic description of the development of cancer. It has been a failing of cancer research that so little emphasis has been placed upon the fact that experimental techniques have permitted the research worker the privilege of observing the sequential development of cancer through various stages compared with the clinician observing human material—invariably at the end point stage.

The initial reaction to the induction of the rabbit ear tumors with coal tar was to question the diagnosis; in this instance, there was essentially no room for argument; many of the lesions induced were unequivocally malignant by any histopathological standards of the time. Subsequent efforts resulted in the demonstration that coal tar was an effective skin cancer inducer in other species including the mouse and the dog. The overall initial reaction in the scientific and medical community was that the prevalent theory that "chronic irritation" gave rise to cancer had been confirmed. Subsequent brilliant studies under the leadership of Kennaway demonstrated (Cook, et al, 1933, Cook and Kenna-way, 1938) that a single component of the carcinogenic coal tar then called 3,4-benzpyrene (subsequently called benzo(a)pyrene) appeared to be the active principle. This isolation of a single compound from literally thousands present in the coal tar was not done fortuitously. First of all, Kennaway and his colleagues made a synthetic tar by passing acetylene and hydrogen through a catalyst and making isoprene tar which proved to be carcinogenic. This estab-lished the fact that the carcinogenic moiety was likely to be a hydrocarbon, thus narrowing down the range of compounds to be examined. Secondly, the polycyclic hydrocarbon then called 1,2,5,6-dibenzanthracene (later called dibenzo(a,h)anthracene) had been independently synthesized and found to be fluorescent in the ultraviolet range. The Kennaway group then proceeded to look for fluorescent fractions of coal tar and were fortunate that benzo(a)pyrene was intensely fluorescent in ultraviolet light. As an aside, it is now quite certain that there are many other carcinogenic compounds—both hydrocarbons and heterocyclic compounds in coal tar—but these need to be categorized more carefully as to their structure and biological activity.

II. Induction of Systemic Tumors

By the time that the isolation of benzo(a)pyrene had been made, a variety of other discoveries in chemical carcinogenesis had occurred. Coal tar carcinogenesis had been observed not only to have a local, but also a systemic, effect. It was observed by Murphy and Sturm that mice painted with coal tar developed skin tumors and also lung adenomas. The prevalence of lung adenomas in mice was not yet known and this first example of enhancement of a tumor present commonly in the controls was not immediately recognized as such.

The polycyclic hydrocarbon carcinogens occupied the first place in the studies of the 1930s. The molecule of benzanthracene fascinated the organic chemists who could make a series of relatively simple methyl derivatives that would vary carcinogenicity and implied that chemical structure and the carcinogenic effect were closely related. The discovery that a related compound, 20-methylcholanthrene, was carcinogenic stimulated a great deal of theoretical speculation that somehow or another steroid metabolism might be involved in the endogenous production of chemical carcinogens. The *in vitro* synthesis of methylcholanthrene from the bile acid, desoxycholic acid, provided a great deal of food for thought; it is of some interest that this possibility has been resurrected recently in studies involving the bile acids as possible "promoters" of colon carcinogenesis. There was a great deal of work done on the relationship of structure to activity during the 1930s that lapped over into the '50s after the Second World War and has, one way or another, continued until the present time. The earlier studies on the metabolism of benzo(a)pyrene were hampered by lack of rapid analytical methods and it is astonishing to see how much was accomplished without liquid, paper or high pressure liquid chromatography and, indeed, even before the invention of spectrophotometers.

The pattern of the problems to come was discerned early in these studies when it became apparent that compounds would always be found to yield a variety of metabolites and it would be necessary to decide which of these was involved in the carcinogenic response and which were merely irrelevant, often just predictable detoxification products. The early metabolites of benzo(a)pyrene to be isolated were mainly hydroxy derivatives and these are now thought to be largely detoxification products. Unlike present day approaches using *in vitro* systems, the testing of metabolites involved the use of animal studies which were long and expensive and often not feasible.

III. Heterocyclic Hydrocarbon Carcinogens

The polycyclic hydrocarbon era resulted in the discovery of a variety of related heterocyclic hydrocarbon carcinogens, some of which had interesting side effects; 7-dibenzo(a,h)0 carbazole, for example, was found to induce both skin and liver tumors in rodents. Interestingly enough, this compound, which occurs in tobacco tars, was later found to induce bronchiogenic carcinomas readily in the hamster lung when introduced directly. The other heterocyclic compounds—notably the benzacridines, have only been studied superficially and probably merit further attention since they are ubiquitous, both in polluted atmospheres, cigarette smoke and certain combustion mixtures associated with occupational cancers. The fact that benzo(a)pyrene was not the only carcinogen in coal tar was reasonably obvious; however, it was clearly established in a series of experiments that there were potent carcinogens present in lower boiling fractions of coal tar that did not contain benzo(a)pyrene that were active on the skin of the rabbit and not the mouse. These compounds have never been identified. Interest in the carcinogenicity of certain catalytically cracked petroleum residues arose as a result of some epidemiological studies. Various carcinogenic fractions were identified with some concomitant fingerprinting of active compounds—again benzanthracenes and benzphenanthrenes. However, both in the case of coal tar and these petroleum residues, complete identification of active materials and particularly pinpointing those compounds responsible for human cancer has not yet been made. The usefulness of such information is obvious in assisting us to control occupational carcinogens without the necessity of undertaking prolonged animal experiments.

The biological characteristics of the carcinogenic response induced by these first carcinogens involved a series of different approaches. Subsequent to the availability of the first inbred mice, various experiments were undertaken to determine the role of genetic background. The fact that these, and subsequently other chemical carcinogens, could enhance the incidence of particular tumors seen in the controls was observed in the case of not only the lung adenomas noted by Murphy and Sturm, but in the instance of various other tumors such as lymphomas, hepatomas and mammary tumors. The obvious problem that this phenomenon might be different from the direct induction of tumors not seen in controls still exists and is unsolved. It now poses a considerable problem to those using chronic studies for practical toxicological purposes.

IV. Mechanism of carcinogenesis, initiation and promotion

The effect on carcinogenesis by polycyclic hydrocarbons and mixtures of associated factors was investigated by several scientists. These studies stemmed in large part from the popular concept that "chronic irritation" and injury played a part in the origin of cancer. Thus, the first notable experiment in the field was that of Deelman (1924) who incised the tar treated area on the skin of a mouse and noted that the wounding increased the numbers of papillomas induced, speeded up their induction time and localized a majority of the tumors to the site of the injury. It was not until almost 20 years later that Peyton Rous and several colleagues (Rous and Kidd, 1941; Mackenzie and Rous, 1941) repeated these studies and using the ear of the rabbit as a test site separated the two phenomena and recognized a two stage process for carcinogenesis in which he named the second stage—produced by the wounding—as "promotion."

4

Berenblum (1941) undertook a series of studies in which he examined a variety of agents in combination with 3,4-benzpyrene and 1,2,5,6-dibenzanthracene. He discovered that mustard gas would inhibit carcinogenesis, whereas croton oil greatly enhanced the process. He also made the interesting observation that has never been exploited that freezing the skin of the mouse with CO_2 snow could cause tumors. Indeed, it has been interesting to note that in some recent studies on bladder carcinogenesis, Cohen et al (1982) have used freezing of the urinary bladder as a non-specific source of "irritation."

In the course of his subsequent studies, Berenblum (1941) stumbled upon the remarkable properties of the irritant vegetable mixture, croton oil, in carcinogenesis. The effects of a weak solution of 3,4-benzpyrene were greatly enhanced by the concomitant application of croton oil. Berenblum immediately seized upon this finding to try and separate the two effects. M. J. Shear (1937) had somewhat earlier discovered that a solution of a non-carcinogenic fraction of creosote had a similar action and named this phenomenon "cocarcinogenesis." It was left to J. C. Mottram to discover that a single application of the carcinogen benzpyrene could be followed by applications of croton oil to produce tumors. Mottram, however, demonstrated that applications of croton oil before, as well as after, the single application of benzpyrene was important in determining the outcome (Mottram, 1944). Subsequently a study by Berenblum and Shubik (1947) demonstrated that a single subeffective dose of a polycyclic hydrocarbon carcinogen could be followed even after a prolonged interval by non-carcinogenic croton oil and that this would give rise to many skin tumors in mice. In these studies, Mottram's report that a prior or sensitizing dose of croton oil had an effect was not confirmed. This has been disputed since and still remains a controversial issue. However, the Berenblum and Shubik experiment established a model experimental situation for studying the stages of chemical carcinogenesis that has been used many times since. The active principle(s) of croton oil have been identified and the compound TPA has been widely studied (Hecker, 1968). Berenblum and Shubik used the Rous terminology of initiation and promotion to describe the stages in the mouse skin study and this terminology has been widely used since that time to describe similar situations, as well as a variety of other situations. Indeed, it is interesting to reflect on the changed attitude to terminology. Enormous care was taken to define terms when these original studies were undertaken; more recently, this approach has given way to a general use of terms such as "promotion" to cover many different situations.

The course of the investigations into the two stages of carcinogenesis in the skin proved to be somewhat disappointing. The studies of Rous and his co-workers concentrated their efforts on the descriptive nature of the tumors induced rather than on mechanisms. It was noted that many of the skin tumors in the rabbit skin would regress even though some were classified as "almost" carcinomas. Rous termed these tumors "carcinomatoid" tumors which have subsequently been called "keratoacanthomas" and "self healing cancers" in humans. The fact that many of the "tumors" occurring in the skin of the mouse following treatment with carcinogen and croton oil also regressed had been recorded initially by Shubik, but largely ignored as of importance since that time. The fact that the pattern of tumor induction by this method seems rather different from that occurring when tumors are induced by a carcinogen alone may obviously be of importance. However, subtle changes of this kind can only be detected in carefully conducted animal experiments and the more recent use of tissue culture systems has made such distinctions difficult to determine.

The extrapolation of these skin studies to other systems was slow in developing, but is now a fashionable area of research. In particular, there is interest in experimental models using the bladder and liver as end points. In none of these instances, however, is the definition of "promotion" made as clear as it was in the original mouse skin studies. The idea that there should be a two stage (at least) mechanism in chemical carcinogenesis involving an initial rapid "mutational" change followed (even after long intervals) by a secondary effect that results in the emergence of tumors is an attractive approach to many experimentalists.

B. NUTRITION AND CANCER

Attention to the problems of nutrition and cancer has become popular in the recent past. The studies undertaken initially by Tannenbaum (1940) and later by Tannenbaum in collaboration with Silverstone (Tannenbaum and Silverstone, 1953) have paved the way to many current views on cancer and nutrition. Tannenbaum's studies, like so many in carcinogenesis, started from clinical observations. Stimulated by the observations of Raymond Pearl derived from actuarial data of the Metropolitan Life Insurance Company in New York that overweight was correlated with a higher cancer incidence, Tannenbaum embarked on a series of carefully planned studies. He investigated the effects of diet on induced, spontaneous and transplanted tumors in animals. For the purpose of this review, it is only necessary to say that he demonstrated with great clarity that caloric restriction resulted in an inhibition of tumor induction by several carcinogenic chemicals; attempts to demonstrate the association of such effects with various dietary components—carbohydrates, fats or proteins or with micronutrients (i.e., minerals or vitamins)—invariably pointed back to caloric restriction as the major factor. Indeed, many of the more recent studies in this field—and most simply repetitive of Tannenbaum's investigations—overlook the need to control caloric intake with great care. In the context of the discovery of initiation and promotion, it is of importance to point out that Tannenbaum discovered that there were two phases in chemical tumor induction from his dietary studies by observing that caloric restriction operated at certain times during tumor induction and not at others.

C. SPECIES AND ORGAN/TISSUE DIFFERENCES IN SENSITIVITY TO CHEMICAL CARCINOGENS

The other biological studies immediately following the initial discovery of the carcinogenicity of coal tar concerned the investigation of the species specificity and tissue specificity of the polycyclic hydrocarbons and subsequently of the various other compounds discovered to have carcinogenic action. Coal tar was soon (Tsutsui, 1918) discovered to have a similar action on the skin of the mouse and later in the dog. After benzpyrene was isolated from tar, it was found to have different potencies in different species. Although it was the presumptive active principle of coal tar, it was more active on the skin of the mouse than coal tar, but less active than coal tar in the rabbit. This fact led to the observation by Berenblum and Schoental (1942) and subsequent unpublished studies by Berenblum and Shubik (1947) that coal tar contained other carcinogens in benzpyrene free fractions that were active in the rabbit. Although benzpyrene induced many sarcomas following intramuscular injection in the mouse, the rat was quite resistant to this action. Later this polycyclic hydrocarbon, as well as several others, were fed to the rat and other rodents. The only tumors induced with regularity were squamous cell carcinomas of the forestomach and tumors of the small intestine. This was frustrating to research workers during the 1940s and 1950s, given the fact that adenocarcinoma of the stomach which was common in both men and women in the U.S. and Europe is a very different type of tumor than that being induced experimentally. Much effort was expended in reproducing this cancer in the laboratory and, in fact, no real success was achieved until nitrosomethylguanidine was discovered by Sugimura (Sugimura, et al, 1966) and found to give rise to some adenocarcinomas of the stomach by Stewart and others at the NCI, but this discovery was not exploited further in any meaningful way.

An animal new to the research laboratory—the Mastomys Nataliensis—was introduced and aroused considerable excitement since it developed adenocarcinoma of the stomach in the natural state. This seemingly minor point is belabored here to point to the greatly different emphasis placed upon such details as the histopathological nature of the induced lesion in man and test animal only 30 years ago. The influence of the pathologist in research has greatly declined since then, although the matter of extrapolation from species to species—particularly from rat to man, remains a major problem to the toxicologist.

D. TOXICOLOGICAL CONCERNS FOR CHEMICAL CARCINOGENESIS

The new interest in carcinogenesis as part of toxicology can best be dated to the discovery of one of the most important experimental carcinogens, acetylaminofluorene, in the course of a chronic toxicity test of a proposed pesticide. This compound, unlike the compounds derived from coal tar, had a systemic effect and was inactive locally. Various tumors occurred following feeding—mammary, liver, bladder and others. As will be discussed later, the biochemical disposition of this compound was responsible for this effect.

Aware of the potential carcinogenicity of various chemicals, the Food and Drug Administration scientists from the U.S.A.—notably, Fitzhugh, Nelson and Lehman, started testing various compounds in 2 year rat studies in the

1940s. In particular, they reported the occurrence of liver tumors with DDT and other chlorinated hydrocarbon pesticides, as well as a range of other interesting results. The discovery of the polycyclic aromatic hydrocarbon carcinogens had provided a field day for the organic chemists. The molecule of benzanthracene was particularly amenable to minor changes and many variants—particularly alkyl benzanthracenes—were synthesized and tested in an effort to establish structure activity relationships. The biological variants that occur when different routes of administration or different species were used did not seem to bother anyone particularly. The Pullmans (Pullman and Pullman, 1955) drew attention to the possible correlation between carcinogenic potency and electron distribution at certain seemingly key points in the molecule. These studies have led the way to the present continued interest in the significance of certain metabolic changes determined by structure in the action of some of these compounds.

The next series of carcinogens to be discovered were the azo dyes—butter yellow—p-dimethylaminoazobenzene—discovered by Yoshida (1932) leading the way and resulting, as with the polycyclic hydrocarbons, in the synthesis of a series of related compounds. These compounds were tested by the oral route and resulted in the development of hepatomas variously in the rat and the mouse and at different levels of potency. Most notably, a major advance was made in approaches to the biochemical investigation of carcinogens using this group of compounds by the Millers (Miller and Miller, 1953) who determined that these compounds were bound to protein and could correlate the level of binding with carcinogenic potency. The Millers later demonstrated the metabolic pathway taken by acetylaminofluorene to the "proximate" carcinogen—the N-hydroxylated derivative (Miller, et al, 1961).

The aromatic amine carcinogens associated with human bladder cancer had been suspect from studies in human occupational groups since the end of the 19th century (Rhen, 1895); however, these effects had not been reproduced effectively in animals until Hueper, Wiley and Wolf succeeded in inducing bladder carcinoma in the dog with B-naphthylamine (1938); for some many years after this, it was believed that it was essential to use the dog for tests of related compounds. These compounds only induced hepatomas in rats and mice. Since it was by then apparent that the aromatic amines were probably metabolized to a proximate carcinogen and that this was concentrated in the urine, various efforts were made to find short cuts to testing these important occupational hazards. A technique was devised to implant these compounds and their potential metabolites directly into the bladder of the mouse. This technique did not prove to be satisfactory since it was found that the vehicle pellets alone, made of either cholesterol or paraffin wax, induced many bladder tumors. This was one of the first examples of probable physical carcinogenesis. More convincing in support of physical carcinogenesis were the studies of Oppenheimer's (Oppenheimer, et al, 1948) who found that tumors could be induced subcutaneously in the rat by implantation of pieces of plastic initially; this was followed by demonstrations that a variety of other materials could do the same, including various metals. In these studies, convincing evidence was found to show that the effect was associated with physical, rather than chemical, characteristics. A disc of a plastic, for example, would result in a sarcoma, whereas powdered plastic of the same kind had no effect. In a study of the effects of implanted paraffin waxes of various kinds (Shubik, et al), it was found that sarcoma inducing ability in the mouse was related to the melting point of the wax rather than to its chemical composition. The mechanism of induction of sarcomas in this way has not been elucidated, although various suggestions have come from different studies, including those with tissue cultures. Although the occurrence of these sarcomas following implantation of inert plastics and other materials is mentioned from time to time, it is difficult to reconcile with current theories of mechanisms of carcinogenesis.

Throughout the history of the study of chemical carcinogens, there has been an understandable desire to have available quick methods for testing these compounds. Studies of metabolism have continuously been hampered by the length of time required to validate the activity of metabolites. The current vogue for short-term testing was preceded by some imaginative studies by J. C. Mottram who introduced Paramecia as test objects; this model was exploited later, but not found adequate. In a study by K. Spencer, G. Pietra and P. Shubik, it was found that the newborn mouse was singularly susceptible to the development of lymphomas following administration by injection of polycyclic hydrocarbons. Efforts were made to exploit this observation as a rapid test for carcinogenicity, but this proved, as might have been expected, to be quite limited as a result of the metabolic inadequacies of the newborn animal. The use of tissue cultures was begun during the early days of the development of the National Cancer Institute by Wilton Earle, who tested methylcholanthrene in fibroblast cultures (Earle and Nettleship, 1943).

Initially, much excitement was generated by the occurrence of various morphological changes in the cultured cells. However, as these studies were pursued, it was found that untreated cultures transplanted subcutaneously to mice became sarcomas. As a result, the use of tissue cultures for the study of chemical carcinogens fell into disrepute for some years, although Earle, Gey and others continued their careful studies for many years. At that time, the occurrence of spontaneous "transformation" would have invalidated a study for most research workers unlike the philosophy of today in which partially transformed cells such as the 3T3 are considered to be most suitable for much fundamental cancer research.

Amongst the other carcinogens discovered early in this saga was urethan or ethyl carbamate. This discovery, made fortuitously, arose from the use of this simple compound as an anesthetic in animal experiments (Nettleship and Henshaw, 1943). Initially, the idea that a compound with this chemical structure could be carcinogenic came as a considerable shock to those research workers contemplating the structure activity relationships primarily of the polycyclic hydrocarbons. However, this concern was to some extent mitigated by the observation that the only effect of this compound was to enhance the incidence of lung adenomas in the mouse—particularly in mice with high lung adenoma incidences. It was not until some years later that it was discovered (Tannenbaum and Silverstone, 1958) that urethan had a much wider spectrum of effects inducing various other tumors and subsequent studies in the hamster, for example, revealed that urethan could give rise to melanocytomas in the dermis. The chemical specificity of urethan (ethyl carbamate) has proved quite remarkable—the methyl carbamate, for example, proving not to be carcinogenic. In spite of much interesting work, no biochemical mechanism of action has been found to be suggestive.

The occurrence of lung adenomas has proved to be of considerable interest to those seeking rapid tests for carcinogenesis. Shimkin has, for some years, suggested testing compounds in mice with a high lung adenoma incidence for a limited period of 6 months or so. Such proposals have received considerable attention, but problems of a high false positive and false negative error rate have prevented their wide application.

It is difficult to know where a historical account of chemical carcinogenesis stops and a review of current work begins. I have decided arbitrarily to carry this account on to the discovery of two additional groups of compounds, the nitrosamines and aflatoxins, since they provide both an illustration of the breadth of vision that must be employed in contemplating these problems in a practical sense and also have so much widened the view of those interested in determining mechanisms.

The discovery of the carcinogenicity of dimethylnitrosamine followed the observation of liver damage occurring in men exposed occupationally to this compound. Barnes and Magee tested this compound in the Medical Research Council Toxicology Unit of the U.K. as a practical toxicological test (Barnes and Magee, 1954). It was, of course, found to be a potent carcinogen inducing liver tumors in rats when fed chronically and kidney tumors when given for a limited period. This discovery has proved to be a landmark; first of all subsequent studies demonstrated that this compound alkylated DNA and that a specific alkylated base—7 methylguanine—could be isolated (Magee and Hultin, 1962). Even though this early work is now considered to provide an unlikely pathway for the carcinogenic action of this compound, it has led to the current series of studies in which nucleic acids are considered to be involved in the initiation stage of carcinogenesis. Secondly, the many studies of Druckrey and his co-workers have resulted in the synthesis of a large number of compounds capable of inducing many tumors not previously seen before in experimental systems. Druckrey has also used these compounds and related compounds in studies of the dose response that might be encountered in carcinogenesis and has laid the foundations for some of the basic concepts underlying the popular regulatory approaches ("risk assessment") to handling carcinogenic chemicals.

The aflatoxins were discovered, again fortuitously, in the pursuit of solutions to practical problems. In this instance, the problem was the killing of many turkeys that had been fed on peanut meals. It was found that this was due to aflatoxin—a fungal metabolite—that additionally has proved to be immensely potent as a carcinogen to several species. It might also have been discovered later in the investigation of an "epidemic" of liver tumors in hatchery trout—an occurrence in which all the fish developed these tumors. The aflatoxin in this instance appears to have come from contaminated cotton seed. The discovery of the aflatoxins illustrated that the occurrence of carcinogenics in the human environment could come just as easily from natural sources as from man-made synthetic processes. It seems not unreasonable to believe that human exposure in underdeveloped countries could play a role in the occurrence of liver cancer—at least as one of the factors.

E. SUMMARY

This brief account of the history of chemical carcinogenesis has drawn attention to the beginnings of some of the studies and to the changing approaches to research that have occurred. Clearly, the account is by no means complete—it would require a book of some length to achieve this aim. However, it is hoped that the main trends are illustrated for the purposes of this volume. Historically, the first occurrence of note was the clinical observation of the carcinogenicity of soot; the subsequent confirmation of the carcinogenicity of coal tar to animals; the isolation of benzpyrene from coal tar and the subsequent synthesis of the many carcinogenic polycyclic hydrocarbons. The early studies of metabolism and on the biological characteristics of the effects of these compounds have paved the way to continued scientific investigation. The discovery of the many other chemical carcinogens has illustrated the ubiquity of these compounds and has formed the basis for cancer prevention.

REFERENCES

Barnes, J.M., and Magee, P.N. Some toxic properties of dimethylnitrosamine. Brit. J. Ind. Med. 11, 167–174 (1954).

Berenblum, I. Mechanism of carcinogenesis; study of significance of cocarcinogenic action and related phenomena. Cancer Res. 1, 807–814 (1941).

Berenblum, I. and Schoental, R. Rate of disappearance of 3:4-benzpyrene from mouse after subcutaneous and intraperitoneal injection. Biochem. J. 36, 92–97 (1942).

Berenblum, I. and Shubik, P. New, quantitative, approach to study of stages of chemical carcinogenesis in mouse's skin. Brit. J. Cancer 1, 383–391 (1947).

Cohen, S.M., Murasaki, G., Fukushima, S., and Greenfield, R.E. Effect of Regenerative Hyperplasia on the Urinary Bladder: Carcinogenicity of Sodium Saccharin and N-[4-(5-nitro-2-furyl)-2-thiazolyl] formamide, Cancer Res. 42, 65–71 (1982).

Cook, J.W., Hewett, C.L., and Hieger, I. The isolation of a cancer-producing Hydrocarbon from coal tar. Parts I, II and III. J. Chem. Soc. 395–405 (1933).

Cook, J.W., and Kennaway, E.L. Chemical compounds as carcinogenic agents; first supplementary report: literature of 1937. Am. J. Cancer 33, 50–97 (1938).

Deelman, H.T. Die Entstehung des experimentellen Teerkrebses und die Bedeutung der Zellenregeneration, Ztschr. f. Krebsforsch 21, 220–226 (1923–24).

Earle, W.R., and Nettleship, A. Production of malignancy in vitro; results of injections of cultures into mice. J. Nat. Cancer Inst. 4, 213–227 (1943).

Hecker, E. Cocarcinogenic principles from the seed oil of Croton tiglium and from other Euphorbiaceae. Cancer Res. 28, 2338–2349 (1968).

Hueper, W.C., Wiley, F.H., and Wolfe, H.D. Experimental Production of Bladder

Tumors in Dogs by Administration of beta-Naphthylamine, J. Indust. Hyg. **20**, 46 (1938).

MacKenzie, I. and Rous, P. Experimental disclosure of latent neoplastic changes in tarred skin. J. Exper. Med. **73**, 391–416 (1941).

Magee, P.N. and Hultin, T. Toxic liver injury and carcinogenesis. Methylation of proteins of rat-liver slices by dimethylnitrosamine in vitro. Biochem. J. **83**, 106–114 (1962).

Miller, J.A. and Miller, E.C. The carcinogenic aminoazo dyes. Advan. Cancer Res. **1**, 339–396 (1953).

Miller, E.C., Miller, J.A., and Hartmann, H.A. N-Hydroxy-2-acetyl-aminofluorene: a metabolite of 2-acetylaminofluorene with increased carcinogenic activity in the rat. Cancer Res. **21**, 815–824 (1961).

Mottram, J.C. Developing factor in experimental blastogenesis. J. Pathol. Bacteriol. **56**, 181–187 (1944).

Nettleship, A. and Henshaw, P.S. Induction of Pulmonary Tumors in Mice with Ethyl Carbamate (Urethane), J. Nat'l Cancer Inst. **4**, 309 (1943).

Oppenheimer, B.S., Oppenheimer, E.T., and Stout, A.P. Sarcomas induced in rats by implanting cellophane. Trans. Assoc. Am. Physicians **51**, 343–348 (1948).

Pullman, A. and Pullman, B. Electronic Structure and Carcinogenic Activity of Aromatic Molecules, Advanc. Cancer Res. **3**, 117 (1955).

Rhen, L. Ueber Blasentumoren bei Fuchsinarbeitern, Arch. Klin. Chir. **50**, 588 (1895).

Rous, P. and Kidd, J.G. Conditional neoplasms and subthreshold neoplastic states; study of tar tumors in rabbits. J. Exper. Med. **73**, 365–390 (1941).

Shear, M.J. Studies in carcinogenesis; production of tumors in mice with hydrocarbons. Am. J. Cancer **26**, 322–332 (1936).

Shear, M.J. Studies in carcinogenesis; development of liver tumors in pure strain mice following injection of 2-amino-5-azotoluene. Am. J. Cancer **29**, 269–284 (1937).

Sugimura, T., Nagao, M., and Okada, Y. Nature **210**, 962 (1966).

Tannenbaum, A. Initiation and growth of tumors; introduction, effects of underfeeding. Am. J. Cancer **38**, 335–350 (1940).

Tannenbaum, A. and Silverstone, H. Nutrition in relation to cancer. Advan. Cancer Res. **1**, 451–501 (1953).

Tannenbaum, A. and Silverstone, H. Urethan (ethyl carbamate) as a multi-potential carcinogen. Cancer Res. **18**, 1225–1231 (1958).

Tsutsui, H. Uber das Kunstlich erzeugte Cancroid bei der Maus, GANN **12**, 17 (1918).

Yamagiwa, K. and Itchikawa, K. Experimental Study of the pathogenesis of carcinoma. J. Cancer Res. **3**, 1–29 (1918).

Yoshida, T. Ueber die experimentelle Erzeugung von Hepatom durch die Futtering mit o-Amido-azotoluol, Proc. imp. Acad. Japan **8**, 464 (1932).

CHAPTER II

PERSPECTIVES ON THE SOMATIC MUTATION MODEL OF CARCINOGENESIS

Brian D. Crawford
University of California
Los Alamos National Laboratory
Genetics Group, LS-3, M886
Los Alamos, New Mexico 87545

A. INTRODUCTION

".... One of the fundamental attributes of a mutation is its sudden appearance. Malignant neoplasms, on the contrary, generally do not arise until after long-continued cellular derangement .... The cytological changes preceding the outbreak of most malignant neoplasms may require a number of years for their evolution. At what moment in the process shall we place the mutation? If at the end, what was the nature of the preceding stages? If at the beginning, not one, but a whole series of successive mutations would have to be acknowledged. And here we fall into absurdity . . ."

Charles Oberling
The Riddle of Cancer, 1952

Cancer remains a horrible enigma—horrible in the pain and suffering it brings to diseased individuals, and an enigma in that despite significant knowledge of its biology, the mechanisms underlying its genesis remain elusive.

As a prelude to other chapters in this volume, this review is designed to emphasize that a critical evaluation of the relationship between mutagenesis and carcinogenesis requires first that each process be quantitated, and the mechanisms underlying each process be defined. Somatic mutation can be studied reliably in the laboratory by examining various heritable phenotypic alterations of mammalian cells, particularly resistance to certain drugs. With the advent of recombinant DNA technology, the molecular basis of gene mutation can now be defined at the DNA level, in biochemical terms. In contrast, neoplastic transformation is less well understood, a fact partially attributable to the lack of a single definitive phenotypic alteration that is characteristic of malignancy. Although tumor formation *in vivo* serves to define neoplastic transformation of cells *in vitro*, tumorigenesis is a multistage, multi-faceted phenomenon which is difficult to analyze at the molecular or cellular level. Several *in vitro* phenotypic characteristics which are associated with neoplastic cells have, however, been studied extensively. Somatic mutation and neoplastic transformation can therefore be investigated by essentially the same experimental approach, by studying heritable alterations of cells in culture. Because this is of necessity an artificial situation, the elucidation of the significance of particular *in vitro* cellular changes to tumorigenicity is crucial to an understanding of neoplastic transformation. As will be described in this chapter, and those which follow in this volume, modern cellular and molecular genetic techniques now are interfacing *in vitro* and *in vivo* studies of neoplasia, and are providing new perspectives on mutational theories of cancer. With these new perspectives come new experimental challenges, and promise for the future.

B. A THEORETICAL PERSPECTIVE: CANCER IS A MULTISTAGE, PROGRESSIVE DEVELOPMENTAL PROCESS

I. Neoplastic Progression

A multistage model of neoplastic development purports that carcinogenesis is not a simple, one-step process. In contrast, most mutational changes can be described by a one-step transition. Before one can evaluate critically the role of mutation in cancer, this complexity of neoplastic transformation must be recognized.

The concept of a progressive nature of neoplastic development was defined best by Leslie Foulds (Foulds, 1969). Histologically distinct stages in the neoplastic development of cancers of the skin, respiratory tract, mammary glands, uterus, and prostate provided pathological evidence that tumors develop through a series of qualitatively different stages (summarized by Foulds, 1954; 1969; 1975). Foulds proposed several principles of neoplastic development, based upon extensive pathological examinations of tumors. These principles emphasized not only the multistage and multifactorial nature of carcinogenesis, but also proposed the *stochastic* emergence of variant sub-populations of cells within a neoplasm. Foulds was limited, however, in his ability to prove conclusively the developmental path of a tumor cell, because his histological studies utilized fixed tissue (the history and future development of which could only be surmised). Nowell (1976) incorporated Foulds' concepts into a clonal evolution hypothesis of neoplasia, which proposed that tumor cell heterogeneity reflects the random generation and proliferation of phenotypic variant stem cell lines, from a single clone of neoplastic cells. Each of these stemlines then exhibit continued growth *in vivo*. Neoplastic progression is thus characterized by the emergence of variant stemlines with selective growth advantage in the host (Fidler, 1978).

In addition to pathological evidence, epidemiologic data support a multistage model of cancer. Certain human cancers, such as retinoblastoma (Knudson, 1971, 1973, 1977; Knudson, *et al.*, 1975; Hethcote and Knudson, 1978; Benedict, *et al.*, 1983), medullary thyroid carcinoma (Baylin, *et al.*, 1978), and carcinoma of the colon and rectum (Ashley, 1969) appear to arise by multiple cellular changes. Epidemiologic and clinical evidence has been presented to support the hypothesis that these diseases, which occur at high frequency in genetically predisposed individuals, arise by at least two mutational events (Knudson, 1971; Knudson, *et al.*, 1975; Hethcote and Knudson, 1978; Baylin, *et al.*, 1978). Additionally, statistical analysis of the age-specific incidence of various kinds of cancer is consistent with a multistage nature of neoplastic development (reviewed by Peto, 1977). Several analyses of epidemiologic data have shown that the logarithm of the incidence of various neoplasms is related linearly to the logarithm of age; the calculated slope of this linear relationship suggests that multiple, independent cellular changes must accumulate before neoplastic transformation is expressed. The number of required events ranges from two or three to seven, according to the type of neoplasm (Ashley, 1969, Armitage and Doll, 1961; Doll, 1978; Peto, 1977).

Finally, experimental systems have demonstrated carcinogenesis to be more than a one-step process. In mice, a two-stage (initiation and promotion) model has been defined in epidermal carcinogenesis (Berenblum, 1954; 1978). Studies of neoplastic transformation of cells in culture, a topic to which much of this volume is addressed, have supported a multistage model of carcinogenesis (Mondal, Brankow, and Heidelberger, 1976; Mondal and Heidelberger, 1977; Fernandez *et al.*, 1980; Kennedy *et al.*, 1980; Barrett and Ts'o, 1978a; 1978b; 1978c; Barrett, *et al.*, 1977; Barrett, *et al.*, 1980; Crawford, *et al.*, 1983; Smith and Sager, 1982). This important parallel of *in vivo* carcinogenesis helps to justify the use of cell culture models in the study of oncogenesis, and provides the rationale for *in vitro* experimental approaches designed to dissect the stages of neoplastic development.

II. Comparing Mutation and Transformation

If one accepts a multistage model of neoplastic development, a simple comparison between single-step mutagenesis and carcinogenesis becomes inadequate. In contrast to conventionally studied somatic mutations, which may be described by a single-step change (wild type → mutant), a multistep process such as tumor progression might be comprised of a number of mutational steps, a number of nonmutational steps, or a combination of both mutational and nonmutational steps. If the latter is the case, then carcinogenesis involves both genetic and so-called epigenetic changes. As described below, the heritable nature of neoplasia, the association of chromosomal abnormalities and inborn genetic disorders with increased susceptibility to malignancy, the documented mutagenicity of most carcinogens, and the demonstration that DNA is a critical target in carcinogenesis all support a role for gene mutation in neoplastic development. However, the relative organ specificity of neoplastic disorders in genetically predisposed individuals (Feinberg and Coffey, 1982), specific hormonal influences on tumor development (Henderson *et al.*, 1977), and the high frequency with which both teratocarcinomas (Mintz, 1978) and certain cellular phenotypic characteristics associated with neoplasia can be induced all emphasize that nonmutational factors in oncogenesis must not be overlooked. Accordingly, any hypothesis on carcinogenesis must acknowledge an array of interacting genetic and epigenetic influences.

Considering the apparent multistage and possibly multifactorial nature of carcinogenesis, understanding the role of mutagenesis in carcinogenesis requires first a dissection of the process of neoplastic development into individual phenotypic transitions, followed by an appraisal of the mutational or nonmutational mechanisms of a particular transition. If neoplastic development can be defined by a series of stages, then hopefully, the contribution of mutagenic changes can be delineated for each step during the transformation of a normal cell to a malignant cell. This rationale has provided the basis for the application of cell culture models for the comparative study of mutagenesis and carcinogenesis (reviewed by Barrett, Crawford, and Ts'o, 1980; Crawford *et al.*, 1983).

In addition to considering whether a step in neoplastic development can be explained by a mutational mechanism, one also must consider the type of mutation involved. If the changes in neoplastic development are mutational, they might involve gene mutations which result in dominant, codominant, X-chromosome-linked recessive, or autosomally-linked recessive phenotypes. The first three types of gene mutations are all expressed phenotypically following a single mutational event, whereas autosomal recessive phenotypes require a two-step mutational mechanism for expression. The gene-dose-dependence and possible mutagenic nature of phenotypic alterations in carcinogenesis are also possibilities to be considered when evaluating the genetic basis of neoplasia. Finally, nonmutational alterations in the genetic material, which nonetheless result in stable phenotypic changes, also must be included as possible genetic mechanisms underlying carcinogenesis.

In summary, the above discussion is meant to illustrate that one must define clearly one of many transitions in neoplastic transformation and study the mechanism of that single step. This requires *a priori* that one define stages of *biological significance* to the neoplastic process—a problem of continuing challenge to oncologists.

C. A CLINICAL PERSPECTIVE

I. Cancer is a Heritable Alteration

Clearly cancer is a stable, heritable cellular alteration. Following isolation from an animal, tumor cells can be maintained in culture, and the progeny of a single tumor cell cloned from the cultured population can reproduce the original disease upon reinjection into a suitable host (Furth and Kahn, 1937). Such observations have indicated that neoplasia is caused by stable alterations in gene structure or gene expression. Analyses of isoenzyme patterns for the X-linked enzyme glucose 6-phosphate dehydrogenase (G6PD) in females heterozygous for this gene have provided strong evidence to indicate that most spontaneous human tumors, both benign and malignant, are clonal in origin (Fialkow, 1969). Baylin and his colleagues (1978) demonstrated that cells from distinct medullary thyroid carcinomas contained one form of G6PD in mosaic females, yet the same individual might have several tumors, each containing cells expressing either G6PD-A or G6PD-B (but not both isozymes). These data likely reflect an inherited defect producing multiple clones of susceptible cells; each tumor arises as a result of subsequent mutation in discrete clones of these cells.

The above observations are consistent with, yet do not require, a mutational etiology for tumors. Although stable heritable traits observed in somatic cells generally have a mutational basis (Siminovitch, 1976), heritability *per se* is not proof of a mutational basis for a phenotype, since nonmutational mechanisms can also explain heritable changes (Mintz and Fleischman, 1981; Pierce and Cox, 1978). Certain properties of differentiated cells are expressed as stable, heritable traits, and have a non-mutational basis. For example, the studies of Mintz and coworkers (see Mintz and Fleischman, 1981) have strongly suggested a nonmutational basis for teratocarcinomas. Neoplastic properties of murine teratocarcinoma cells can be suppressed when the cells are injected into a normal blastocyst. These blastocysts develop into normal mice whose tissues are composed partially of cells derived from the tumor cells. Such "normalization" of tumor cells has been interpreted as signifying altered control of gene expression, rather than alteration of gene structure in the tumorigenic teratocarcinoma cells (Mintz and Fleischman, 1981). Pierce also has emphasized that cancer cells do not lose the capacity to differentiate (Pierce and Cox, 1978; Gray and Pierce, 1964). These documented instances of spontaneous regression/differentiation in tumors emphasize the need to consider tumors as developmentally dynamic entities.

Although one must acknowledge the need to consider non-mutational alterations in gene expression as mechanisms in neoplastic development, it remains possible that results obtained in the above experiments can be explained by the altered phenotypic expression, or "reprogramming," so to speak, of a mutated gene. For example, a tumor cell may arise by a mutational mechanism(s), but during development, the expression of this mutation might be suppressed by providing the proper environment for terminal differentiation. An example of a genetic disease in which the molecular defect is a point (base-substitution) mutation, but can be "masked" by differentiation are certain hemoglobinpathies in fetal hemoglobin (Bunn et al., 1977). Here, mutant γ-globin genes can result in pathological phenotypes at birth, but this disorder is "cured" when γ-chain synthesis is repressed and normal β-chain synthesis is induced. The reverse situation is true with β-chain mutations, such as the sickle-cell anemias; here, the mutant phenotype is observed only after development has progressed to allow β-chain synthesis. One might argue, then, that the observation that some tumor cells can undergo terminal differentiation, and that such differentiation is accompanied by cessation of proliferation, does not exclude a mutational involvement in carcinogenesis. One must ask *at what step* in the transformation process the mutation affects the cellular phenotype; if an alteration at this step does not preclude terminal differentiation, the transformed phenotype may be overridden, in a sense, by the process of differentiation. This concept may gain additional interest as our understanding of the role of cellular proto-oncogenes in embryogenesis increases (Muller et al., 1982; 1983).

II. Studies in Human Genetics are Suggestive of a Mutational Basis for Certain Cancers

1. Syndromes Involving Chromosomal Instability or Deficiencies in DNA Repair

Although it is difficult to prove that the observed aneuploidy of many cancer cells is related causally to the development of the tumor, there are examples of conditions where the chromosome disorder predisposes an individual to cancer. In certain congenital autosomally-linked recessive syndromes (such as Fanconi's anemia (FA), Bloom's syndrome, and Ataxia telangiectasia (AT)) wherein there is a high frequency of chromosome breakage and karyotypic abnormalities in somatic cells, there is a greatly increased incidence of cancer (Knudson, 1973; Hecht and McCaw, 1977, Huang and Sheridan, 1981; Setlow, 1978; Swift, 1971; Swift and Henderson, 1966). In these cases, the chromosomal disorders are not secondary effects of the cancer, because they occur in normal cells from these individuals; it is thus possible that the observed aneuploidy is causally related to the tumor development. Patients with FA and AT have been observed to contain clones of cells with specific chromosome aberrations. Hecht and McCaw (1977) have proposed that some clones may have a selective advantage *in vivo*; gradual increase of such clones has been observed to accompany leukemia in AT patients. AT and FA are associated for Bloom's syndrome (Setlow, 1978). Although the increased frequency of chromosome aberrations in individuals with these syndromes is likely a factor in tumorigenesis, other factors, such as immune deficiency (observed in AT) may also be involved.

Xeroderma pigmentosum (XP) represents a class of recessive genetic disorders in humans which involve deficiency in DNA repair, usually in the excision repair pathway (Cleaver and Bootsma, 1975; Cleaver, 1977; Setlow, 1978). Patients with XP develop multiple skin tumors in areas exposed to UV light. Unrepaired thymine dimers in DNA have thus been implicated in skin cancer. Additional evidence linking pyrimidine dimers to carcinogenesis was provided by model experiments in fish (*Poecilia formosa*). Thyroid cells of these gynogenetic fish irradiated with UV formed thyroid tumors when transplanted in isogeneic recipients (Hart, Setlow, and Woodhead, 1977). If UV irradiation was followed by photoreactivating illumination, the yield of tumors was decreased. These data suggested that as a premutational lesion, an unrepaired pyrimidine dimer can result in tumorigenic transformation.

The general significance of DNA repair deficiency syndromes in carcinogenesis has been questioned (Cairns, 1981), largely due to the paucity of fatal tumors observed at sites other than the skin in XP individuals. Cairns suggested that UV light is the main source of mutagenic lesions in DNA, and that internal cancers in the general population were unlikely to be the result of single gene mutation. The high frequency of early morbidity in patients with DNA repair disorders complicates this analysis, however. Feinberg and Coffey (1982) have reviewed epidemiologic data in connection with this issue. By examining the age- and sex-adjusted cancer incidence ratios by organ site for several chromosomal instability disorders (XP, Bloom's syndrome, and dyskeratosis congenita), these authors found a surprising organ-site specificity for cancer, at sites which are not the most common sites for cancer in the general population (within the age range of patients examined in this study). Whether this observation was linked to tissue-specific differences in mutagen susceptibility remains unclear.

Recent studies concerning the chromosomal mapping of cellular homologs of retroviral oncogenes have supported the significance of several clinically-observed cytogenetic abnormalities in cancer (reviewed by Yunis, 1983 and Rowley, 1980; 1983). These findings, addressed in a later section of this chapter, support a role for specific chromosome alterations in neoplastic disorders.

2. Other Genetic Disorders

Certain tumor syndromes are inherited with a high degree of penetrance. The best studied example of such syndromes is retinoblastoma. Persons who carry the gene for susceptibility to this disease have a 95% probability of developing retinoblastoma, and the probability that their offspring will be carriers and affected is 50% (Knudson, 1973). The individuals who carry this gene will be affected bilaterally, whereas noncarriers will often be affected only unilaterally. Knudson and his colleagues have explained these observations on the basis of a two-hit model, in which the expression of this tumor requires two steps to convert a normal cell into a neoplastic cell (Knudson, 1971; Knudson, 1977; Hethcote and Knudson, 1978). In hereditary cases, the first step is an inherited germ-line mutation and the second step, possibly a secondary mutation, occurs in a somatic cell. In the nonhereditary cases, two events are necessary in the somatic cell. Since only the second step is necessary in the hereditary case, the incidence is much higher than in the nonhereditary cases, and retinoblastoma occurs in both eyes (Knudson, 1971; 1973; 1977; Hethcote and Knudson, 1978).

Age-specific incidence data have provided substantial evidence that this disease occurs by two mutational steps. Moolgovkar and Knudson (1981) have extended this analysis to explain other hereditary tumors by multistep mechanisms.

Patients with hereditary bilateral retinoblastoma are at increased risk for osteogenic sarcoma, and this risk is further increased by irradiation (Abramson *et al.*, 1982; Sagerman *et al.*, 1969; Strong and Knudson, 1973). This finding indicates that the hereditary lesion affects tissues other than the retina, and suggests that the second (somatic) event is mutational. A number of independent cases of retinoblastomas have been reported in which the affected individual has an interstitial deletion of the long arm of chromosome 13. Sparkes *et al.*, (1980; 1983) provided a regional assignment (to 13q14) for the gene for susceptibility to retinoblastoma, based on close linkage to human esterase-D. Benedict and colleagues (1983) recently have extended Knudson's two-step hypothesis in proposing retinoblastoma to be an autosomally-linked recessive disorder at the cellular level, expressed only when both alleles at 13q14 are mutated. By this hypothesis, the retinoblastoma "gene" functions to *maintain* the normal cellular phenotype; when a homozygous mutant genotype is achieved, the neoplastic phenotype is expressed. Such a hypothesis is distinct from models of tumorigenesis based on dominant oncogene activation (discussed below), and emphasizes the diverse genetic mechanisms which may be involved in neoplasia.

Another well-accepted genetically-based tumor is Wilms' tumor (Matsunaga, 1981). Aniridia-Wilms' tumor syndrome is often associated with a deletion in the short arm of chromosome 11 (11p13); it has been proposed that the gene(s) associated with aniridia and Wilms' tumor are closely linked on chromosome 11 (Bader *et al.*, 1979). Like retinoblastoma, this finding is significant in identifying chromosome regions as sites where mutation may give rise to specific types of tumors in predisposed individuals. Interestingly, in identical twins with deletion of 11p13 and aniridia, one sibling may develop Wilms' tumor, whereas the other may not. Thus, deletion of 11p13 may predispose an individual to neoplasia, but tumorigenesis may require a subsequent cellular alteration (Yunis, 1983). Cohen *et al.* (1979) have similarly described a family in which inheritance of a balanced 3:8 chromosomal translocation predisposes individuals to renal cell carcinoma.

There are also cancers showing no particular familiar aggregation, which appear to be correlated with what have been termed "non-random" chromosome changes (Rowley, 1980; 1982). The best known among these is the so-called "Philadelphia chromosome" (Nowell and Hungerford, 1960; 1961), which is found in a high proportion of patients with chronic myelocytic leukemia. This chromosome anomaly usually is described as a translocation between chromosome 22 and another autosome, frequently chromosome 9 (Rowley, 1980). Rowley (1982) and Yunis (1983) have summarized several nonrandom chromosome alterations in other hematologic cancers.

As discussed in a subsequent section of this review, specific chromosome abnormalities may have significance with regard to recent hypotheses concerning the activation of cellular oncogenes as a step in carcinogenesis.

D. AN EXPERIMENTAL PERSPECTIVE

I. Carcinogens as Mutagens

The work of Ames and colleagues (McCann and Ames, 1976; McCann, *et al.*, 1975; Ames, Lee and Durston, 1973; Ames, *et al.*, 1973) established clearly that most carcinogens are mutagens. These results implicate DNA as a susceptible target in neoplastic transformation. Using special strains of Salmonella in the presence of a microsomal activation system, McCann and colleagues (1975) demonstrated a 90% correlation between the carcinogenicity and mutagenicity of tested chemicals. Of the carcinogens that are inactive in the Salmonella mutagenesis assay, many are either mutagenic in other systems or produce mutagenic metabolites (McCann and Ames, 1975). Hollstein, *et al.* (1979) and Purchase *et al.* (1978) evaluated the reliability of the Ames testing procedures in comparison to other short-term tests for carcinogens; in summary, the current philosophy is that a battery of *in vitro* tests can, with reliability, predict the carcinogenicity of suspect chemicals. Purchase *et al.* emphasized, however, that no single *in vitro* test procedure is devoid of false positive or false negative results. The use of appropriate chemical-class controls and structural analogy may be needed for the rapid screening of chemical carcinogens. Moreover, *in vitro* detection methods should not rely solely on mutagenesis as an endpoint (Purchase *et al.*, 1978).

There are stark exceptions to the correlation between chemical mutagenicity and carcinogenicity. There are compounds which are extremely potent mutagens in procaryotes, such as nitrous acid, hydroxylamine, and base analogs, which are noncarcinogens in animals (Miller, 1978; Miller and Miller, 1971; 1977). In contrast to mutagens which are noncarcinogens, there are compounds for which carcinogenic potential has been clearly demonstrated, whereas mutagenicity has not. For example, ethionine, a potent hepatocarcinogen (Farber, 1963) has not been shown to be mutagenic. Some evidence suggests, however, that this compound, a known inducer of cellular differentiation in several *in vitro* systems (Mendelsohn, *et al.*, 1980; Christman *et al.*, 1977) may act by altering the pattern of the methylation of DNA, perhaps by interfering with methylation reactions which utilize 5-adenosylmethionine as the methyl group donor (Mendelsohn, *et al.*, 1980; Jones and Taylor, 1980; Wilson and Jones, 1983). This hypothesis, while non-mutational in nature, still involves an alteration in cellular DNA, and if true, also may provide new insights regarding an alternative mechanism by which carcinogenesis might be induced by mutagenic alkylating agents (Cox, 1980; Wilson and Jones, 1983). The role of DNA methylation in aging, differentiation, and cancer has been discussed in a speculative review by Holliday (1979), and is discussed in more detail in a subsequent section of this review.

Another interesting exception to the correlation between mutagenicity and carcinogenicity is diethylstilbestrol (DES), a synthetic steroidal hormone known to be a carcinogen in humans and rodents (IARC monograph, 1979). DES and its metabolites are inactive as mutagens in the Ames test, even with a variety of metabolic activating systems (see Barrett, *et al.*, 1981; Metzler, *et al.*, 1980). Although such studies of DES indicate a nonmutational basis for its action, the ability of DES to induce aneuploidy in a number of cellular systems, (Sawada and Ishidate, 1978; Ishidate and Odashima, 1977) as well as the demonstrated aneuploidy of dysplastic lesions in women exposed to DES prenatally (Fu, *et al.*, 1979), lends support to the hypothesis that mutation at the chromosomal level (e.g., nondisjunction or translocation) is involved in carcinogenesis (Barrett, *et al.*, 1981; Tsutsui, *et al.*, 1983). This hypothesis would explain the ability of DES to induce neoplastic transformation in Syrian hamster embryo cells without measurable somatic mutation (Barrett, *et al.*, 1981), since mutants such as those affected at the Na+/K+ ATPase (Ouabain resistant) or HPRT (6-thioguanine resistant) loci would not be detectable as the result of changes in ploidy in mammalian cells. A high frequency of chromosomal lesions has been reported in carcinogen-treated Syrian hamster cells (Benedict *et al.*, 1972); this might explain the high frequency of morphological transformation seen in experiments with rodent cells.

The involvement of chromosome-type mutations in carcinogenesis, in contrast to only base-substitution mutations, might also explain the reported differences in the ratio of morphological transformation and mutation frequencies (Barrett and Ts'o, 1978; Chan and Little, 1978; Landolph and Heidelberger, 1979). Chemicals (e.g., DES) which induce aneuploidy at a high frequency, but not single-locus mutation would have a high ratio of transformation to mutation, whereas chemicals which are effective inducers of single gene mutations would have a lower ratio of transformation to mutation. Compounds which induce both gross chromosomal alterations and single gene mutations likely would fall somewhere in the middle of this hypothetical spectrum (see Tsutsui *et al.*, 1983 and Barrett and Elmore, elsewhere in this volume).

In conclusion, there is an accumulating body of evidence which is consistent with a role of mutation in carcinogenesis. Unfortunately, none of the evidence is definitive, a fact partially attributable to the paucity of systems in which somatic mutation and neoplastic transformation can be examined concomitantly. The mutagenicity of chemical carcinogens primarily has been studied in either bacterial systems or systems employing neoplastic mammalian cells, neither of which is suitable for studying the induction of neoplastic transformation. Unless somatic mutation and neoplastic transformation can be studied quantitatively in the same cellular system, a direct comparison of the two processes is not possible. To this end, the laboratory of Paul Ts'o successfully implemented a mammalian cellular system, utilizing early passage, diploid Syrian hamster embryo cells (DiPaolo *et al.*, 1969; 1971; Berwald and Sachs, 1963; 1965), for concomitant studies of progressive neoplastic transformation and somatic mutation (Barrett, Bias, and Ts'o, 1978; Barrett, *et al.*, 1977; Barrett and Ts'o, 1978b; Crawford *et al.*, 1983). Some significant results with this system are summarized in the following section.

II. DNA is a Critical Target in Chemical Carcinogenesis

There is much circumstantial evidence that DNA is a critical target in carcinogenesis. The ultimate forms of most carcinogens are electrophiles which interact with DNA (Miller and Miller, 1971; Miller, 1978). The extent of interaction with DNA correlates with carcinogenic potential of chemicals, whereas the extent of interaction with RNA or protein does not correlate (Brookes, 1966; Brookes and Lawley, 1964). Individuals with inborn genetic defects affecting the ability to repair DNA damage are prone to cancer (Setlow, 1978). Tissue-specific induction of cancer has been correlated with the ability (or lack thereof) to repair DNA damage (Goth and Rajewski, 1974; Laerum and Rajewski, 1975). Hart, Setlow, and Woodhead (1977) as described above, demonstrated that unrepaired pyrimidine dimers in DNA can give rise to tumors in fish. These observations are consistent with DNA being a critical target in neoplastic transformation, but do not prove this hypothesis. Unfortunately, this hypothesis is difficult to prove with most chemical carcinogens, since they are good electrophiles and interact with a variety of cellular macromolecules.

Barrett, Tsutsui, and Ts'o (1978) approached this problem from a different perspective. They reasoned that if DNA is a critical target in carcinogenesis, then a direct perturbation of DNA should be sufficient to initiate neoplastic transformation. To induce damage directly to DNA, Syrian hamster embryo cells were treated with 5-bromodeoxyuridine (BrdU), which is incorporated exclusively into cellular DNA in place of its analog, thymidine. Such BrdU-substituted DNA has an ultraviolet absorption spectrum which is shifted towards longer wavelengths; consequently, irradiation with light of wavelengths greater than 300 nm (near UV) produces a significantly higher number of photochemical lesions in BrdU-substituted DNA than occurs in nonsubstituted DNA. The major photochemical reaction is an initial photodissociation of the bromine atom, producing a uracil radical, followed by decomposition of the radical. In alkaline conditions, DNA single-strand breaks are observed (Barrett, *et al.*, 1978). Irradiation of BrdU-treated cells with near UV light induces cytotoxicity, DNA strand breakage, and single-locus somatic mutation in Syrian hamster cells (Barrett, Tsutsui, and Ts'o, 1978; Tsutsui, *et al.*, 1978, 1979, 1981). Barrett, *et al.*, demonstrated that treatment of normal Syrian hamster embryo cells with BrdU and near UV also resulted in morphologic and ultimate neoplastic transformation, whereas treatment with BrdU alone or near UV alone did not. This effect was specific for DNA, since in synchronous cultures, only cells in S phase were transformed (Tsutsui, *et al.*, 1979; Tsutsui and Ts'o, unpublished observations). These results demonstrate that DNA is a critical susceptible target in carcinogenesis, since a perturbation directed to DNA is sufficient to induce neoplastic transformation *in vitro*. Recently, Little and colleagues (LeMotte *et al.*, 1982) obtained similar results in studies of mouse 3T3 cells transformed by incorporation of ^{125}I-IUDR into DNA. These important results in rodent cells have not yet been extended to human cell systems, wherein the incidence of spontaneous transformation is less a complicating factor.

A demonstration that DNA is a critical target in carcinogenesis is strong support for a mutational basis of cancer, but does not prove that a somatic mutation is the immediate cause of neoplastic transformation. Agents which perturb DNA may cause somatic mutations, yet they may also induce epigenetic changes in the presence or absence of stable somatic mutations. It should be cautioned, therefore, that no study has excluded the possibility that in addition to DNA, other macromolecules (such as RNA and protein) can be susceptible cellular targets for chemically-induced neoplastic transformation.

III. Cell Fusion and the Analysis of Genetic Determinants of the Neoplastic Phenotype

If somatic mutation of a single structural gene is the basis of neoplastic transformation, in principle, the examination of hybrid cells formed between normal and neoplastically transformed cells should allow a distinction between two alternative, simplistic genetic models of carcinogenesis. In one model, cells become transformed as the result of the new, inappropriate expression of a dominantly acting cellular transforming gene. In some cases, this expression might result from genes encoded by an exogenous virus, but the expression of an altered or previously silent cellular gene is the primary mechanism considered here. This model predicts that hybrids will show dominant (or co-dominant) expression of the properties of neoplastically transformed cells, since the newly expressed or altered gene(s) will be expressed in the hybrid cells. By an alternative model, cells become neoplastically transformed because cellular genes essential to the maintenance of the normal phenotype are no longer expressed. This could result from a somatic mutation, or from non-mutational alterations in gene expression (examples of which are discussed in a subsequent section). This model predicts that hybrid cells formed between normal and neoplastically transformed cells would have the properties of normal cells; that is, suppression of neoplastic phenotype occurs as the result of providing the necessary genetic information from the normal cell. These basic models have been discussed extensively (see Ringertz and Savage, 1976; Ozer and Jha, 1977; and Stanbridge et al., 1982 for reviews) and serve only as a general basis for the following discussion of previous experimental observations.

Somatic cell genetic studies have produced seemingly contradictory results on the genetic mechanisms that regulate the neoplastic phenotype. In early experiments on tumor production by normal x tumor cells, the hybrid cell inocula produced tumors; such results were interpreted as indicating that tumorigenicity is expressed dominantly (Barski and Cornegert, 1962; Defendi, et al., 1967; Scaletta and Ephrussi, 1965). It was demonstrated subsequently, however, that such an interpretation was erroneous, because tumors arose from normal x tumor cell hybrids by the selective outgrowth of variant, segregant tumorigenic cells within the inoculated population (Harris, 1979; Harris, et al., 1969). An extensive series of experiments by Harris, Klein, Wiener and co-workers demonstrated that intraspecies cell hybrids between highly tumorigenic and non-tumorigenic or low tumorigenic mouse cells were nearly always suppressed for tumorigenicity; tumors did not develop until segregant cells were produced by chromosome elimination (reviewed by Ringertz and Savage, 1976; Ozer and Jha, 1977). Confirmatory results regarding this suppression of tumorigenicity were reported by Stanbridge (1976) and Stanbridge and Wilkinson (1978; 1980) using cell hybrids between normal human cells and HeLa subclones that are tumorigenic in athymic mice. Sager and colleagues (Sager and Kovac, 1978; 1979; Howell and Sager, 1978; 1979; Kitchin and Sager, 1980a; 1980b) also reported detailed studies using Chinese hamster intraspecies cell hybrids formed between closely related, highly tumorigenic and non-tumorigenic cell strains, with similar results. These studies form the basis for the view that cellular tumorigenicity behaves as a recessive phenotype; i.e., is suppressible in cell hybrids (Stanbridge et al., 1982).

In contrast to these studies, other investigators studying intraspecies cell hybrids generated in vitro (Croce and Koprowski, 1974) or in vivo (Aviles et al., 1977), or interspecies hybrids between normal mouse cells and SV40-transformed human cells (Croce, Aden, and Koprowksi, 1975) have concluded that cellular tumorigenicity can behave as a dominant trait. While several studies were concerned with virus-mediated transformation, dominance was also observed in fusions of non-viral transformants. Kucherlapati and Shin (1979) described a series of intraspecies mouse-human hybrids formed between highly tumorigenic, but genetically distinct, spontaneously-derived mouse cell lines and human diploid fibroblasts. These investigators reported failure to obtain complete suppression of tumorigenicity of these cells in athymic mice; this was observed regardless of the extent and composition of the human chromosome complements retained in the hybrid clones. Although not proved, the results of cytological and isoenzyme analyses made it improbable that the lack of suppression was attributable to cellular selection in vivo for a more tumorigenic subpopulation in the injected hybrid cells. These results were deemed to be consistent with the view that either suppression of cellular tumorigenicity demonstrated in intraspecies cell hybrids does not occur in interspecies (mouse x human) cell hybrids or, alternatively, genetic determinants located on two or more human chromosomes are required simultaneously to suppress tumorigenicity in these cells. The latter interpretation was supported by studies in the laboratory of Stanbridge (Stanbridge et al., 1981; 1982), which analyzed four related nontumorigenic and tumorigenic HeLa x fibroblast intraspecific human hybrid cell lines for specific chromosome(s) associated with the control of tumorigenicity. The loss of one copy each of both chromosome 11 and 14 was associated with the expression of tumorigenicity. Together, these results suggest complex, multigenic control of neoplastic expression.

When the properties of hybrid cells have been determined by tests for in vitro characteristics, a non-coordinate expression of tumorigenicity and in vitro phenotype characteristics associated with neoplastic cells has been shown (Howell and Sager, 1979; Stanbridge and Wilkinson, 1978). Moreover, upon characterization of biochemically isolated hybrid cells, both expression and suppression of markers of neoplastic transformation have been reported in different experimental systems (Jha and Ozer, 1976; Jha et al., 1978; Marin,

1971; Wiblin and MacPherson, 1973; Croce and Koprowski, 1974; Sager and Kovac, 1978; 1979; see also Ringertz and Savage, 1976; and Stanbridge *et al.*, 1982). Such results emphasize the possibly multigenic nature of the transformed phenotype. It has not always been clear, however, whether these findings reflect different mechanisms of neoplastic transformation, or a discrepancy between tests *in vivo* for tumor production and *in vitro* for the transformed phenotype.

This summary is not intended to provide an in-depth review of the literature in this area. Rather, it serves to emphasize that studies of cell hybrids have shown seemingly disparate results, ranging from full expression to full suppression of tumorigenicity, and including not only partial or non-coordinate expression of the transformed phenotype, but also segregation of subpopulations of cells which have either re-expressed or suppressed particular transformed phenotypes. Reconciliation of these apparently paradoxial results has plagued somatic cell geneticists interested in carcinogenesis. The question which emerges from this apparently contradictory literature is whether the methods of cell culture and somatic cell genetics are even adequate to permit meaningful genetic analysis of the complex problem of carcinogenesis. The difficulties can be discussed in terms of both the design and the interpretation of cell fusion studies to examine the expression of the neoplastic phenotype.

Among the principal difficulties in design of cell fusion studies to examine the expression of tumorigenicity have been: 1) *the use of established, heteroploid cell lines that are heterogeneous in karyotype.* Such cells, by virtue of their continuous passaging in cell culture, may have undergone additional events *secondary* to the alteration controlling the tumorigenic phenotype. Such secondary alterations complicate and may prevent straightforward genetic complementation analysis; 2) *the inability to correlate, with tumorigenicity, in vitro traits at the individual cell rather than the cell population level.* Failure to recognize this problem has often led to the disregard of segregant cell populations which may arise from the initial cell hybrids even of intra-species origin. Typically, hybrid cells have been examined only after their biochemical selection, isolation, and growth to a large population size (usually involving 20 or more cell divisions). During this time, segregant cells distinct from the original hybrid cell type can arise. Preferably, one should employ methods to examine, at the cellular level, the *in vitro* expression of phenotypic characteristics in hybrid cells as soon as possible after fusion; 3) *the interference of the host immune response in the assessment of tumorigenicity.* In early studies, this complication was addressed by using large inocula (e.g., 10^6 or more) of parental or hybrid cells in the evaluation of cellular tumorigenicity. Unfortunately, this makes the degree of tumorigenicity of the parental cells used for fusion questionable. For example, if only one out of 10^6 "transformed" cells is truly tumorigenic, the probability of such a cell engaging in cell fusion with a normal cell is negligible, and one might really isolate non-tumorigenic x non-tumorigenic cell hybrids rather than the desired tumorigenic x non-tumorigenic cells. Furthermore, the host immune response might result in an erroneous underestimation of the tumorigenicity of cells; in this case, cells deemed to be non-tumorigenic might really be capable of tumor formation. Upon isolation of clonal hybrid strains, purified from less tumorigenic (and perhaps more anti-genic) cells within the population, these cells might give apparent 'dominance' of tumorigenicity in cell hybrids. These arguments serve to illustrate that the *heterogeneity* of the tumorigenicity of the cell populations has been a problem in many cell fusion analyses of the neoplastic phenotype. This problem is exacerbated by the difficulties in dealing with the host's immune response when assessing tumorigenicity. To some extent, this problem can be circumvented by the use of the athymic nude mouse for tumorigenicity studies. Sager and Kovac (1979) addressed the accurate quantitative assessment of tumorigenicity in the context of cell fusion analysis of tumorigenicity. By a co-injection assay (where-in mixed suspensions of lethally x-irradiated normal cells were injected with serial dilutions of cell lines to be tested for tumorigenicity), these investigators demonstrated that as few as ten transformed cells used in cell fusion were tumorigenic, whereas cells used as the non-tumorigenic parent for fusion pro-vided no tumors upon inoculation of 10^6 cells. Thus, the availability of the nude mouse for the testing of cellular tumorigenicity, regardless of the strain or background of the cells to be tested, makes it possible to study quantitatively the tumorigenicity of both intra- and interspecies cell hybrids. 4) *Finally, cell fusion studies of the genetic basis for the neoplastic phenotype will always be compli-cated by the presence of cytoplasmic factors donated by the fused cells.* The existence of cytoplasmic regulatory control, or mitochondrially-linked genetic control of the neoplastic state cannot, therefore, easily be excluded. Only if supported by careful studies using cellular reconstitution, and chromosome or DNA-mediated gene transfer, can cell fusion analysis provide a meaningful, critical evaluation of the genetic control of the transformed state. To date, no study has encompassed all these approaches in a single comprehensive analysis.

The interpretation of cell fusion studies designed to examine the expression of transformation is hampered by the methodological considerations discussed above, which too often have been disregarded. Perhaps equally important, however, is the difficulty in interpreting these experiments and their designs with respect to a multistep model of carcinogenesis. *A multistep process would not be expected to be amenable to straightforward genetic complementation analysis*, if only the "end products," so to speak, of this process are examined. The early cell fusion experiments of Weiner, Klein, and Harris (1974) empha-sized this point. From 42 clonal populations derived from 12 different crosses between different mouse tumor cells, only one type of fusion generated hybrid cells with reduced tumorigenicity; in all other cases, the hybrid cells were highly malignant. It appeared that in a wide range of tumor types, the recessive lesions controlling tumorigenicity failed to complement each other. This unexpected finding was explained by postulating that either the gene(s) controlling malig-nancy consist of only one or at most two complementation group(s), or cells comprising the noncomplementary tumor combinations may originally have arisen by independent genetically complementable, cellular mechanisms, but underwent irreversible secondary changes which prevented straightforward genetic complementation (Weiner, *et al.*, 1974, Klein, 1976). The first hypothe-sis is consistent with an autosomally-linked recessive single-gene mutation controlling neoplasia, whereas the second explanation would be in accord with one of the principles of tumor progression (i.e., independent progression of characters in a tumor) (Founds, 1969). Thus, *genetic analyses of the mutational nature of neoplasia will be complicated by the possibility that the cancer cell may have more than one pathway to the same phenotypic endpoint*. A multistep and multifactorial model for neoplastic development would predict precisely the apparently discordant types of results which cell fusion analyses have provided. Only by separating the process of carcinogenesis into discrete phenotypic transitions, and evaluating the dominance or recessiveness of the expression of the phenotypic alteration corresponding to each step, can cell fusion analysis provide meaningful information regarding the genetic control of neoplasia. If tumorigenicity is the result of heritable alterations in one or more genes regulating a number or series of biochemical processes, it can be expected that individual tumor cell lines will behave differently in different hybrid cell combinations. This concept might explain the apparently discrepant results obtained in so many laboratories, and emphasizes the complexities inherent in Mendelian approaches to this problem.

IV. Cellular Transforming Genes

Despite the contradictory evidence obtained from cell fusion studies, the observation that cells stably inherit the transformed phenotype supports a genetic basis for carcinogenesis. Although this is certainly true for cells transformed by oncogenic viruses (where it can be demonstrated that specific viral genes are required for the maintenance of the transformed state), most tumors, especially those in man, are not known to have a viral etiology. The question of whether cancer can result from an alteration in endogenous cellular genes has been given a new focus, however, with the discovery that oncogenes of retroviruses are transduced copies of cellular genes, known as "proto-oncogenes" or "cellular oncogenes" (Weinberg, 1980; Bishop, 1978; 1983; Cooper, 1982). Several experimental strategies have now converged to expand the catalog of known oncogenes, and implicate their expression in carcinogenesis.

1. Cellular Homologs of Retroviral Transforming Genes

Retroviruses are a family of RNA viruses that replicate by way of a DNA provirus integrated into cellular DNA. Acute transforming viruses are highly oncogenic; they efficiently transform cells in culture, and induce neoplasia with a short latent period in infected animals. At least seventeen distinct retroviral oncogenes have been identified within the genomes of such viruses, whose expression is associated with oncogenesis (see Bishop, 1983; Varmus and Levine, 1983 for reviews).

The transforming genes of acute transforming retroviruses are homologous to DNA sequences present in normal cells. These normal cell homologs are highly conserved in vertebrate evolution, and appear not to be linked to viral DNA (reviewed by Weinberg, 1980; Bishop, 1978; 1983). Transcription of most of these genes has been detected in normal cells, and normal cell proteins that are related to proteins encoded by the homologous virus oncogene have been identified. With the exception of the *ras* genes, which clearly constitute a multigene family in some species (Chang *et al.*, 1982; Ellis *et al.*, 1981; Chatto- padhyay *et al.*, 1982), the respective cellular proto-oncogenes typically have been reported to represent single-copy sequences in cellular DNA. The charac- terization of oncogenic viruses has thus advanced our knowledge of several candidate cellular genes involved in carcinogenesis.

In summary, acute transforming retroviruses represent *in vivo* recombinants in which a gene, normally resident in the cellular genome, has been transduced into a retroviral genome. As a consequence of its association with viral se- quences regulating transcription, the gene is expressed at augmented levels in infected cells and elicits cellular transformation. It is thus possible that aug- mented or inappropriate expression of a normal, endogenous cellular proto- oncogene might result in oncogenic transformation. Alternatively, trans- formation might result from structural differences in viral and cellular proteins, attributable to gene mutation which occurs as a consequence of gene transduc- tion. Several lines of experimentation have addressed these hypotheses. These experiments underscore how the fields of viral and chemical carcinogenesis are now converging.

2. DNA-Mediated Gene Transfer of the *in vitro* Transformed Phenotype

Transfer of biologically active eucaryotic DNA typically is accomplished by the calcium phosphate precipitate method of Graham and Van der Eb (1973). This method has been demonstrated to provide stable genetic transformants, for biochemically-selectable single copy genes, at frequencies ranging to as high as 0.1-1 genetic transformants per microgram of total genomic DNA (Wigler *et al.*, 1978). The advent of this technique allowed direct examination of the transforming potential of tumor cell DNA.

The hypothesis that cellular genes can impart properties associated with neoplastic cells was first supported by DNA transfection experiments using NIH 3T3 cells as recipients (Cooper *et al.*, 1980; Shih *et al.*, 1979). These heteroploid cells likely represent a late stage in multistep transformation (an issue addressed below), yet have served as a convenient and extensively used test system to detect cellular sequences capable of inducing focal transformation, a cellular alteration indicative of loss of contact inhibition of growth.

High molecular weight DNA from a variety of neoplastic cells has been shown to induce focal transformation of NIH 3T3 cells (reviewed by Cooper,

1982; Bishop, 1983). This assay has been used to detect transforming potential in a wide variety of neoplasms, including spontaneously-occurring as well as chemically-induced tumors from a variety of tissues and vertebrate species. Carcinogenesis thus appears to have been accompanied by, or to have involved directly, the acquisition of dominantly-acting genetic alterations, reflected in the activation of cellular transforming genes detectable by transfection. Several caveats should be mentioned at this point, however:

- *Not all DNA's obtained from neoplastic cells have induced transformation upon transfection to NIH 3T3 cells* (Shih *et al.*, 1979; Perucho *et al.*, 1981; Murray *et al.*, 1981). Carcinogenesis in such neoplasms may have involved epigenetic changes, or genetic (perhaps recessive mutational) changes not detectable by transfection. Alternatively, these cells might contain dominantly-acting genes which simply are not detectable by the NIH 3T3 focus assay. Although not yet demonstrated, the possibility of host- or tissue-specificity of gene expression cannot be overlooked. Furthermore, exceptionally large genes may not be detected in this assay, simply due to their inefficient transfer and integration. It is noteworthy that the majority of neoplastic cells which have been examined do not exhibit dominantly-acting transforming genes in the NIH 3T3 system.

- *NIH 3T3 cells likely represent a preneoplastic, "late-stage" recipient cell type.* As a consequence, this assay appears suitable only for genes which induce focal transformation; the relevance of this growth alteration to multistage transformation remains unclear. It is unlikely that all important steps in carcinogenesis can be delineated with this cell system. This point is addressed in greater detail below.

- *"Dominance" has not been defined in a Mendelian sense.* Although expression of focal transformation has been interpreted as reflecting dominantly-activated oncogenes in the donor cell genome, no study has examined the dominance/recessiveness of expression of an oncogene by, for example, cell fusion analysis *in conjunction* with gene transfer. Furthermore, the genetic background (homozygous mutant, or heterozygous mutant—which would theoretically show co-dominant or dominant expression of a mutant trait) of the donor tumor cell has not been examined in detail. Such investigations have been hampered in most cases by the obscure culture history and frank aneuploidy of established cell lines used as a source of donor DNA (O'Toole *et al.*, 1983). Moreover, the aneuploid genetic background of the NIH 3T3 cell precludes strict Mendelian interpretations of dominance or recessiveness of phenotypic expression. Consequently, the term "dominantly-acting transforming gene" most accurately reflects the potential to form foci in NIH 3T3 cells. As discussed below, the finding that augmented expression of a normal cellular proto-oncogene can elicit focus formation also complicates straightforward Mendelian interpretations of dominance using this assay system. This point has been underscored by the recent report (Capon *et al.*, 1983) for one donor cell examined, that the activated oncogene is functionally homozygous.

3. Molecular Cloning Experiments Have Revealed a Role for Somatic Mutation in Oncogene Activation

Despite the considerations outlined above, the convergence of cellular carcinogenesis and retrovirology has been emphasized in a most surprising way by molecular cloning experiments.

First, the biological activities of active cellular oncogenes detected by the focal transformation assay were demonstrated to display characteristic sensitivity to inactivation by restriction endonuclease cleavage of donor cell DNA (Shilo and Weinberg, 1981; Lane et al., 1981; Perucho et al., 1981). This indicated that the same or related oncogene(s) might be activated in tumors of diverse origin. In several cases, the pattern of retention of flanking repetitive DNA sequences in donor DNA was interpreted as indicating the existence of related or distinct genes in different tumor DNAs (Perucho et al., 1981; Murray et al., 1981).

In subsequent experiments, by use of co-transfection with biologically selectable or identifiable markers, or alternatively, by reliance on the identification of repetitive human DNA sequences which flanked active oncogenes transfected into NIH 3T3 cells, several investigators achieved the molecular cloning of cellular oncogenes (Goldfarb et al., 1982; Shih and Weinberg, 1981; Pulciani et al., 1982). These molecularly cloned sequences were clearly abnormal, in that they transformed cells with efficiencies that were orders of magnitude above the background frequencies displayed by their counterparts cloned from normal cells.

Although it was expected that such cloning experiments would lead to the isolation of new oncogenes, several laboratories undertook investigations to examine the relationship between cellular oncogenes and previously characterized oncogenes transduced by retroviruses. The first such comparative study yielded surprising results: the cellular oncogene cloned from a bladder carcinoma line, T24/EJ, was found to be a member of the *ras* family of oncogenes, conserved in vertebrate evolution (Der and Cooper, 1982; Santos et al., 1982; Parada et al., 1982). Several genes homologous to the transforming genes of the Harvey- and Kirsten-strains of murine sarcoma virus had been molecularly cloned and characterized from normal human DNA (Chang et al., 1982). In an elegant series of experiments, Tabin et al. (1982) and independently. Reddy et al. (1982) demonstrated that a point mutation, resulting in a single amino acid substitution, was responsible for the acquisition of transforming properties by the oncogene cloned from the bladder carcinoma, in contrast to its normal cellular counterpart.

Although the demonstration of a point mutation responsible for activation of this *ras* proto-oncogene supports a somatic mutation model of carcinogenesis, the generality of this finding has been questioned. Feinberg et al. (1983) demonstrated, by examining a wide variety of spontaneously-arising human tumors, that the particular mutation at amino acid 12 described for the bladder carcinoma *ras* oncogene was not a requisite alteration in human cancer. Furthermore, experiments by Chang and colleagues (1982) demonstrated that the normal, wild-type human gene homologous to the *ras* oncogene of Harvey murine sarcoma virus would induce focal transformation when ligated to a transcriptional control element (the long terminal repeat) from a murine or feline retrovirus. These results indicated that abnormally high levels of a gene product encoded by a normal human oncogene can induce transformation. Similar results had been presented previously for cellular oncogenes cloned from rodent genomes (Blair et al., 1981; Defeo et al., 1981; Oskarsson et al., 1980). This "quantitative" mechanism of transformation seems paradoxial when juxtaposed to the "qualitative" mutational mechanism proposed for the transforming activity of the mutant ras oncogene. Recently, a model has been proposed to account for the consequences of a mutation at residue 12 in the p21 ras protein (Pincus et al., 1983). By examining the energetically allowed conformations of the hydrophobic decapeptide surrounding this substitution site, it was proposed that the most favorable form of the ras gene product exists when the normal peptide (containing glycine at residue 12) is in a left-handed bend conformation. This favorable conformation cannot be achieved when valine, for example, is substituted at residue 12. However, inspection of energy differences for different conformational states revealed that perhaps 20% of the normal peptide should exist in a conformation like that found for the mutant protein (Pincus et al., 1983). In light of this favorable partitioning to the alternative conformation (which seemed inconsistent with the high levels of normal p21 ras protein required to achieve transformation) these authors proposed a model where p21 ras protein interacts with another cellular element. Any mutation leading to amino acid substitution at position 12 would abolish the conformation required for interaction of p21 ras with this cellular element. By this model, mass-action considerations also were invoked to explain how an excess of normal p21 ras protein could lead to transformation.

Santos and colleagues (1983) described results which emphasize the role mutation in p21 ras can play in activating this gene. These authors found that the normal ras gene could induce focal transformation, but only when multiple (30-50) copies of the gene become integrated in the NIH 3T3 cell genome. Such transformation was not faithfully transmitted in secondary transfection assays. During their experiments, they observed, however, that DNA from one of the normal proto-oncogene derived transformants did induce focal transformation upon secondary transfection. The nucleotide sequence of the human ras oncogene was determined for this donor DNA and revealed a new (G → A) transition mutation at the same position as the transversion mutation (G → T) previously found in the T24/EJ bladder carcinoma cell line. This result does not eliminate the possibility that other structural changes might confer transforming properties to this protein, but does underscore the significance of the single amino acid substitution at position 12 in producing 21 ras protein which elicits focus formation in mouse NIH 3T3 cells.

4. Tumorigenic Conversion of Primary Cells May Require the Action of More Than One Oncogene

As discussed in a subsequent section, neoplasia induced by certain weakly oncogenic retroviruses (whose mode of action appears to be gene activation by

32

insertion mutagenesis) is consistent with a multistep model of oncogenesis (Cooper, 1982). This observation, together with the accepted limitations of the NIH 3T3 cell transformation assay, has stimulated research on the role of oncogene expression in the transformation of normal cells. Lane *et al.* (1982) emphasized the possible existence of stage-specific transforming genes in B- and T-lymphocyte neoplasms. Two groups have presented data which indicate further that tumorigenic conversion of primary embryo fibroblast cells requires at least two cooperating oncogenes. Land *et al.* (1983) demonstrated that transfection of the rat embryo fibroblasts by a mutant human *ras* oncogene did not yield tumor cells unless the fibroblasts were first immortalized as established cell lines prior to transfection. The pre-crisis embryo fibroblasts could evolve to tumorigenic lines if a second oncogene, such as the viral of cellular *myo* gene, or gene for polyoma large-T antigen, was co-transfected with the *ras* gene. Similarly, Ruley (1983) reported that adenovirus early region 1A provides functions required for subsequent *ras* transformation of primary cells. These results were interpreted to suggest that separate establishment and transforming functions are required for the oncogenic transformation of cells in culture. This offers the hope that the number of steps in carcinogenesis can in some cases be few, and amenable to dissection at the molecular level.

E. A NEW PERSPECTIVE—DIVERSE TYPES OF DNA ALTERATIONS MAY BE INVOLVED IN CARCINOGENESIS

I. Single-Locus (Point) Mutation

Point mutations induced by carcinogens could act either in *cis* or *trans*. Such alterations could be defined by cell fusion studies, in conjunction with gene transfer. For example, mutations in a coding region of a gene might confer dominant transforming activity such as that detected by DNA transfection. Mutations within or adjacent to a gene might also affect the ability of a gene, or its gene product, to respond to negative regulators. Such alterations also could be dominant lesions detectable by DNA transfection or cell fusion analyses. Alternatively, structural gene mutations might be recessive, and require homozygosity for phenotypic expression. Mutations in regulatory genes also can be envisioned, which might release oncogenes from their normal control. Such alterations would likely be recessive, reversible upon cell fusion, and not detectable by a transfection assay. Benedict and colleagues (1983) have emphasized the importance of recessive alterations in the genesis of retinoblastoma, a hereditary eye tumor.

As discussed above, the demonstration that a single base-substitution mutation in cellular *ras* genes can confer dominant focus-forming ability to the altered p21 *ras* gene product has lent credence to a role for point mutation at some step in carcinogenesis. Similarly, mutation in the same position (amino acid 12) has been evoked to account for the oncogenicity of the viral forms of *ras*. In a test of this hypothesis, Capon and colleagues (1983) placed the coding elements of mutant c-Ki-ras genes under the transcriptional control of a heterologous expression system. Such plasmids induced focal transformation of Rat-1 cells, in contrast to the absence of detectable transforming activity of the wild-type c-Ki-ras gene. Their findings provide additional support for the hypothesis that single amino acid substitutions are capable of conferring transforming ability on the c-Ki-ras gene product. Interestingly, these investigators reported that at least one human tumor cell line is functionally homozygous for the mutant gene—thus emphasizing the question of whether mutant *ras* genes are truly active dominantly in a Mendelian sense.

Although demonstration of a point mutation in a defined gene such as the *ras* oncogenes may help to explain the carcinogenic action of point mutagens, one must ask how other mutagens, whose mode of action may be frameshift or deletion in nature, can exhibit carcinogenicity. Moreover, one wonders how other agents, for which no mutagenic potential can be defined, can induce neoplastic transformation. Perhaps some hints at answers to these questions can be found by considering other types of alterations in the DNA.

II. DNA Rearrangement/Transposition

In a speculative review, John Cairns (1981) proposed that the process of neoplastic transformation might be best explained by gross DNA rearrangement and perhaps, the transposition of specific DNA sequences. By this hypothesis, either gene activation or inactivation can be envisioned to occur as a result of insertional mutagenesis or position effect. Such ideas were encompassed by Klein (1981) in describing how altered chromosome or gene dosage and specific chromosome rearrangements might be causally involved in neoplasia. Recently, the molecular characterization of oncogene structure and expression in neoplastic cells has provided evidence in support of these theories.

1. Origin of Retroviruses from Cellular Moveable Genetic Elements

There are striking similarities between retroviral proviruses and both bacterial and eucaryotic moveable genetic elements (Shapiro and Cordell, 1982; Temin, 1980; Ju and Skalka, 1980). In the case of spleen necrosis virus, by molecular cloning of cell-virus junctions, a 5bp direct repeat of cellular DNA was found next to a 3bp inverted repeat of viral DNA (Shimotohno *et al.*, 1980). Similar findings were reported for studies of proviral integrations of moloney murine sarcoma virus (Dhar *et al.*, 1980) and mouse mammary tumor virus (Majors and Varmus, 1981). Interestingly, the topology of integrated moveable genetic elements of yeast (TY1) and Drosophila (copia) is similar: a 5bp direct repeat of cellular DNA next to a 2-5bp inverted repeat of mobile element DNA (see Shapiro and Cordell, 1982 for a review). Additional structural and sequence similarities among retroviruses and characterized mobile genetic elements have fueled speculation that mobile elements have served as the precursors to retroviruses (Flavell, 1981). Retroviruses have so far been found, however, only in vertebrates. In contrast, moveable genetic elements have been documented in maize, bacteria, yeast, and Drosophila, but not in vertebrate species (see Shapiro and Cordell, 1982). It has been proposed, nonetheless, that certain repetitive sequence families in higher eucaryotes might be capable of transposition (Haynes et al., 1981; Sharp, 1983; Kominami et al., 1983). Fahmy and Fahmy have proposed (1980), by analogy with observations in Drosophila (Green, 1977), that carcinogens may act to induce gross DNA rearrangement/transposition, and thereby alter gene expression in mammalian cells. This hypothesis is consistent with Cairns' hypothesized role for gene transposition in cancer (Cairns, 1981).

2. Insertional Mutagenesis, Oncogene Activation, and Multistep Models of Cancer

The best documented examples of insertional mutagenesis in higher eucaryotic cells are those found as a consequence of retrovirus infection. The integration of viral DNA into the host genome to give a provirus occurs randomly as a consequence of infection by retroviruses. Such integration is potentially mutagenic: genes may be inactivated as a result of their disruption, and regulatory regions of the virus, if in the proximity of cellular genes, may alter gene expression. Proof for this hypothesis was provided by the study of bursal lymphomas induced by avian retroviruses (Payne et al., 1981; Hayward et al., 1981). Avian leukosis viruses (ALV's) do not possess oncogenes, yet lymphomas induced by ALV contain integrated viral DNA in a common host domain in different tumors (Hayward et al., 1981). Molecular cloning studies revealed that within this common domain could be found a cellular proto-oncogene (c-myc) whose expression was augmented as a result of the insertion of viral DNA (Hayward et al., 1981). Interestingly, the topology of the insertion events which can generate such activation can be either 5' or 3' to the cellular myc locus (Payne et al., 1981). These findings emphasize how augmented expression of a cellular gene, normally expressed at low levels, can lead to tumorigenesis without mutation in the coding region of that locus. If other retroviruses without oncogenes can induce transformation, study of the sites of their integration in cellular DNA can in theory lead to the identification of cellular genes which may be involved in carcinogenesis. In this regard, attempts have been made to implicate the rearrangement of LTRs of endogenous retroviruses in transformation induced by chemical carcinogens (Kirschmeier et al., 1982). In one case, the spontaneous activation of the cellular mos gene in a mouse tumor has been correlated with the juxtaposition of the LTR (long terminal repeat) of an intracisternal A-particle gene, so as to provide augmented transcription of the c-mos locus (Rechavi et al., 1983). Intracisternal A-particle genes are represented as a family of repetitive sequences in mouse and Syrian hamster

DNA, and bear striking structural similarities to classically-defined transposable elements in lower organisms (Kuff *et al.*, 1983). The activation of c-*mos* by IAP gene insertion may reflect the ability of such sequences to transpose in the genome. This suggests that the rearrangement of other, as yet uncharacterized, repetitive sequence families in higher vertebrates might play a similar role in mutagenesis and carcinogenesis.

The pathogenesis of neoplasms induced by weakly oncogenic retroviruses which do not carry specific viral transforming genes also supports a multistep model for carcinogenesis. Such neoplasms include chicken B-cell lymphomas and a nephroblastoma induced by avian lymphoid leukosis virus, mouse mammary carcinomas induced by mouse mammary tumor virus, and mouse T cell neoplasms induced by murine leukemia viruses (see Cooper, 1982). These weakly transforming viruses do not transform cells in culture, and require long latent periods before tumor formation *in vivo*. The long latent period and pathogenesis of neoplasms induced by these viruses is consistent with a multistep process occuring *in vivo*. In several tumors, insertion of viral DNA was shown to activate the cellular *myc* gene; increased transcription of this gene may thus be the direct consequence of LLV infection. However, when NIH 3T3 cells were transformed with DNA from LLV-induced B cell lymphomas, the avian *myc* gene was not transferred to foci that were detected and isolated. This result indicated that LLV-induced B-cell lymphomas contain at least two transforming genes—the cellular *myc* activated by proviral DNA insertion, and a distinct cellular gene, not linked to viral DNA, that acts as a dominantly transforming gene in NIH 3T3 cells. Similar observations were reported by the laboratory of Weinberg for promyelocytic leukemia cells (HL-60) and an American Burkitt's lymphoma: in each case, the tumor cells carried altered versions of the c-*myc* gene, as well as altered versions of a second cellular oncogene, termed N-*ras*, which has dominant transforming activity in NIH 3T3 cells (see Land *et al.*, 1983).

III. Specific Chromosomal Alterations Associated with Cancer

Although aneuploidy is a characteristic frequently observed in cancer cells, it is difficult to discern whether chromosomal abnormalities are the primary cause or secondary effects of neoplastic transformation. Chromosome disorders were the original basis of the somatic mutation theory as proposed by von Hansemann (1890; 1893) and Boveri (1914). Alterations in chromosome structure may be considered mutational, because they involve disruption of the primary structure of DNA. At the chromosome level, these alterations might be in the form of deletions, or rearrangements which, by "position effects," might alter the phenotypic expression of affected genes. Thus, chromosome rearrangements can have consequences analogous to insertional mutagenesis by retroviruses. Additionally, chromosome abnormalities such as nondisjunction or mitotic recombination might permit the expression of recessive phenotypes ordinarily unexpressed in the heterozygous state. These concepts are discussed in more detail in the sections which follow.

1. Chromosome Changes and Gene Dosage Effects

a) Background

Following the hypothesis by Boveri (1914) and von Hansemann (1890) that chromosome imbalance may lead to neoplastic development, elucidation of the relationship between chromosome changes and malignancy has been one of the most persistent and frustrating challenges in oncology. Experimental efforts have focused primarily upon two aspects of this problem: 1) examination of the chromosomal rearrangements exhibited by established tumor cell populations, and 2) attempted study of the karyotypic changes occurring early in neoplastic transformation. The lack, however, of reliable indicators of discrete preneoplastic stages in the transformation process has hampered the latter approach. Consequently, although chromosome changes have been associated with malignant cells, it is difficult to discern whether these alterations are a cause, or result of carcinogenesis (see German, 1974 for a review). Moreover, until the past decade or so, the inadequacy of chromosome resolution and the inefficiency of conventional cytological methods precluded meaningful analyses of the role of specific chromosome alterations in primary cancer.

Advances in the *in vitro* culturing of mammalian cells, as well as the development of improved methods for chromosome preparation, have permitted a more critical evaluation of Boveri's hypothesis. Several studies have suggested that non-random chromosomal changes may be associated with certain specific neoplastic disorders (Rowley, 1980; 1982; 1983; Yunis, 1983). The predominant appearance of a karyotypically distinct cell type within a tumor cell population gave rise to the concept of clonal evolution of tumor cells (Nowell, 1976). This concept envisioned a predominant subpopulation of the clonally-derived tumor cell population as having a specific karyotype, but as being the source of variant cells capable of indefinite growth as a neoplasm. Recent theories thus regard tumor cells as being in a constant state of flux, heterogeneous in both karyotype and phenotype (Nowell, 1976; Fidler, 1978).

Observations of karyotypic and phenotypic heterogeneity may have relevance with respect to observations concerning gene dosage in carcinogenesis. Karyotypic analyses of transformed Syrian hamster cell lines led Sachs and co-workers (Yamamoto *et al.*, 1973; Bloch-Shtacher and Sachs, 1976) to postulate that in this system, the *balance* of certain specific "expressor" chromosomes to "suppressor" chromosomes, was highly correlated with phenotypic transformation. These studies were later supported by the work of Benedict *et al.* (1975) in the study of a chemically transformed Syrian hamster cell line and its revertants. These studies were seminal in the later development of a gene dosage model of carcinogenesis (Klein, 1981).

b) Recent Findings

Chromosome abnormalities recently have been implicated causally in carcinogenesis by virtue of 1) specific rearrangements which occur in the vicinity of defined cellular oncogenes, and 2) specific alterations in gene dosage which would occur as the consequence of non-disjunction events. Both of these observations are encompassed by Klein's gene dosage model of carcinogenesis (Klein, 1981).

Specific, common, karyotypic rearrangements in tumor cells may place identifiable oncogenes under altered transcriptional control. Rowley (1982; 1983) and Yunis (1983) have summarized some of the commonly found rearrangements in human tumor cells. The general pattern of these findings bears an interesting similarity to the pathogenesis of B-cell lymphomas induced by avian retroviruses. For example, the B-cell tumors of Burkitt's lymphoma frequently show translocations involving chromosome 8 and the region of a chromosome which bears an immunoglobulin gene: chromosome 2 (kappa chains), chromosome 14 (heavy chains), or chromosome 22 (lambda chains) (see Rowley or Yunis, 1983). In rearrangements involving chromosomes 8 and 14, the c-*myc* locus has been shown to be directly involved at the translocation breakpoint, purportedly resulting in c-*myc* transcriptional activation (Dalla-Favera *et al.*, 1982). Similar observations have been reported for translocations between chromosomes 12 and 15 in mouse plasmacytomas, where the juxtaposition of c-*myc* (on chromosome 15) near the constant region for alpha heavy chains results in augmented *myc* transcription (Taub *et al.*, 1983). This finding was a direct confirmation of George Klein's (1981) earlier hypothesis based on cytogenetic observations.

Other karyotypic abnormalities show tantalizing correlations with the chromosomal locations of cellular proto-oncogenes. Examples include: c-*myb* on chromosome 6 (deletions in T cell leukemias, and acute lymphatic leukemia, and translocations in some ovarian adenocarcinomas); c-*fes* on chromosome 15 (translocations in acute promyelocytic leukemia); c-*sis* on chromosome 22 (translocations in chronic myelogenous leukemia and B-cell tumors); c-Harvey *ras* 1 on chromosome 11 (deletions in Wilms' tumor); and c-*abl* on chromosome 9 (chronic myelogenous leukemia). It should be noted that chromosome deletion can achieve the same result, in theory, as a translocation event (i.e., the transcriptional activation of an oncogene by juxtaposition of the gene to a strong promoter of transcription). Combined cytogenetic and molecular genetic studies may thus help in explaining the carcinogenic action of many clastogenic agents, including ionizing radiations (the primary mechanism of which is to induce gross chromosomal alterations rather than point mutation). It should be cautioned, however, that accepting the role of chromosomal duplications and rearrangements in oncogene activation presumes that the increased dosage of a cellular proto-oncogene is related to tumorigenesis—a hypothesis that remains equivocal. Moreover, in the absence of demonstrated transcriptional activation, it can be argued that the rearrangement of oncogene loci could reflect merely the result of chance alone, particularly in light of the dispersion of these genes in the human karyotype.

A gene dosage hypothesis of carcinogenesis also can accommodate another well-documented property of tumor cells—karyotypic *heterogeneity*. The extreme variability in chromosome content in tumor cells (presumably as the result of extensive nondisjunction) can be envisioned to generate a variety of stemlines with selective advantage (Deaven *et al.*, 1981)—perhaps as the result of increasing the gene dosage for particular cellular proto-oncogenes, or creating situations where mutant cellular genes become functionally homozygous (as the result of loss of the normal homolog). To date, the importance of mitotic nondisjunctive error, and the possible effects certain chemicals may have in inducing this process, have received little attention.

2. Alternative Roles for Chromosomal Variability in Carcinogenesis

Although specific translocations activating oncogenes and the gene dosage hypothesis of carcinogenesis currently are receiving great experimental attention, chromosome variability can be accommodated into other models of neoplastic evolution. For example, it has been proposed (Ohno, 1974; Comings, 1973) that one pathway in neoplastic development is the transition of a heterozygous to a homozygous recessive mutant cell. Support for this hypothesis was provided by studies with tumor promoters. When cells initiated with a suboptimal dose of chemical carcinogen are treated with promoters, which alone are neither mutagenic or carcinogenic (Berenblum, 1954; 1978), the lag time for tumor expression is shortened and the frequency of tumor appearance is increased. Kinsella and Radman (1978) reported that the promoter TPA (12-0-tetradecanoyl phorbol-13-acetate) increases the frequency of sister chromatid exchange, and postulated further that induced mitotic recombination could result in homozygosity of a recessive mutant allele. By this hypothesis, sister chromatid exchange is merely a reflection of more generalized recombination occurring within the cell. It has been proposed alternatively that tumor promoters might induce aneuploidy in mammalian cells, and result in the segregation of mutant phenotypes by nondisjunction. Support for this hypothesis was provided by Parry and colleagues (1981), who demonstrated that a variety of tumor promoters (but not structurally related non-promoting compounds) were capable of inducing aneuploidy in yeast. Compounds were assayed for their abilities to induce mitotic aneuploidy and crossing over in the D6 strain of yeast *Saccharomyces cerevisiae*. This diploid strain carries a series of recessive, coupled markers on chromosome VII which makes it amenable to studies of both induced aneuploidy and mitotic recombination (Parry and Sharp, 1981). All tumor promoters tested for the ability to induce aneuploidy were positive, whereas nonpromoters were negative. In contrast, none of the tumor promoting compounds were capable of inducing detectable mitotic recombination.

Since segregation and expression of autosomally-linked recessive phenotypes can occur by chromosomal mechanisms, aneuploidy, as well as chromosomal rearrangement, might facilitate this type of gene segregation during neoplastic development. Aneuploidy is the hallmark of cancer, and although there are exceptions which are (or appear) diploid, most tumor cells are aneuploid with a tendency towards hyperdiploidy. There are several genetic disorders (discussed above) which feature both chromosomal abnormalities and increased frequency of malignancy. There is also a correlation among increased age and increased frequencies of chromosomal abnormalities and malignancy (Tice, 1978). Any of these abnormalities might permit, by nondisjunctive errors, an expression of recessive allelic mutations localized on autosomes. Thus, Boveri's (1914) original somatic mutation theory of cancer, which was based on changes in ploidy, may be important in a mutational theory of cancer involving the expression of a recessive autosomally-linked gene mutation.

IV. Gene Amplification

Gene amplification is a well-documented mechanism by which cells can meet the demand for increased quantities of particular gene products (Brown and Dawid, 1968; Alt et al., 1978; Spradling and Mahowald, 1981). In somatic cells, gene amplification may permit cells to overcome deficiencies in specific enzyme activities. Such deficiencies may be the result of specific metabolic inhibition (Alt et al., 1978; Wahl et al., 1979), mutations in the gene itself (Roberts and Axel, 1982; Brennand et al., 1982), or the consequence of less direct toxic stress (Hildebrand et al., 1983). During development, gene amplification may occur for specific genes or sets of genes at precise stages (Spradling and Mahowald, 1981; and see Schimke, 1982 for several examples).

In most cases examined, an increase in gene copy number corresponds to a proportionate increase in mRNA and protein. Perhaps the most extensively studied locus which amplifies in response to specific metabolic stress is that which encodes dihydrofolate reductase (dhfr). Numerous studies (consult Schimke, 1982) have shown that dhfr gene copy number can increase in cells resistant to methotrexate, an antifolate agent used extensively in cancer chemotherapy. In cultured cells, amplified genes may exist stably within the chromosome, often as a homogeneously staining region (HSR) detected in G-banded chromosomes (Biedler and Spengler, 1976; Nunberg et al., 1978) or unstably as presumably autonomously replicating units (double minutes) which lack centromenes and kinetochores (Kaufman et al., 1981; Brown et al., 1981; Haber and Schimke, 1981; Schimke, 1982). In the cases examined, the amplified unit of DNA is quite large (up to 2000 kilobase pairs) and can extend into sequences for which cloned probes are not available (Nunberg et al., 1978; Hamlin et al., 1982). Such observations have demonstrated that the precise definition of an amplified unit would be an arduous task. Consequently, model systems have been used to generate and characterize amplified sequences in mammalian DNA (Roberts et al., 1983).

What role might gene amplification play in carcinogenesis, and how might these alterations in DNA structure be elicited by carcinogens? Several investigations have provided information concerning these questions, and have suggested that DNA amplification may indeed be involved in the process of carcinogenesis.

Lavi (1981) demonstrated that exposure of SV40-transformed Chinese hamster embryo cells to various chemical and physical carcinogens could induce SV40 DNA synthesis. Such amplification of SV40 DNA sequences did not result in the production of infectious virus, but rather, was characterized by the presence of heterogeneous DNA molecules from the integrated SV40 locus. Lavi discussed these results in the context of general gene amplification being induced at random by carcinogens. Similarly, Varshavsky (1981) suggested that one mechanism of tumor promotion and carcinogenesis may operate by an increase in the frequency of extra illegitimate rounds of DNA replication (replicon misfiring). Varshavsky further postulated that such replicon misfiring might not only lead to increased gene copy number, but also might facilitate gene segregation and the expression of recessive phenotypes (Varshavsky, 1981). Such random misfiring of replicons might be detectable using a marker locus for which gene dosage mutants can be detected.

To test the above hypothesis, Varshavsky examined whether tumor promoters might act by facilitating gene amplification. By a series of single-step selections for resistance to methotrexate, the tumor promoter TPA (12-0-tetradecanoyl-phorbol-13 acetate) was shown to induce dhfr gene amplification (Varshavsky, 1981). Phorbol (a non-tumor-promoting analog of TPA) did not exhibit such activity. Barsoum and Varshavsky (1983) demonstrated further that certain mitogenic hormones which are involved in the regulation of cell proliferation also can induce gene amplification at the dhfr locus. These results suggest that agents which affect DNA replication (many chemical and physical carcinogens would fall into this category) might be effective in inducing gene amplification. This has profound implications for the use of antimetabolites in cancer chemotherapy, since the generation of drug-resistant variant tumor stemlines could occur as a consequence of such treatment (Brown et al., 1983).

The observation that generalized gene amplification might occur as a random event after exposure of cells to chemical or physical carcinogens raises the possibility that a given cell will amplify a gene (e.g., a proto-oncogene) related to carcinogenesis, and thereby gain a proliferative advantage, and perhaps escape growth control. Pall (1981) proposed that a crucial, perhaps early, step in carcinogenesis might be a DNA alteration producing a duplicated proto-oncogene. This hypothesis is consistent with the gene dosage model of carcinogenesis discussed by Klein (1981). Observations of specific oncogene copy number in certain neoplastic cells have provided support for this proposal.

Karyotypic evidence of gene amplification has been found in a variety of human tumors, in the form of HSRs or double minutes (Biedler et al., 1973; Brodeur et al., 1977; 1981; Gilbert et al., 1981). Cellular oncogenes can be included in these amplifications. Double minutes and HSRs in the mouse adrenocortical tumor Y-1 and an HSR in the colon carcinoma line COLO 320 contain amplified copies of the oncogenes c-Ki-*ras* and c-*myc*, respectively (Schwab et al., 1983; Alitalo et al., 1983). The c-*myc* gene also is amplified in a promyelocytic leukemia cell line (Collins and Groudine, 1982). Amplified DNA with limited homology to the *myc* cellular oncogene (called N-*myc*) is shared by human neuroblastoma cell lines and a neuroblastoma tumor (Schwab et al., 1983). Double minutes and HSRs are found commonly in cells of human neuroblastomas (Brodeur *et al.*, 1981). By *in situ* hybridization, Schwab *et al.* (1983) demonstrated that HSRs are the site of amplified N-*myc* sequences. Other investigators have shown, by DNA transfection studies using NIH 3T3 cells, that one neuroblastoma cell line carries an additional gene (termed N-*ras*) homologous to the *ras* family of oncogenes, which confers focal transformation on NIH 3T3 cells (Shimizu *et al.*, 1983). It is thus possible that the amplification of the N-*myc* proto oncogene is only one of several genetic changes involved in the evolution of the neuroblastoma. Alternatively, the amplification of N-*myc* and/or alteration of N-*ras* sequences may be inconsequential to the neoplastic process, and merely a reflection of the inherent karyotypic instability of tumor cells, or their prolonged *in vitro* culture history in some cases.

In summary, the amplification of specific gene sequences can be envisioned as an additional mechanism by which neoplastic evolution can occur. By virtue of the selective advantage specific gene amplification might confer on a particular cell, one can easily imagine that this genetic alteration may play a role in neoplastic progression particularly in the generation of tumor cell heterogeneity. This should justify additional studies designed to examine the mechanisms and consequences of this genetic alteration, and stimulate research on amplified sequences in tumor cells.

V. DNA Methylation

Another alteration in the structure of DNA which is receiving increased attention in the context of carcinogenesis induced by chemicals is that affecting the methylation pattern in DNA. Alterations in DNA methylation were proposed to be causally related to neoplasia by Holliday (1979). Riggs (1975) proposed a model based on DNA methylation to explain the initiation and maintenance of X-inactivation and other aspects of gene expression during differentiation.

The pattern of 5-methylcytosine residues in DNA is thought to be associated with gene expression in eucaryotic cells (reviewed by Razin and Riggs, 1980; Erlich and Wang, 1981; Doerfler, 1983). Methylation patterns are often tissue specific: structural genes and/or flanking sequences are hypomethylated in tissues actively expressing globin (Waalwijk and Flavell, 1978; McGhee and Ginder, 1979), ovalbumin and conalbumin (Mandel and Chambon, 1979), immunoglobulin (Yagi and Koshland, 1981), metallothionein (Compere and Palmiter, 1981) and σ-crystallin genes (Jones *et al.*, 1981), to cite several examples. These same DNA sequences are hypermethylated in tissues which do not express the genes. The correlation between hypomethylation and gene expression has been described for viral DNA integrated in infected cells (see Doerfler, 1983 for a review).

Furthermore, results with 5-azacytidine-induced differentiation (Jones and Taylor, 1980; Venolia *et al.*, 1981) also support a relationship between DNA methylation and gene activity. Landolph and Jones (1982) reported that 5-

azacytidine and related cytosine analogs are negligibly mutagenic in mammalian cells. Such analogs of cytosine are capable, however, of causing focal transformation of mouse cells in culture (Benedict et al., 1977). This suggests that alterations in DNA methylation may be one mechanism by which certain steps in neoplastic progression can occur. What evidence supports such a hypothesis?

Considerable evidence has been obtained to show that methylation patterns can be stable over many passages in eucaryotic cells (Wigler et al., 1981), although clonal variation in methylation patterns has been described in cultured cells (Shmookler-Reis and Goldstein, 1982). It is generally accepted that cells contain "maintenance" methyltransferase activity which provides modification of hemimethylated sites in DNA formed during the semiconservative replication of DNA (Riggs, 1975). The natural substrate for this enzymatic activity is hemimethylated DNA, in which the parental strand of DNA contains 5-methylcytosine residues, and the daughter strand does not (Jones and Taylor, 1980; 1981).

If methylation patterns in DNA can control gene expression, one might suppose that alterations in the normal pattern of methylation are involved in the altered phenotype of neoplastic cells. Jones and Taylor (1981) and Wilson and Jones (1983) have demonstrated that a diverse range of carcinogens can inhibit the methyltransferase reaction. Certain carcinogens were capable of direct inactivation of the methyltransferase enzyme; the inhibitory action of other compounds presumably occurred through DNA adduct formation, the induction of apurinic sites and single-strand breaks. This study demonstrated that a broad range of DNA damaging agents significantly inhibit methyltransferase activity. The inhibition of cytosine methylation by such compounds might therefore be related to their oncogenic potential. Thus, although the documented mutagenicity of many compounds may be correlated with their carcinogenicity, mutagenicity may not be the mechanistic *basis* for transformation by such agents. Moreover, the inhibition of methyltransferase activity may help to explain the carcinogenicity of chemicals which are not mutagenic *per se*: L-ethionine, a potent hepatocarcinogen, but non-mutagen, may be an example of such a compound (Mendelsohn et al., 1980).

Interestingly, *de novo* methylation activity may be an important characteristic of gene regulation in embryogenesis (Jahner et al., 1982). Early-stage mouse embryos and embryonal carcinoma cells have been shown to be non-permissive for DNA virus as well as retrovirus gene expression (see Jahner et al., 1982); such is not the case for post-implantation embryos. Breznik and Cohen (1982) reported altered methylation of endogenous mouse mammary tumor virus promoter sequences during mammary carcinogenesis. Since hypomethylation correlates with gene expression, the demethylation observed in spontaneous Balb/c tumors suggests that promoter derepression (and attendant gene activation) may be involved in the evolution of mammary carcinomas. Harbers et al. (1981) reported similar correlations between the methylation state of integrated moloney murine leukemia virus and gene activity. By analogy, alterations in the methylation of promoter regions of endogenous cellular genes, or even the structural regions of genes conceivably could activate cellular proto-oncogenes, or cellular genes involved in growth control. Feinberg *et al.* (1983) have recently reported hypomethylation of a surprisingly large number of gene loci which were examined in tumor cells in an unbiased fashion. Such findings may reflect a generalized defect in the fidelity of methyltransferase activity in tumor cells in comparison to normal cells, thus resulting in random alterations in DNA methylation. If specific changes in gene expression confer a selective advantage on the cell, changes in DNA methylation may be one of the mechanisms generating tumor cell heterogeneity. Dissection of carcinogenesis into various stages should allow a definition of when specific changes in gene methylation might occur in neoplastic progression. Furthermore, transcriptional *inactivation* of gene loci by changes in methylation also may be involved in carcinogenesis; examples of such alterations remain to be discovered. The development of model systems to detect compounds capable of altering DNA methylation should aid in defining how many such agents are indeed also carcinogenic. Such studies are just now beginning (Wilson and Jones, 1983).

F. A Retrospective: The Origin of the Somatic Mutation Theory of Cancer

> "... Having arrived now at the end of our journey, we have to confess that the problem of cancer has not been solved, though highly significant facts accumulated during the past few years suggest that it is not insoluble.... To those who may be inclined to reproach the author for a too enthusiastic partisanship, he would reply that it is never ill-judged to be guided by a hypothesis, so long as it does no violence to the known facts, and that the best proof of value is the amount of research stimulated ...."
>
> Charles Oberling
> *The Riddle of Cancer*, 1952

Theodor Boveri generally is acknowledged as the first to postulate that somatic mutation is the basis of the heritable alteration in neoplastic cells. Boveri studied the development of sea urchins, and noted a correlation between abnormal development of these organisms and aneuploidy, which he considered to be analogous to cancer (1892). In *Zur frage der entstehung maligner tumoren* (1914), he stated "... the essence of my theory is not the abnormal mitoses, but a certain abnormal chromatin complex, no matter how it arises. Every process which brings about this condition would lead to a malignant tumor." Actually, von Hanseman (1890) previously had described, in a carcinoma of the larynx, a great abundance of mitotic figures with large numbers of tripolar and multipolar divisions, and remarked on many "hyperchromatic" and "hypochromatic" mitoses. He described this hypochromatism to consist not merely of a reduction of the amount of chromatin in the chromosomes, but rather, in actual reduction in the number of the chromosomes. In describing cancer, von Hansemann first used the term "anaplasia" to refer to the "redifferentiation" of the cell. By abnormal, pluripolar mitoses (and what we now know as nondisjunction), a new, cancerous cell type was thus produced (von Hansemann, 1893). That von Hansemann recognized nondisjunction is evidenced by his cytological observations of mitotic "lag," whereby a chromosome was seen to adhere to the mitotic spindle. He emphasized that the whole process of anaplasia is a gradual and progressive one, and that the loss of differentiated function increases as the anaplasia progresses.

It seems that oncology has come full circle. Boveri's hypothesis can now be examined in a new context. Modern cell and molecular biology can provide many additional tools required to dissect carcinogenesis into discrete stages. But clearly, we still do not know all of the steps, or even all of the alternative paths in neoplasia. In searching for answers, we hope we are asking the important questions—and at least are following some of the correct paths the cell shows us.

Certainly, by many of the studies described in this review, valuable information has been gained concerning the biology and genesis of neoplasia, and the role of DNA alterations in this process. To see cancer as a multistep process is to recognize this disease as a problem in cellular differentiation and development. Accordingly, any attempt to describe such a complex process by simplistic, Mendelian-type genetics using cultured cells of fibroblast origin will necessarily be inadequate. Consequently, we continue to be deficient in explaining mechanistically the entire developmental process of carcinogenesis. Hopefully, the ideas and experimental approaches presented in this chapter have provided an indication of the types of molecular genetic and biochemical approaches which, if coupled with advances in tumor cell biology and somatic cell genetics, and knowledge of cell differentiation, can offer new insights to the enigma we call cancer.

> ... The water continually flowed and flowed and yet, it was always there; it was always the same, and yet, every moment it was new ....
>
> Hermann Hesse, *Siddhartha*

ACKNOWLEDGMENTS

At the time this review was completed (1983), the author was supported by a J. Robert Oppenheimer Fellowship from the Los Alamos National Laboratory, and research contracts administered through the Department of Energy, Office of Health and Environmental Research.

I gratefully acknowledge the editorial assistance of Monica Fink in the preparation of this manuscript.

BIBLIOGRAPHY

Abramson, D.H., Ellsworth, R.M., Roseblatt, M., Tretter, P., Jereb, B., Kitchin, F.D.: Arch. Opthamol. (in press).

Alitalo, K., Schwab, M., Lin, C.C., Varmus, H.E., Bishop, J.M.: Homogeneously staining chromosomal regions contain amplified copies of an abundantly expressed cellular oncogene (c-myc) in malignant neuroendocrine cells from a human colon carcinoma. Proc. Natl. Acad. Sci. USA **80**, 1707–1711 (1983).

Alt, F.W., Kellems, R., Bertino, J., Schimke, R.T.: Selective multiplication of dihydrofolate reductase genes in methotrexate resistant variants of cultured murine cells. J. Biol. Chem. **253**, 1357–1370 (1978).

Ames, B.N., Durston, W.E., Yamasaki, E., Lee, F.D.: Carcinogens are mutagens: A simple test system combining liver homogenates for activation and bacteria for detection. Proc. Nat. Acad. Sci. USA **70**, 2281–2285 (1973).

Ames, B.N., Lee, F.D., Durston, W.E.: An improved bacterial test system for the detection and classification of mutagens and carcinogens. Proc. Nat. Acad. Sci. USA **70**, 782–786 (1973).

Armitage, P., Doll, R.: Stochastic models for carcinogenesis. In: Proceedings of the 4th Berkeley Symposium on Mathematical Statistics and Probability: Biology and problems of health, Vol. 4, University of California Press: Berkeley; p. 19 (1961).

Ashley, D.J.B.: The two "hit" and multiple "hit" theories of carcinogenesis. British Journal of Cancer **23**, 313–328 (1969).

Aviles, D., Jami, J., Rousset, J.P., Ritz, E.: Tumor x host cell hybrids in the mouse: chromosomes from the normal cell parent in malignant hybrid tumors. J. Natl. Cancer Inst. **58**, 1391–1399 (1977).

Bader, J.L., Li, F.P., Gerald, P.S., Leikin, S.L., Randolph, J.G.: 11p chromosome deletion in four patients with aniridia and Wilms' tumor. Proc. Am. Assoc. Cancer Res. **20**, 210 (1979).

Barski G., Cornefert, F.: Characteristics of 'hybrid'-type clonal cell lines obtained from mixed cultures in vitro. J. Natl. Cancer Inst. **28**, 801–821 (1962).

Barrett, J.C., Bias, N.E., Ts'o, P.O.P.: A mammalian cellular system for the concomitant study of neoplastic transformation and somatic mutation. Mutation Research **50**, 121–136 (1978).

Barrett, J.C., Crawford, B.D., Grady, D.L., Hester, L.D., Jones, P.A., Benedict, W.F., Ts'o, P.O.P.: The temporal acquisition of enhanced fibrinolytic activity by Syrian hamster embryo cells following treatment with benzo(a)pyrene. Cancer Res. **37**, 3815–3812 (1977).

Barrett, J.C., Ts'o, P.O.P.: Evidence for the progressive nature of neoplastic transformation in vitro. Proc. Nat. Acad. Sci. U.S.A. **75**, 3761–3765 (1978a).

Barrett, J.C., Ts'o, P.O.P.: The relationship between somatic mutation and neoplastic transformation. Proc. Nat. Acad. Sci. USA **75**, 3297–3301 (1978b).

Barrett, J.C., Ts'o, P.O.P.: Mechanistic studies of neoplastic transformation of cells in culture. In: Polycyclic Hydrocarbons and Cancer, Vol. 2, H. Gelboin and P.O.P. Ts'o, Eds., Academic Press: New York; p. 235–267 (1978c).

Barrett, J.C., Tsutsui, T., Ts'o, P.O.P.: Neoplastic transformation induced by a direct perturbation of DNA. Nature **274**, 229–232 (1978).

Barrett, J.C.: Cell transformation, mutation, and cancer. Gann monogr. **27**, 195–206 (1981).

Barrett, J.C., Wong, A., McLachian, J.A.: Diethylstilbestrol induces neoplastic transformation without measurable gene mutation at two loci. Science **212**, 1402–1404 (1981).

Barrett, J.C., Crawford, B.D., Ts'o, P.O.P.: The role of somatic mutation in a multistage model of carcinogenesis. In: Mammalian Cell Transformation by Chemical Carcinogens, N. Mishra, V. Dunkel, and M. Mehlman, eds. Adv. Mod. Environ. Tox. **1**, 467–501 (1981).

Barsoum, J., Varshavsky, A.: Mutagenic hormones and tumor promoters greatly increase the incidence of colony-forming cells bearing amplified dihydrofolate reductase genes. Proc. Nat. Acad. Sci. USA **80**, 5330–5334 (1983).

Baylin, S., Hus, S., Gann, D., Smallridge, R.C., Wells, S.A.: Inherited thyroid medullary carcinoma: a final monoclonal mutation in one of multiple clones of susceptible cells. Science **199**, 429–431 (1978).

Benedict, W.F., Gielen, V.E., Nebert, D.W.: Polycyclic hydrocarbon-produced toxicity, transformation, and chromosomal aberrations as a function of aryl hydrocarbon hydroxylase activity in cell cultures. Int. J. Cancer **9**, 435–451 (1972).

Benedict, W.F.: Early changes in chromosomal number and structure after treatment of fetal hamster cultures with transforming doses of polycyclic hydrocarbons. J. Natl. Cancer Inst. **49**, 585–590 (1972).

Benedict, W.F., Rucker, N., Mark, C., *et al*: Correlation between balance of specific chromosomes and expression of malignancy in hamster cells. J. Natl. Cancer Inst. **54**, 157–162 (1975).

Benedict, W.F., Banerjee, A., Gardner, A., Jones, P.A.: Induction of morphological transformation in mouse C3H/10T 1/2 clone 8 cells and chromosomal damage in hamster $A(T_1)C1-3$ cells by cancer chemotherapeutic agents. Cancer Res. **37**, 2202–2208 (1977).

Benedict, W.F., Murphree, A.L., Banerjee, A., Spina, C.A., Sparkes, M.C., Sparkes, R.S.: Patient with 13 chromosome deletion: evidence that the retinoblastoma gene is a recessive cancer gene. Science **219**, 973–975 (1983).

Berenblum, I.: A speculative review; the probable nature of promoting action and its significance in the understanding of the mechanism of carcinogenesis. Cancer Res. **14**, 471–477 (1954).

Berenblum, I.: Historical perspective. In: Carcinogenesis, Vol. 2, T.J. Slaga, A. Sivak and R.K. Boutwell, Eds., Academic Press: New York (1978).

Berwald, Y., Sachs, L.: In vitro cell transformation with chemical carcinogens. Nature **200**, 1182–1184 (1963).

Berwald, Y., Sachs, L.: In vitro transformation of normal cells to tumor cells by carcinogenic hydrocarbons. J. Natl. Cancer Inst. **35**, 641–661 (1965).

Biedler, J.L., Helson, L., Spengler, B.A.: Morphology and growth, tumorigenicity, and cytogenetics of human neuroblastoma cells established in continuous culture. Cancer Res. **33**, 2643–2652 (1973).

Biedler, J.L., Spengler, B.: Metaphase chromosome anomaly: association with drug resistance and cell-specific products. Science **191**, 185–187 (1976).

Biedler, J.L., Ross, R.A., Shanske, S., Spengler, B.A.: Human neuroblastoma cytogenetics: search for significance of homogeneously staining regions and double minute chromosomes. In: A.E. Evans (ed.), Advances in Neuroblastoma Research, pp. 81–96. New York, Raven Press (1980).

Biedler, J.L. Spengler, B.A.: A novel chromosome abnormally in human neuroblastoma and antifolate-resistant Chinese hamster cell lines in culture. J. Natl. Cancer Inst. **57**, 683–695 (1976).

Bishop, J.M.: Retroviruses. Ann. Rev. Biochem. **47**, 35–88 (1978).

Bishop, J.M.: Cellular oncogenes and retroviruses. Ann. Rev. Biochem. **53**, 301–354 (1983).

Blair, D.G., Oskarsson, M., Wood, T.G., McClements, M.L., Fischinger, P.J., Van de Woude, G.G.: Activation of the transforming potential of a normal cell sequence: A molecular model for oncogenesis. Science **212**, 941–942 (1981).

Bloch-Shtacher, N., Sachs, L.: Chromosome balance and the control of malignancy. J. Cell Physiol. **87**, 89–100 (1976).

Boveri, T.H.: Zur frage der entstehung maligner tumoren. Fisher, Jena (1914).

Boveri, T.H.: Uber die entstehung des gegensatzes zwischen der geschlechtszellen und der somatischen zellen bie *Ascaris*. S.B. Ges Morph. Physiol. Munch. **8**, 114–125 (1892).

Brennand, J., Chinault, A.C., Konecki, D.S., Melton, D.W., Caskey, C.T.: Cloned cDNA sequences of the hypoxanthine/guanine phosphonbosyltransferase gene from a mouse neuroblastoma cell line found to have amplified genomic sequences Proc. Nat. Acad. Sci. USA **79**, 1950–1054 (1982).

Breznik, T., Cohen, J.C.: Altered methylation of endogenopus viral promoter sequences during mammary carcinogenesis. Nature **295**, 255–257 (1982).

Brodeur, G.M., Sekhon, G.L., Goldstein, M.N.: Chromosomal aberrations in human neuroblastomas. Cancer (Phila.), **40**, 2256–2263 (1977).

Brodeur, G.M., Green, A.A., Hayes, F.A., Williams, K.J., Williams, D.L., Tsiatis, A.A.: Cytogenetic features of human neuroblastomas and cell lines. Cancer Res. **41**, 4678–4686 (1981).

Brookes, P.: Quantitative aspects of the reaction of some carcinogens with nucleic acids and the possible significance of such reactions in the process of carcinogenesis. Cancer Res. **26**, 1994–2003 (1966).

Brookes, P., Lawley, P.D.: Evidence for the binding of polynuclear aromatic hydrocarbons to the nucleic acids of mouse skin: Relation between carcinogenic power of hydrocarbons and their binding to deoxyribonucleic acid. Nature **202**, 781–784 (1964).

Brown, D, David, I.: Specific gene amplication in oocytes. Science **160**, 272–280 (1968).

Brown, P., Beverley, S., Schimke, R.: Relationship of amplified dihydrofolate reductase genes to double minute chromosomes in unstably resistant mouse fibroblast cell lines. Mol. Cell. Biol. **1**, 1077–1083 (1981).

Brown, P.C., Tlsty, T.D., Schimke, R.T.: Enhancement of methotrexate resistance and dihydrofolate reductase gene amplification by treatment of mouse 3T6 cells with hydroxyurea. Mol. Cell. Biol. **3**, 1097–1107 (1983).

Bunn, H.F., Forget, G.B., Ranney, H.M.: Human Hemoglobins. Philadelphia, PA. W.B. Saunders Co. (1977).

Cairns, J.: The origin of human cancers. Nature **289**, 353–357 (1981).

Capon, D.J., Seeburg, P.H., McGrath, J.P., Hayflick, J.S., Edman, U., Levinson, A.D., Goeddel, D.V.: Activation of Ki-ras2 gene in human colon and lung carcinomas by two different point mutations. Nature **304**, 507–513 (1983).

Chan, G.L., Little, J.B.: Induction of ouabain-resistant mutations in C3H/10T 1/2 mouse cells by ultraviolet light. Proc. Nat. Acad. Sci. **75**, 3363–3366 (1978).

Chang, E.H., Ellis, R.W., Scolnick, E.M., Lowy, D.R.: Transformation by cloned harvey murine sarcoma virus DNA: efficiency increased by long terminal repeat DNA. Science **210**, 1249–1251 (1980).

Chang, E.H., Furth, M.E., Scolnick, E.M., Lowy, D.R.: Tumorigenic transformation of mammalian cells induced by a normal human gene homologous to the oncogene of Harvey murine sarcoma virus. Nature **297**, 479–483 (1982).

Chang, E.H., Gonda, M.A., Ellis, R.W., Scolnick, E.M.: Human genome contains four

48

genes homologous to transforming genes of Harvey and Kirsten murine sarcoma viruses. Proc. Nat. Acad. Sci. USA **79**, 4848–4852 (1982).

Chattopadhyay, S.K., Chang, E.H., Lander, M.R., Ellis, R.W., Scolnick, E.M., Lowy, D.R.: Amplification and rearrangement of onc genes in mammalian species. Nature **296**, 361–363 (1982).

Christman, J.K., Price, P., Pedrinan, L., Acs, G.: Correlation between hypomethylation of DNA and expression of globin genes in Friend erythroleukemia cells. Eur. J. Biochem. **81**, 53–61 (1977).

Cleaver, J.E.: Human diseases with in vitro manifestations of altered repair and replication of DNA. In: Genetics of Human Cancer, J.J. Mulvihill, R.W. Miller and J.F. Fraumeni, Eds., Raven Press: New York; p. 355–363 (1977).

Cleaver, J.E., Bootsma, D.: Xeroderma pigmentosum: Biochemical and genetic characteristics. Ann. Rev. Genet. **9**, 19–38 (1975).

Cohen, A.J., Li, F.P., Berg, S., Marchetto, D.J., Tsai, S., Jacobs, S.C., Brown, R.S.: Hereditary renal-cell carcinoma associated with a chromosomal translocation. N. Eng. J. Med. **301**, 592–595 (1979).

Collins, S., Groudine, M.: Amplification of endogenous myc-related DNA sequences in a human myeloid leukaemia cell line. Nature **298**, 679–681 (1982).

Comings, D.E.: A general theory of carcinogenesis. Proc. Nat. Acad. Sci. **70**, 3324–3328 (1973).

Compere, S.J., Palmiter, R.D.: DNA methylation controls and inducibility of the mouse metallothionein-I gene in lymphoid cells. Cell **25**, 233–240 (1981).

Cooper, G.M., Okenquist, S., Silverman, L.: Transforming activity of DNA in chemically transformed and normal cells. Nature **284**, 418–421 (1980).

Cooper, G.M.: Cellular transforming genes. Science **218**, 801–806 (1982).

Cox, R.: DNA methylase inhibition in vitro by N-methyl-N-mitro-N-nitrosoguanidine. Cancer Res. **40**, 61–63 (1980).

Crawford, B.D., Barrett, J.C., Ts'o, P.O.P.: Neoplastic conversion of preneoplastic Syrian hamster cells: rate estimation by fluctuation analysis. Molec. Cell. Biol. **3**, 931–945 (1983).

Croce, C., Aden, D., Koprowski, H.: Somatic cell hybrids between mouse peritoneal macrophages and SV-40 transformed human cells. II. Presence of human chromosome 7 carrying simian virus-40 genome in cells of tumors induced by hybrid cells. Proc. Nat. Acad. Sci. **72**, 1397–1400 (1975).

Croce, C.M., Koprowski, H.: Positive control of the transformed phenotype in hybrids between normal and SV-40 transformed human cells. Science **184**, 1288–1289 (1974).

Dalla-Favera, R., Bregni, M., Erikson, J., Patterson, D., Gallo, R.C., Croce, C.M.: Human c-myc onc gene is located on the region of chromosome 8 that is translocated in Burkitt lymphoma cells. Proc. Nat. Acad. Sci. USA **79**, 7824–7827 (1982).

Deaven, L.L., Cram, L.S., Wells, R.S. et al: Relationships between chromosome complement and cellular DNA content in tumorigenic cell populations. In: Arrighi, F.E., Rao, P.N., Stubblefield, E. (eds.), MD Anderson Hospital and Tumor Institute. Genes, Chromosomes and Neoplasia. New York, Raven Press, pp. 419–452 (1981).

Defendi, V., Lehman, J., Kraemer, P.: Morphologically normal hamster cells with malignant properties. Virology **19**, 592–598 (1963).

Defendi, V., Ephrussi, B., Koprowski, H. et al: Properties of hybrids between polyoma-transformed and normal mouse cells. Proc. Nat. Acad. Sci. **57**, 299–305 (1967).

DeFeo, D., Gonda, M.A., Young, H.A., Chang, E.H., Lowy, D.R., Scolnick, E.M., Ellis, R.W.: Analysis of two divergent rat genomic clones homologous to the transforming gene of Harvey murine sarcoma virus. Proc. Nat. Acad. Sci. USA **78**, 3328–3332 (1981).

Der, C.J., Krontiris, T.G., Cooper, G.M.: Transforming genes of human bladder and lung carcinoma cell lines are homologous to the ras genes of Harvey and Kirsten sarcoma viruses. Proc. Nat. Acad. Sci. USA **79**, 3637–3640 (1982).

Der, C.J., Cooper, G.M.: Altered gene products are associated with activation of cellular ras_k genes in human lung and colon carcinomas. Cell **32**, 201–208 (1983).

Dhar, R., McClements, W.L., Enquist, L.W., Vande Woude, G.F.: Nucleotide sequences of integrated Moloney sarcoma provirus long terminal repeats and their host and viral junctions. Proc. Nat. Acad. Sci. U.S.A. **77**, 3937–3941 (1980).

Dhar, R., Ellis, R.W., Shih, T.Y., Oroszlan, S., Shapiro, B., Maizel, J., Lowy, D., Scolnick, E.: Nucleotide sequence of the p21 transforming protein of harvey murine sarcoma virus. Science **217**, 934–937 (1982).

DiPaolo, J.A., Donovan, P., Nelson, R.: Quantitative studies of in vitro transformation by chemical carcinogens. J. Nat. Cancer Inst. **42**, 867–874 (1969).

DiPaolo, J.A., Nelson, R.L., Donovan, P.J.: Morphological, oncogenic, and karyological characteristics in Syrian hamster embryo cells transformed in vitro by carcinogenic polycyclic hydrocarbons. Cancer Res. **31**, 1118–1127 (1971).

Doerfler, W.: DNA methylation and gene activity. In: Ann. Rev. of Biochem. **52**, 93–124 (1983).

Doll, R.: An epidemiological perspective of the biology of cancer. Cancer Res. **38**, 3573–3583 (1978).

Ehrlich, M., Wang, R.Y.H.: 5-methycytosine in eukaryotic DNA. Science **212**, 1350–1357 (1981).

Ellis, R.W., DeFeo, D., Shih, T.Y., Gonda, M.A., Young, H.A., Tsuchida, N., Lowy, D.R., Scolnick, E.M.: The p21 src genes of Harvey and Kirsten sarcoma viruses originate from divergent members of a family of normal vertebrate genes. Nature **292**, 506–511 (1981).

Fahmy, M.J., Fahmy, O.G.: Intervening DNA insertions and the alteration of gene expression by carcinogens. Cancer Res. **40**, 3374–3382 (1980).

Farber, E.: Ethionine carcinogenesis. Adv. Cancer Res. **7**, 383–474 (1963).

Feinberg, A.P., Vogelstein, B.: Hypomethylation distinguishes genes of some human cancers from their normal counterparts. Nature **301**, 89–92 (1983).

Feinberg, A.P., Vogelstein, B., Droller, M.J., Baylin, S.B., Nelkin, B.D.: Mutation affecting the 12th amino acid of the c-Ha-ras oncogene product occurs infrequently in human cancer. Science **220**, 1175–1177 (1983).

Feinberg, A.P., Coffey, D.S.: Organ site specificity for cancer in chromosomal instability disorders. Cancer Res. **42**, 3252–3254 (1982).

Fernandez, A., Mondal, S., Heidelberger, C.: A probabilistic view of the transformation of cultured C3H/10T 1/2 mouse embryo fibroblasts by 3-methylcholanthrene. Proc. Natl. Acad. Sci. **77**, 7272–7276 (1980).

Fidler, I.J.: Tumor heterogeneity and the biology of cancer invasion and metastasis. Cancer Res. **38**, 2651–2660 (1978).

Filalkow, P.J.: Clonal origin of human tumors. Ann. Rev. Med. **30**, 135–143 (1979).

Finnegan, D.J.: Retroviruses and transposable elements—which came first? Nature **302**, 105–106 (1983).

Flavell, A.: Did retroviruses evolve from transposable elements? Nature **289**, 10–11 (1981).

Foulds, L.: The experimental study of tumor progression: A review. Cancer Res. **14**, 327–339 (1954).

Foulds, L.: Neoplastic development, Vol. 2, Academic Press: London (1975).

Francke, U., Holmes, L.B., Atkins, L., Riccardi, V.M.: Aniridia–Wilms' tumor association: Evidence for specific deletion of 11p13. Cytogenet. Cell Genet. **24**, 185–192 (1979).

Fu, Y.S., Reagan, J.W., Richart, R.M., Townsend, D.E.: Nuclear DNA and histologic studies of genital lesions in diethylstibestrol-exposed progeny. I. Intraepithelial squamous abnormalities. Am. J. Clin. Pathol. **72**, 503–514 (1979).

Furth, J., Kahn, M.C.: The transmission of leukemia of mice with a single cell. Amer. J. of Cancer **31**, 276–282 (1937).

German J., Ed.: Chromosomes and Cancer, John Wiley and Sons, Inc., New York (1974).

Gilbert, F., Balaban, G., Breg, W.R., Gallie, B., Reid, T., Nichols, W.: Homogeneously staining region in a retinoblastoma cell line. Relevance to tumor initiation and progression. J. Natl. Canc. Inst. **67**, 301–306 (1981).

Goldfarb, M., Shimizu, K., Perucho, M., Wigler, M.: Isolation and preliminary characterization of a human transforming gene from T24 bladder carcinoma cells. Nature **296**, 404–409 (1982).

Goth, R., Rajewsky, M.F.: Persistance of O^6-ethylguanine in rat brain DNA: Correlation with nervous system specific carcinogenesis by ethyl-nitrosourea. Proc. Nat. Acad. Sci. USA **71**, 639–643 (1974).

Graham, F.L., van der Eb, A.J.: A new technique for the assay of infectivity of human adenovirus 5 DNA. Virology **52**, 456–467 (1973).

Gray, J.M., Pierce, G.B.: Relationship between growth rate and differentiation in vivo. J. Natl. Cancer Inst. **32**, 1201–1212 (1964).

Green, M.M.: The case for DNA insertion mutations in Drosophila. In: Bukhari, A.I., Shapiro, J.A., Adhya, S.L. (eds.), DNA Insertion Elements, Plasmids and Episomes. New York, Cold Spring Harbor Laboratory, pp. 437–445 (1977).

Haber, D.A., Schimke, R.T.: Unstable amplification of an altered dihydrofolate reductase gene associated with double-minute chromosomes. Cell **26**, 355–362 (1981).

Hamlin, J., Montoya–Zavala, M., Heintz, N., Millbrandt, J., Azizkahn, J.: Studies on the mechanism of dihydrofolate reductase gene amplification in Chinese hamster ovary cells. In: *Gene Amplification*. R. Schimke, ed. Cold Spring Harbor, New York, Cold Spring Harbor Laboratory Press. pp. 155–159 (1982).

Harbers, K., Schnieke, A., Stuhlmann, H., Jahner, D., Jaenisch, R.: DNA methylation and gene expression: endogenous retroviral genome becomes infectious after molecular cloning. Proc. Natl. Acad. Sci. USA **78**, 7609–7613 (1981).

Harnden, D.G.: Ataxia Telangiectasia Syndrome: Cytogenetic and cancer aspects. In: Chromosomes and Cancer, J. German, Ed., John Wiley and Sons: New York; p. 616–636 (1974).

Harnden, D.G.: Cytogenetics of human neoplasia. In: Genetics of HUman Cancer, J.J. Mulvihill, R.W. Miller and J.F. Fraumeni, Eds., Raven Press: New York; p. 87–104 (1977).

Harris, H., Klein, G.: Malignancy of somatic cell hybrids. Nature **224**, 1315–1316 (1969).

Harris, H., Miller, O.J., Klein G., Worst, P., Tachibana, T.: Suppression of malignancy by cell fusion. Nature **223**, 363–368 (1969).

Harris, H.: Some thoughts about genetics, differentiation, and malignancy. Somat. Cell Genet. **5**, 923–930 (1979).

Hart, R.W., Setlow, R.B., Woodhead, A.D.: Evidence that pyrimidine dimers in DNA can give rise to tumors. Proc. Natl. Acad. Sci. USA **74**, 5574–5578 (1977).

Haynes, S., Toomey, T., Leinwand, L., Jelinek, W.: The Chinese hamster Alu-equivalent sequence: a conserved highly repetitious interspersed DNA sequence in mammals has the structure suggestive of a transposable element. Mol. Cell Biol. **7**, 573–583 (1981).

Hayward, W.S., Neel, B.G., Astrin, S.M.: ALV-induced lymphoid leukosis: activation of a cellular *onc* gene by promoter insertion. Nature **290**, 475–479 (1981).

Hecht, F., McCaw, B.K.: Chromosome instability syndromes. In: Genetics of Human Cancer, J.J. Mulvihill, R.W. Miller and J.F. Fraumeni, Eds., Raven Press: New York; p. 105–123 (1977).

Henderson, B.E., Gerkins, V.R., Pike, M.C., Casagrande, J.T.: Endocrine function and breast cancer. In: Genetics of Human Cancer, J.J. Mulvihill, R.W. Miller and J.F. Fraumeni, Eds., Raven Press: New York; p. 291–295 (1977).

Hethcote, H.W., Knudson, A.G.: Model for the incidence of embryonal cancers: Application to retinoblastoma. Proc. Natl. Acad. Sci. USA **75**, 2453–2457 (1978).

Hildebrand, C.E., Crawford, B.D., Enger, M.D., Griffith, B.B., Griffith, J.K., Hanners, J.L., Jackson, P.J., Longmire, J.L., Munk, A.C., Tesmer, J.G., Walters, R.A.: Coordinate amplification of metallothionein I and II gene sequences in cadmium-resistant CHO variants. UCLA Symposia on Molecular and Cellular Biology, D. Hamer and M. Rosenberg (eds.) Vol. 8, (1982).

Holliday, R., Pugh, J.E.: DNA modification mechanisms and gene activity during development. Science **187**, 226–232 (1975).

Holliday, R.: A new theory of carcinogenesis. Br. J. Cancer **40**, 513–522 (1979).

Hollstein, M., McCann, J., Angelosanto, F.A., Nichols, W.W.: Short term tests for carcinogens and mutagens. Mutat. Res. **65**, 133–226 (1979).

Howell, N., Sager, R.: Noncoordinate expression of SV-40-induced transformation and tumorigenicity in mouse cell hybrids. Somat. Cell Genet. **5**, 129–143 (1979).

Howell, N., Sager, R.: Tumorigenicity and its suppression in hybrids of mouse and Chinese hamster cell lines. Proc. Natl. Acad. Sci. USA **75**, 2358–2362 (1978).

Huang, P.C., Sheridan, R.B.: Genetic and biochemical studies with ataxia telangiectasia. Hum. Genet. **59**, 1–9 (1981).

IARC monographs on the evaluation of the carcinogenic risk of chemicals to man, Vol. 21. p. 173, Lyon, France: International Agency for Research on Cancer (1979).

Ishidate, M., Odashima, S.: Chromosome tests with 134 compounds on Chinese hamster cells in vitro. A screening for chemical carcinogens. Mutation Res. **48**, 337–354 (1977).

Jahner, D., Stuhlmann, H., Stewart, C.L., Harbers, K., Lohler, J., Simon, I., Jaenisch, R.: De novo methylation and expression of retroviral genomes during mouse embryogenesis. Nature **298**, 623–628 (1982).

Jha, K.K., Cacciapuoti, J., Ozer, H.L.: Expersion of transformation in cell hybrids. II. Nonsuppression of the transformed phenotype in hybrids between a chemically transformed and nontransformed derivatives of Balb/3T3. J. Cell Physiol. **97**, 147–152 (1978).

Jha, K.K., Ozer, H.L.: Expersion of transformation in cell hybrids. I. Isolation and application of density-inhibited Balb/3T3 cells deficient in hypoxanthine phosphoribosyl-transferase and resistant to ouabain. Somat. Cell Genet. **2**, 215–223 (1976).

Jones, P.A., Benedict, W.F., Baker, M.S., Mondal, S., Rapp, W., Heidelberger, C.: Oncogenic transformation of C3H/10T 1/2/clone 8 mouse embryo cells by halogenated pyrimidine nucleosides. Cancer Res. **36**, 101–107 (1976).

Jones, P.A., Taylor, S.M.: Cellular differentiation, cytidine analogs and DNA methylation. Cell **20**, 85–93 (1980).

Jones, P.A., Taylor, S.M.: Hemimethylated duplex DNAs prepared from 5-azacytidine-treated cells. Nucl. Acids Res. **9**, 2933–2947 (1981).

Jones, R.E., DeFeo, D., Piatigorisky, J.: Transcription and site-specific hypomethylation of the γ-crystallin in gene embryonic chicken lens. J. Biol. Chem. **256**, 8172–8176 (1981).

Ju, G., Skalka, A.M.: Nucleotide sequence analysis of the long terminal repeat (LTR) of avian retroviruses: structural similarities with transposable elements. Cell **22**, 379–386 (1980).

Kaufman, R., Brown, P., Schimke, R.: Loss and stabilization of amplified dihydrofolate reductase genes in mouse sarcoma S-180 cell lines. Mol. Cell Biol. **1**, 1084–1093 (1981).

Kennedy, A.R., Fox, M., Murphy, G., Little, J.B.: Relationship between X-ray exposure and malignant transformation in C3H 10T 1/2 cells. Proc. Natl. Acad. Sci. USA **77**, 7262–7266 (1980).

Kinsella, A.R., Radman, M.: Tumor promoter induces sister chromatid exchanges: Relevance to mechanisms of carcinogenesis. Proc. Natl. Acad. Sci. USA **75**, 6149–6153 (1978).

Kirschmeier, P., Gattoni-Celli, S., Dina, D., Weinstein, I.B.: Carcinogen- and radiation-transformed C3H 10T 1/2 cells contain RNAs homologous to the long terminal repeat of murine leukemia virus. Proc. Natl. Acad. Sci. USA **79**, 2773–2777 (1982).

Kitchin, R., Sager, R.: Genetic analysis of tumorigenesis. V. Chromosomal analysis of tumorigenic and nontumorigenic diploid Chinese hamster cell lines. Somat. Cell Genet. **6**, 75–87 (1980a).

Kitchin, R., Sager, R.: Genetic analysis of tumorigenesis. VI. Chromosome rearrangement in tumors derived from diploid premalignant Chinese hamster cells in nude mice. Somat. Cell Genet. **6**, 615–630 (1980b).

Klein, G., Bregula, U., Weiner, F., Harris, H.: The analysis of malignancy of cell fusion. I. Hybrids between tumor cells and L cell derivatives. J. Cell Sci. **8**, 659–672 (1971).

Klein, G.: Analysis of malignancy and antigen expression by cell fusion. Federation Proceedings **35**, 2202–2204 (1976).

Klein, G.: The role of gene dosage and genetic transpositions in carcinogenesis. Nature **294**, 313–318 (1981).

Knudson, A.G.: Mutation and cancer: Statistical study of retinoblastoma. Proc. Natl. Acad. Sci. USA **68**, 820–823 (1971).

Knudson, A.G.: Mutation and human cancer. Adv. in Cancer Res. **17**, 317–352 (1973).

Knudson, A.G.: Genetic and environmental interactions in the origin of human cancer. In: Genetics of Human Cancer, J.J. Mulvihill, R.W. Moller and J.F. Fraumeni, Eds., Raven Press: New York; p. 391–399 (1977).

Knudson, A.G., Hethcote, H.W., Brown, B.W.: Mutation and childhood cancer: A probabilistic model for the incidence of retinoblastoma. Proc. Natl. Acad. Sci. USA **72**, 5116–5120 (1975).

Kominami, R., Muramatsu, M.: A mouse type 2 Alu sequence (M2) is mobile in the genome. Nature **301**, 87–89 (1983).

Krontiris, T.G., Cooper, G.M.: Transforming activity of human tumor DNAs. Proc. Natl. Acad. Sci. USA **78**, 1181–1184 (1981).

Kucherlapati, R., Shin, S.I.: Genetic control of tumorigenicity in interspecific mammalian cell hybrids. Cell **16**, 639–648 (1979).

Kuff, E.L., Feenstra, A., Lueders, K., Smith, L., Hawley, R., Hozumi, N., Shulman, M.: Intracisternal A-particle genes as movable elements in the mouse genome. Proc. Natl. Acad. Sci. USA **80**, 1992–1996 (1983).

Laerum, D.D., Rajewsky, M.F.: Neoplastic transformation of fetal rat brain cells in culture after exposure to ethylnitrosourea in vivo. J. Natl. Cancer Inst. **55**, 1177–1187 (1975).

Land, H., Parada, L.F., Weinberg, R.A.: Tumorigenic conversion of primary embryo fibroblasts requires at least two cooperating oncogenes. Nature **304**, 596–602 (1983).

Landolph, J.R., Heidelberger, C.: Chemical carcinogens produce mutations to ouabain resistance in transformable C3H 10T 1/2 Cl 8 mouse fibroblasts. Proc. Natl. Acad. Sci. USA **76**, 930–934 (1979).

Landolph, J.R., Jones, P.A.: Mutagenicity of 5-azacytidine and related nucleosides in C3H/10T 1/2 clone 8 and V79 cells. Cancer Res. **42**, 817–823 (1982).

Lane, M.-A., Sainten, A., Cooper, G.M.: Activation of related transforming genes in mouse and human mammary carcinomas. Proc. Natl. Acad. Sci. USA **78**, 5185–5189 (1981).

Lane, M.-A., Neary, D., Cooper, G.M.: Activation of a cellular transforming gene in tumours induced by Abelson murine leukemia virus. Nature **300**, 659–661 (1982).

Lane, M.-A., Sainten, A., Cooper, G.M.: Stage-specific transforming genes of human and mouse B- and T-lymphocyte neoplasms. Cell **28**, 873–880 (1982).

Lavi, S.: Carcinogen-mediated amplification of viral DNA sequences in simian virus 40-transformed Chinese hamster embryo cells. Proc. Natl. Acad. Sci. USA **78**, 6144–6148 (1981).

Majors, J.E., Varmus, H.E.: Nucleotide sequences at host-proviral junctions for mouse mammary tumor virus. Nature **289**, 253–258 (1981).

Mandel, J.L., Chambon, P.: DNA methylation: specific variations in the methylation pattern within and around ovalbumin and other chicken genes. Nucl. Acids Res. **7**, 2081–2103 (1979).

Marin, G.: Segregation of morphological revertants in polyoma-transformed hybrid clones of hamster fibroblasts. J. Cell Sci. **9**, 61–69 (1971).

Matsunaga, E.: Genetics of Wilms' tumor. Hum. Genet. **57**, 231–246 (1981).

McCann, J., Ames, B.N.: Detection of carcinogens as mutagens in the Salmonella/microsome test: Assay of 300 chemicals. Discussion. Proc. Natl. Acad. Sci. USA 950–954 (1976).

McCann, J., Choi, E., Yamasaki, E., Ames, B.N.: Detection of carcinogens as mutagens in the Salmonella/microsome test: Assay of 300 chemicals. Proc. Natl. Acad. Sci. USA **72**, 5135–5139 (1975).

McGhee, J.D., Ginder, G.D.: Specific DNA methylation sites in the vicinity of the chicken β-globin genes. Nature **280**, 419–420 (1979).

McLachlan, J.A., Wong, A., Degen, G.H., Barrett, J.C.: Morphological and neoplastic transformation of Syrian hamster embryo fibroblasts by diethyistilbestrol and its analogs. Cancer Res. **42**, 3040–3045 (1982).

Mendelsohn, N., Michl, J., Gilbert, H.S., Acs, G., Christman, J.K.: L-ethionine as an inducer of differentiation in human promyelocytic leukemia cells (HL-60). Cancer Res. **40**, 3206–3210 (1980).

Metzler, M., Gottschlich, R., McLachlan, J.A.: Oxidative metabolism of stilbene estrogens. In: J.A. McLachlan (ed.), Estrogens in the Environment, pp. 293–303. Amsterdam: Elsevier-North Holland, Inc. (1980).

Miller, E.C.: Some current perspectives on chemical carcinogenesis in humans and experimental animals: Presidential address. Cancer Res. **38**, 1479–1496.

Miller, E.C., Miller, J.A.: The mutagenicity of chemical carcinogens: Correlations, problems and interpretations. In: Chemical Mutagens; Principles & Methods for their Detection. Vol. 1, A. Hollaender, Ed., Plenum Press: New York; p. 83–119 (1971).

Miller, J.A., Miller, E.C.: Ultimate chemical carcinogens as reactive mutagenic electrophiles. In: H.H. Hiatt, J.D. Watson, J.A. Winsten, eds. Origins of Human Cancer. Cold Spring Harbor, New York: Cold Spring Harbor Laboratory; 605–627 (1977).

Mintz, B.: Genetic mosaicism and in vitro analysis of neoplasia and differentiation. In:

Cell Differentiation and Neoplasia, G.F. Saunders, Ed., Raven Press: New York; p. 27–53 (1978).

Mintz, B., Fleischman, R.A.: Teratocarcinomas and other neoplasms as developmental defects in gene expression. Adv. Cancer Res. **34**, 211–278 (1981).

Mohandas, T., Sparkes, R.S., Shapiro, L.J.: Reactivation of the inactive human X chromosome: evidence for X-inactivation by DNA methylation. Science **211**, 393–396 (1981).

Mondal, S., Brankow, D.W., Heidelberger, C.: Two-stage chemical oncogenesis in cultures of C3H/10T 1/2 cells. Cancer Res. **36**, 2254–2260 (1976).

Mondal, S., Heidelberger, C.: Transformation of C3H/10T 1/2 C18 mouse embryo fibroblasts by ultraviolet radiation and a phorbol ester. Nature **260**, 710–711 (1977).

Moolgavkar, S.H., Knudson, A.G., Jr.: Mutation and cancer: a model for human carcinogenesis. N.M.C.I. **66**, 1037–1052 (1981).

Muller, R., Slamon, D.J., Tremblay, J.M., Cline, M.J., Verma, I.M.: Differential expression of cellular oncogenes during pre- and postnatal development of the mouse. Nature **279**, 640–644 (1982).

Muller, R., Slamon, D.J., Adamson, E.D., Tremblay, J.M., Muller, D., Cline, M.J., Verma, I.M.: Transcription of c-onc genes c-ras^{Ki} and c-fms during mouse development. Molec. Cell. Biol. **3**, 1062–1069 (1983).

Murray, M.J., Shilo, B-Z., Shih, C., Cowing, D., Hsu, H.W., Weinberg, R.A.: Three different human tumor cell lines contain different oncogenes. Cell **25**, 355–361 (1981).

Neel, B.G., Hayward, W.S., Robinson, H.L., Fang, J., Astrin, S.: Avian leukosis virus-induced tumors have common proviral integration sites and synthesize discrete new RNAs: oncogenesis by protor insertion. Cell **23**, 323–334 (1981).

Nowell, P.C., Hungerford, D.A.: A minute chromosome and human granulocytic leukemia. Science **132**, 1497 (1960).

Nowell, P.C., Hungerford, D.A.: Chromosome studies in human leukemia. II. Chronic granulocytic leukemia. J. Natl. Cancer Inst. **27**, 1013–1035 (1961).

Nowell, P.C.: The clonal evolution of tumor cell populations. Science **194**, 23–28 (1976).

Nunberg, J., Kaufman, R., Schimke, R., Urlaub, G., Chasin, L.: Amplified dihydrofolate reductase genes are localized to a homogeneously staining region of a single chromosome in a methotrexate resistant Chinese hamster ovary cell line. Proc. Natl. Acad. Sci. USA **75**, 5553–5556 (1978).

Oberling, C.: The riddle of cancer. New Haven, Connecticut, Yale University Press (1952).

Ohno, S.: Aneuploidy as a possible means employed by malignant cells to express recessive phenotypes. In: German J. (ed.), Chromosomes and Cancer. New York, John Wiley and Sons, pp. 77–94 (1974).

Oskarsson, M., McClements, W.L., Blair, D.G., Maizel, J.V., Vande Woude, G.F.: Properties of a normal mouse cell DNA sequence (sarc) homologous to the src sequence of moloney sarcoma virus. Science **207**, 1222–1224 (1980).

O'Toole, C.M., Povey, S., Hepburn, P., Franks, L.M.: Identity of some human bladder cancer cell lines. Nature **301**, 429–431 (1983).

Ozer, H.L., Jha, K.K.: Malignancy and transformation: expression in somatic cell hybrids and variants. Adv. Cancer Res. **25**, 53–93 (1977).

Pall, M.I.: Gene-amplification model of carcinogenesis. Proc. Natl. Acad. Sci. USA **78**, 2465–2468 (1981).

Parada, L.F., Tabin, C.J., Shih, C., Weinberg, R.A.: Human EJ bladder carcinoma oncogene is homologue of Harvey sarcoma virus ras gene. Nature **297**, 474–478 (1978).

Parry, J.M., Parry, E.M., Barrett, J.C.: Tumor promoters induce mitotic aneuploidy in yeast. Nature (Lond.) **294**, 263–265 (1981).

Parry, J.M., Sharp, D.: The induction of mitotic aneuploidy of the 42 coded compounds using yeast culture D6. In: F.J. deSerres, and J. Ashby (eds.), Evaluation of Short-Term Tests for Carcinogens: Report of the International Collaborative Program, pp. 468–481. New York: Elsevier-North Holland (1981).

Payne, G.S., Bishop, J.M., Varmus, H.E.: Multiple arrangements of viral DNA and an activated host oncogene in bursal lymphomas. Nature **295**, 209–217 (1982).

Perucho, M., Goldfarb, M., Shimizu, K., Lama, C., Fogh, J., Wigler, M.: Human-tumor-derived cell lines contain common and different transforming genes. Cell **27**, 467–476 (1981).

Peto, R.: Epidemiology, multistage models, and short-term mutagenicity tests. In: Origins of Human Cancer, H. Hiatt, J.D. Watson and J.A. Winsten, Eds., Cold Spring Harbor Laboratory Press: New York; p. 1403–1428 (1977).

Pierce, G.B., Cox, W.F.: Neoplasms as caricatures of tissue renewal. In: Cell Differentiation and Neoplasia, G.F. Saunders, Ed., Raven Press: New York; p. 57–66 (1978).

Pincus, M.R., van Renswoude, J., Harford, J.B., Chang, E.H., Carty, R.P., Klausner, R.D.: Prediction of the three-dimensional structure of the transforming region of the EJ/T24 human bladder oncogene product and its normal cellular homologue. Proc. Natl. Acad. Sci. USA **80**, 5253–5257 (1983).

Pulciani, S., Santos, E., Lauver, A.V., Long, L.K., Aaronson, S.A., Barbacid, M.: Oncogenes in solid human tumours. Nature **300**, 539–542 (1982).

Pulciani, S., Santos, E., Lauver, A.V., Long, L.K., Robbins, K.C., Barbacid, M.: Oncogenes in human tumor cell lines: molecular cloning of a transforming gene from human bladder carcinoma cells. Proc. Natl. Acad. Sci. USA **79**, 2845–2849 (1982).

Purchase, I.F.H., Longstaff, E., Ashby, J., Styles, J.A., Anderson, D., Lefevre, P.A., Westwood, F.R.: An evaluation of 6 short-term tests for detecting organic chemical carcinogens. Br. J. Cancer **37**, 873–903 (1978).

Razin, A., Riggs, A.D.: DNA methylation and gene function. Science **210**, 604–610 (1980).

Rechavi, G., Givol, D., Canaani, E.: Activation of a cellular oncogene by DNA rearrangement: possible involvement of an IS-like element. Nature **300**, 607–611 (1982).

Reddy, E.P., Reynolds, R.K., Santos, E., Barbacid, M.: A point mutation is responsible for the acquisition of transforming properties by the T24 human bladder carcinoma oncogene. Nature **300**, 149–152 (1982).

Riggs, A.D.: X-inactivation, differentiation and DNA methylation. Cytogenet. Cell Genet. **14**, 9–25 (1975).

Ringertz, N.R., Savage, R., Eds.: Analysis of malignancy by cell fusion. In: Cell Hybrids, Academic Press: New York; p. 245–270 (1976).

Roberts, J.M., Buck, L.B., Axel, R.: A structure for amplified DNA. Cell **33**, 53–63 (1983).

Roberts, J.M., Axel, R.: Gene amplification and gene correction in somatic cells. Cell **29**, 109–119 (1982).

Rowley, J.D.: Chromosome abnormalities in cancer. Cancer Genet. Cytogenet. **2**, 175–198 (1980).

Rowley, J.D.: Human oncogene locations and chromosome aberrations. Nature **301**, 290–291 (1983).

Rowley, J.D.: Identification of the constant chromosome regions involved in human hematologic malignant disease. Science **216**, 749–751 (1982).

Ruley, H.E.: Adenovirus early region 1A enables viral and cellular transforming genes to transform primary cells in culture. Nature **304**, 602–606 (1983).

Sager, R., Kovac, P.E.: Genetic analysis of tumorigenesis: I. Expression of tumor-forming ability in hamster hybrid cell lines. Somatic Cell Genetics **4**, 375–392 (1978).

Sager, R., Kovac, P.E.: Genetic analysis of tumorigenesis. IV. Chromosome reduction and marker segregation in progeny clones from Chinese hamster cell hybrids. Somat. Cell Genet. **5**, 491–502 (1979).

Sager, R., Kovac, P.E.: Genetic analysis of tumorigenesis. I. Expression of tumor-forming ability in hamster hybrid cell lines. Somat. Cell Genet. **4**, 375–392 (1978).

Sagerman, R.H., Cassady, J.R., Tretter, P., Ellsworth, R.M.: Radiation induced neoplasia following external beam therapy for children with retinoblastoma. Am. J. Roentgenol **105**, 529–535 (1969).

Santos, E., Tronick, S.R., Aaronson, S.A., Pulciani, S., Barbacid, M.: T24 human bladder carcinoma oncogene is an activated form of the normal human homologue of BALB- and Harvey-MSV transforming genes. Nature **298**, 343–347 (1982).

Santos, E., Reddy, E.P., Pulciani, S., Feldmann, R.J., Barbacid, M.: Spontaneous activation of a human proto-oncogene. Proc. Natl. Acad. Sci. USA **80**, 4679–4683 (1983).

Sawada, M., Ishidate, M.: Colchicine-like effects of diethylstilbestrol (DES) on mammalian cells in vitro. Mutation Res. **57**, 175–182 (1978).

Scaletta, L.J., Ephrussi, B.: Hybridization of normal and neoplastic cells in vitro. Nature **205**, 1169–1171 (1965).

Schimke, R.: Gene amplification, Cold Spring Harbor, New York, Cold Spring Harbor Laboratory (1982).

Schwab, M., Alitalo, K., Klempnauer, K–H., Varmus, H.E., Bishop, J.M., Gilbert, F., Brodeur, G., Goldstein, M., Trent, J.: Amplified DNA with limited homology to myc cellular oncogene is shared by human neuroblastoma cell lines and a neuroblastoma tumour. Nature **305**, 245–248 (1983).

Setlow, R.B.: Repair deficient human disorders and cancer. Nature **27**, 713–717 (1978).

Shapiro, J.A., Cordell, B.: Eukaryotic mobile and repeated genetic elements. Biol. Cell **43**, 31–54 (1982).

Sharp, P.A.: Conversion of RNA to DNA in mammals: Alu-like elements and pseudogenes. Nature **301**, 471–472 (1983).

Shih, C., Shilo, B.–Z., Goldfarb, M.P., Dannenberg, A., Weinberg, R.A.: Passage of phenotypes of chemically transformed cells via transfection of DNA and chromatin. Proc. Natl. Acad. Sci. USA **76**, 5714–5718 (1979).

Shih, C., Weinberg, R.A.: Isolation of a transforming sequence from a human bladder carcinoma cell line. Cell **29**, 161–169 (1982).

Shilo, B.–Z., Weinberg, R.A.: Unique transforming gene in carcinogen-transformed mouse cells. Nature **289**, 607–609 (1981).

Shimizu, K., Goldfarb, M., Suard, Y., Perucho, M., Li, Y., Kamata, T., Feramisco, J., Stavnezer, E., Fogh, J., Wigler, M.H.: Three human transforming genes are related to the viral ras oncogenes. Proc. Natl. Acad. Sci. USA **80**, 2112–2116 (1983).

Shimizu, K., Birnbaum, D., Ruley, M.A., Fasano, O., Suard, Y., Edlund, L., Taparowsky, E., Goldfarb, M., Wigler, M.: Structure of the Ki-ras gene of the human lung carcinoma cell line Calu-1. Nature **304**, 497–500 (1983).

Shimotohno, K., Mizutani, S., Temin, H.M.: Sequence of retrovirus provirus resembles that of bacterial transposable elements. Nature **285**, 550–554 (1980).

Shmookler-Reis, R.J., Goldstein, S.: Interclonal variation in methylation patterns for expressed and non-expressed genes. Nuc. Acids Res. **10**, 4293–4304 (1982).

Siminovitch, L.: On the nature of hereditable variation in cultured somatic cells. Cell **7**, 1–11 (1976).

Smith, B.L., Sager, R.: Multistep origin of tumor-forming ability in Chinese hamster embryo fibroblast cells. Cancer Res. **42**, 389–396 (1982).

Sparkes, R.S., Sparkes, M.C., Wilson, M.G., et al: Regional assignment of genes for human esterase D and retinoblastoma to chromosome band 13q14. Science **208**, 1042–1044 (1980).

Sparkes, R.S., Murphree, A.L., Lingua, R.W., Sparkes, M.C., Field, L.L., Funderburk, S.J., Benedict, W.F.: Gene for hereditary retinoblastoma assigned to human chromosome 13 by linkage to esterase D. Science **219**, 971–973 (1983).

Spradling, A.C., Mahowald, A.P.: A chromosome inversion alters the pattern of specific DNA replication in Drosophila follicle cells. Cell **27**, 203–209 (1981).

Stanbridge, E.J.: Suppression of malignancy in human cells. Nature **260**, 17–20 (1976).

Stanbridge, E.J., Wilkinson, J.: Analysis of malignancy in human cells: malignant and transformed phenotypes are under separate genetic control. Proc. Natl. Acad. Sci. USA **75**, 1466–1469 (1978).

Stanbridge, E.J., Wilkinson, J.: Dissociation of anchorage independence from tumorigenicity in human cell hybrids. Int. J. Cancer **26**, 1–8 (1980).

Stanbridge, E.J., Glandermeyer, R.R., Daniels D.W., Nelson–Rees, W.A.: Specific chromosome loss associated with the expression of tumorigenicity in human cell hybrids. Somatic Cell Genet. **7**, 699–712 (1981).

Stanbridge, E.J., Der, C.J., Doeson, C.J., Nishimi, R.Y., Peehl, D.M., Weisman, B.E., Wilkinson, J.E.: Human cell hybrids: analysis of transformation and tumorigenicity. Science **215**, 252–259 (1982).

Strong, L.C., Knudson, A.G.: Second cancers in retinoblastoma. Lancet **2**, 1086 (1973).

Swift, M.: Fanconi's anemia in the genetics of neoplasia. Nature (London) **230**, 370–373 (1971).

Swift, M., Hirschorn, K.: Fanconi's anemia: Inherited susceptibility to chromosome breakage in various tissues. Annal. Inter. Med. **65**, 496–503 (1966).

Tabin, C.J., Bradley, S.M., Bargmann, C.I., Weinberg, R.A., Papageorge, A.G., Scolnick, E.M., Dhar, R., Lowy, D.R., Chang, E.H.: Mechanism of activation of a human oncogene. Nature **300**, 143–149 (1982).

Taub, R., Kirsch, I., Morton, C., Lenoir, G., Swan, D., Tronick, S., Aaronson, S., Leder, P.: Translocation of the c-myc gene into the immunoglobin heavy chain locus in human Burkitt lymphoma and murine plasmacytoma cells. Proc. Natl. Acad. Sci. USA **79**, 7837–7841 (1982).

Taylor, S.M., Jones, P.A.: Multiple new phenotypes induced in 10T 1/2 and 3T3 cells treated with 5-azacytidine. Cell **17**, 771–779 (1979).

Temin, H.M.: Origin of retroviruses from cellular moveable genetic elements. Cell **21**, 599–600 (1980).

Tice, R.R.: Aging and DNA-repair capability. In: The Genetics of Aging, E.L. Schneider, Ed., Plenum Press: New York; p. 53–89 (1978).

Tsutsui, T., Barrett, J.C., Ts'o, P.O.P.: Induction of 6-thioguanine resistant and ouabain resistant mutations in synchronized Syrian hamster cell cultures during different periods of the S phase. Mutation Res. **52**, 255–264 (1978).

Tsutsui, T., Barrett, J.C., Ts'o, P.O.P.: Chromosomal aberrations, DNA damage and morphological transformation of synchronized Syrian hamster embryo cells: Effect of 5-bromodeoxyuridine and near ultraviolet radiation. Cancer Res., **39**, 2356–2365 (1979).

Tsutsui, T., Crawford, B.D., Ts'o, P.O.P., Barrett, J.C.: Comparison between mutagenesis in normal and transformed Syrian hamster fibroblasts: difference in the temporal order of HPRT gene replication. Mutation Res. **80**, 357–371 (1981).

Tsutsui, T., Maizumi, H., McLachlan, J.A., Barrett, J.C.: Aneuploidy induction and cell transformation by diethylstilbestrol: A possible chromosomal mechanism in carcinogenesis. Cancer Res. **43**, 3814–3821 (1983).

Varmus, H. and Levine, A.J. (eds). Readings in Tumor Virology. Cold Spring Harbor Press, N.Y. (1983).

Varmus, H.E., Quintrell, N., Ortiz, S.: Retroviruses as mutagens: insertion and excision of a nontransforming provirus alter expression of a resident forming provirus. Cell **25**, 23–36 (1981).

Varshavsky, A.: Phorbol ester dramatically increases incidence of methotrexate-resistant mouse cells: possible mechanisms and relevance to tumor promotion. Cell **25**, 561–572 (1981).

Venolia, L., Gartler, S.M., Wassman, E.R., Yen, P., Mohandas, T., Shapiro, L.J.: Transformation with DNA from 5-azacytidine-reactivated X chromosomes. Proc. Natl. Acad. Sci. USA **79**, 2352–2354 (1982).

von Hansemann: Studien uber die spezificitat, den altruismus, und die anaplasie der zellen. Berlin (1893).

von Hansemann: Ueber asymmetyrische zelltheilung in epithelkrebsen und deren biologische bedeutung. Virchows Arch **119**, 299–326 (1890).

Waalwijk, C., Flavell, R.A.: DNA methylation at a CCGG sequence in the large intron of the rabbit β-globin gene: tissue specific variations. Nucl. Acids Res. **5**, 4631–4641 (1978).

Wahl, G., Padgett, R., Stark, G.: Gene amplification causes overproduction of the first three enzymes of UMP synthesis in N-(phosphoroacetyl)-L-asparate resistant hamster cells. J. Biol. Chem. **254**, 8679–8689 (1979).

Weinberg, R.A.: Origins and roles of endogenous retroviruses. Cell **22**, 643–644 (1980).

Weinber, F., Klein, G., Harris, H.: The analysis of malignancy by cell fusion. III. Hybrids between diploid fibroblasts and other tumor cells. J. Cell Sci. **8**, 681–692 (1971).

Weiner, F., Klein, G., Harris, H.: The analysis of malignancy by cell fusion. V. Further evidence of the ability of diploid cells to suppress malignancy. J. Cell Sci. **15**, 177–183 (1974a).

Weiner, F., Klein, G., Harris, H.: The analysis of malignancy by cell fusion. VI. Hybrids between different tumor cells. J. Cell Sci. **16**, 189–198 (1974b).

Wiblin, C.N., MacPherson, I.A.: Reversion in hybrids between SV-40-transformed hamster and mouse cells. Int. J. Cancer **12**, 148–161 (1973).

Wigler, M., Sweet, R., Sim, G.K., Wold, B., Pellicer, A., Lacy, E., Maniatis, T., Silverstein, S., Axel, R.: Transformation of mammalian cells with genes from procaryotes and eucaryotes. Cell **16**, 777–785 (1979).

Wigler, M., Pellicer, A., Silverstein, S., Axel, R.: Biochemical transfer of single-copy eucaryotic genes using total cellular DNA as donor. Cell **14**, 725–731 (1978).

Wigler, M., Levy, D., Perucho, M.: The somatic replication of DNA methylation. Cell **24**, 33–40 (1981).

Wilson, V.L., Jones, P.A.: Inhibition of DNA methylation by chemical carcinogens in vitro. Cell **32**, 239–246 (1983).

Yagi, M., Koshland, M.E.: Expression of the J chain gene during B cell differentiation is inversely correlated with DNA methylation. Proc. Natl. Acad. Sci. USA **78**, 4907–4911 (1981).

Yamamoto, T., Rabinowitz, A., Sachs, L.: Identification of the chromosomes that control malignancy. Nature New Biol. **243**, 247–250 (1973a).

Yunis, J.J., Ramsay, N.K.: Familial occurrence of the aniridia-Wilms' tumor syndrome with deletion 11p13–14.1. J. Pediatr. **96**, 1027–1030 (1980).

Yunis, J.J.: The chromosomal basis of human neoplasia. Science **221**, 227–236 (1983).

CHAPTER III

PERSPECTIVES ON DETECTION OF CHEMICAL CARCINOGENS AS MUTAGENS

Virginia C. Dunkel, Ph.D.
Food and Drug Administration
Center for Food Safety and Applied Nutrition
Washington, D.C. 20204

A. HISTORICAL PERSPECTIVE

In 1915, Yamagiwa and Itchikawa reported their findings on the induction of carcinomas on the ears of rabbits after long continued topical applications of coal tar. One year prior to this discovery, Boveri (1914) published, in German, his ideas about the etiology of cancer. His observations on the irregular distribution of chromosomes to daughter cells of sea urchin eggs and the related atypical growth of such aneuploid cells led him to hypothesize that cancer was related to abnormal chromosomes. He wrote "The essence of my theory is not abnormal mitosis but in general a definite abnormal chromosome-complex. However this may arise, the results would always be a definite tumor." Essentially the work of Yamagiwa and Itchikawa opened the field of experimental chemical carcinogenesis and led to the search for other tumor inducing agents while the hypothesis proposed by Boveri was the fore-runner of the somatic mutation theory of cancer and stimulated efforts to correlate carcinogenic and mutagenic activity of chemicals.

Between 1915 and 1933 considerable effort was directed to experimental studies on induction of skin tumors with tars and their crude fractions. This in turn led to a search for the active agents. The eventual identification and isolation of the carcinogenic component 3,4-benzypyrene from coal tar (Cook, *et al.*, 1933) proved not only to be the culmination of an extensive effort headed by E.L. Kennaway but also the starting point for the synthesis and testing of a variety of other polycyclic aromatic hydrocarbons.

As studies were continuing with the hydrocarbons, other reports began to appear about the carcinogenic activity of compounds in other chemical classes. In 1933, Yoshida reported that 2'3-dimethyl-4-aminoazobenzene, an intermediate used in the synthesis of azo dyes, was a systematically acting liver carcinogen, and in 1938 Heuper reported the successful induction of bladder tumors in dogs fed β-napthylamine. This was followed by the discovery that

61

2-acetylaminofluorene (Wilson, et al., 1941), a chemical originally intended for use as a pesticide, was a potent carcinogen, and the fortuitous observation by Nettleship and Henshaw (1943) that urethane, a chemical used for anaesthetic purposes, induced lung adenomas in mice. During the 1950's and 1960 there were further additions to the growing array of chemicals showing carcinogenic activity. Magee and Barnes (1955) showed that dimethylnitrosamine, a chemical with demonstrated hepatotoxicity, was also a liver carcinogen and the discovery was also made that naturally occurring products of plants (Cook et al., 1950) and fungi (Kraybill and Shimkin, 1964) possessed carcinogenic activity.

As advances were being made in the identification of chemical carcinogens, the somatic mutation theory of cancer was also proceeding through a developmental process. Boveri's theory as he proposed it never gained wide acceptance. Observations on tumors showed that chromosomal aberrations were seen in only a small percentage of cells in a tumor, and cells showing gross abnormalities in most cases were end stage cells and not the precursors of additional generations of tumor cells (Berenblum, 1974).

Nevertheless, in the 1920's several German investigators expressed the view that a normal cell might be converted to a tumor cell as a result of mutation, and it was at this time that Baer published a monograph in which he incorporated mutations of genes into the somatic mutation hypothesis (Reviewed in Burdette, 1955). This concept of somatic mutation then began to gain more support and was cited in some early publications on the etiology of cancer. In 1933, Murray, in a discussion on experimental production of malignant tumors, included the "genetical hypothesis originating with Boveri and modified by Bauer" together with the viral hypothesis and the chronic irritation theory as contemporary concepts. Boycott (1933) who also participated in the same discussion considered somatic mutation a convenient hypothesis to explain the fact that tumor cells apparently breed true through successive generations. At approximately the same time Lochart-Mummery (1932), after reviewing numerous characteristics of tumors cells, concluded that the somatic mutation hypothesis was a promising explanation for the origin of cancer.

The idea that the carcinogenic process might involve a mutagenic event led to a number of early studies attempting to correlate mutagenic and carcinogenic activites of chemicals. Auerbach and Robson (1944) provided a basis for such attempts through their demonstration of chemical induction of mutations in Drosophila. They reported that allyl isothiocyanate (mustard oil) (1944) and dichloro-diethyl-sulfide (mustard gas) (1946) produced mutations as effectively as x-irradiation. Demerec (1948), following the current feeling among geneticists that chemical carcinogens should also be mutagens, tested both polycyclic aromatic hydrocarbons and azo compounds in Drosophila and reported induction of x-chromosome lethals and chromosomal aberrations. He concluded from the data that there was a definite correlation between mutagenicity and carcinogenicity. The correlation however was not complete; of the seven carcinogens tested six were mutagenic and of the nine non-carcinogens, two were mutagenic and one was "classified as doubtful." Barratt and Tatum (1951), using *Neurospora crassa* as the test organism, also reported successful mutation induction by several carcinogenic hydrocarbons and azo dyes including 1,2,5,6-dibenz-anthracene and 20-methylcholanthrene. They pointed out, however, that even the most active mutagenic carcinogens, among those they tested, were much less active than nitrogen mustard and radiation. Other early efforts were directed to studies on mutation induction in animals. Carr (1947), for example, treated mice with 1,2,5,6-dibenzanthracene and reported induction of germinal mutations, and Strong (1949) using 20-methylcholanthrene likewise reported induction of germinal mutations in mice.

In other studies, however, results were obtained indicating that there was no correlation between carcinogenic and mutagenic activity. For example, Berenblum and Shubik (1949), in studies on the initiating phase of carcinogenesis, tested the mutagen mustard gas for its capacity to initiate mouse skin and found it to be inactive as an initiator. Latarjet *et al.* (1950) treated *Escherichia coli* with 20-methylcholanthrene and obtained no increase in mutation rate even through fluorescence studies indicated that the chemical had entered the cell. Burdette and Haddox (1954) also reported no increase in mutants in *Neurospora crassa* after treatment with 20-methylcholanthrene or 1,2,5,6-dibenzanthracene.

There were many other efforts to show a correlation between mutagenicity and carcinogenicity and in 1955, Burdette reviewed the experimental data available to that time and concluded that there was no general correlation between the mutagenicity and carcinogenicity of chemicals tested for both activities. He also noted that a number of reasons could be offered to explain the discrepancies between the results obtained. Among these he included species differences, unsuitable routes of injection or unsuitable solvents, lack of appropriate parameters for judging quantitative relationships, differences in the types of cells tested for mutagenicity and carcinogenicity and, finally, inadequate information on the metabolic fate of carcinogens and the forms in which they are active.

It was not however until further studies indicated that many chemical carcinogens required "metabolic activation" to exert their effect that consideration was given to the possibility that the lack of mutagenicity of certain carcinogens might be related to the inability of test organisms, such as bacteria and fungi, to convert such chemicals to reactive forms. Malling (1966) using the nonenzymatic hydroxylation system of Undenfriend was able to convert both dimethylnitrosamine and diethylnitrosamine into mutagens for *Neurospora crassa*. It had been previously reported that these carcinogens were not mutagenic in bacteria (Geissler, 1962), yeast (Marquardt *et al.*, 1964) and Neurospora (Marquardt *et al.*, 1963) but were mutagenic for Drosophila (Pasternak, 1962). At approximately the same time, Smith (1966) reported that methylaxozymethanol, prepared by enzymatic deglucosylation of crystalline cycasin, induced a mutagenic response in several mutant strains of *Salmonella typhimurium*. The cycasin itself did not cause any mutant induction and it was suggested that the Salmonella lacked the necessary deglucosylating enzyme to convert it to its active form. Gabridge and Legator (1969), recognizing that bacterial systems tended to give negative results for compounds meabolized to an active state by the whole animal, developed a host-mediated assay. In this assay the bacteria were injected into the peritoneal cavity of a mouse and DMN was given by intramuscular injection. The bacteria were then removed and the number of mutants determined. Through the use of this procedure they demonstrated the need for mammalian metabolism for induction of mutations in bacteria with this compound. Subsequently, Malling (1971) reported that a liver extract rather than the whole animal could be used for conversion of DMN to a mutagen for Salmonella. This was a key event in the development of *in vitro* mutagenicity procedures and the use of liver enzyme preparation was adapted by Ames and co-workers (1973, 1975) for use with specially constructed strains of *Salmonella typhimurium* (Ames, 1971). The development of this methodology and the subsequent demonstration (McCann *et al.*, 1975) that there was a high correlation between the mutagenicity and the reported carcinogenicity of a large series of compounds stimulated further evaluation of carcinogenic chemicals for mutagenic activity.

B. TEST SYSTEMS

The endpoints that are now used to determine the mutagenic activity of chemicals include gene mutation, chromosomal damage, DNA damage and repair and cell transformation. These can be measured in a number of different systems including bacteria, lower eukaryotes such as fungi and yeast, mammalian cells in culture as well as whole animal systems such as Drosophila and rodents.

A large number of assays using bacteria and fungi as test organisms can be used to measure mutation induction. The mutations are detected as phenotypic changes and can result from alterations in the structure of DNA such as base substitutions, frameshifts, large deletions, insertions and translocations. The most extensively studied and widely used microbial gene mutation assay is the Ames Salmonella/mammalian microsome test (Ames *et al.*, 1975; Maron and Ames, 1983). The test utilizes specially constructed mutants of *Salmonella typhimurium* blocked at various steps in histidine biosynthesis to detect reverse mutations. In general, the test chemical and cells of the different tester strains, both with and without liver S-9 mix for metabolic-activation, are incorporated into soft agar and plated on a base of selective agar. The assay is sensitive and versatile and can be used to evaluate many types of substances including liquids, solids, gases and highly toxic substances.

Other microorganisms which have been used for testing but to a much lesser degree include other strains of bacteria such as *Escherichia coli* (Mohn *et al.*, 1980), the yeast *Saccharomyces cerevisiae* (Zimmerman, 1973) and the mold *Neurospora crassa* (deSerres and Malling, 1971). A general problem encountered in using both yeasts and mold however is the permeability of the cell wall which can restrict entry of certain chemicals into the cell. In addition, the eukaryotic microorganisms usually require higher concentrations of chemicals for induction of mutations than do bacteria, possibly because yeasts and molds exhibit more powerful detoxification mechanisms and have more DNA repair pathways.

Gene mutation can also be conveniently measured in several mammalian cell systems. The systems most frequently utilized in these assays include V79 (Chu and Malling, 1968; Huberman and Sachs, 1976; Kuroki *et al.*, 1977) and CHO (Hsie *et al.*, 1979) Chinese hamster cells and L5178Y mouse lymphoma cells (Clive *et al.*, 1979; Amacher *et al.*, 1979). The markers commonly used in V79 and CHO cells to detect the mutagenic events are resistance to the purine analogues 8-azaquanine or 6-thioguanine which arises from a loss of hypoxanthineguanine phosphoribosyl transferase (HGPRT) activity or resistance to ouabain which results from a mutation affecting a membrane-associated sodium/potassium ATPase. In L5178Y mouse lymphoma cells the marker generally used is resistance to bromodeoxyuridine (BUdR) or trifluorothymidine (TFT) which results from a loss of thymidine kinase activity. Since all of these cell lines have limited capacity to metabolize chemicals to their ultimate reactive form, exogenous metabolic activation is provided either by liver enzyme S-9 preparations or intact cells; both primary fibroblasts (Huberman and Sachs, 1974) and liver epithelial cells (Langenbach *et al.*, 1978) have been used. Cell mediated mutagenesis appears to be a better indicator of in vivo metabolic pathways (Bigger *et al.*, 1980; Dybing *et al.*, 1979; Schmeltz *et al.*, 1978; Selkirk, 1977) and may also reflect the organ specificity of the chemicals tested.

The sex linked recessive lethal test (Vogel, 1981) is the most widely used test for mutation in Drosophila. Recessive lethals are a heterogeneous class and consist of point mutations, deletions and small and large rearrangements. It has been estimated that the number of loci which can mutate to a lethal condition on the x-chromosome is in the order of 600 to 800 loci (Abrahamson *et al.*, 1980). Two generations are required for detection of mutation induction which is determined by the absence of one entire class of males in the F2 generation. The test is usually performed by treating wild-type males and then mating them to a tester strain of female homozygous for markers that affect the shape and color of the eyes. The F_1 females from this mating are then pair mated to F_1 males and in the F_2 generation four genotypes can be identified by their different phenotypes. Induced lethals are detected by the absence of one phenotypic class of F_2 males.

A number of different assays can be used for detecting chromosomal damage and include those measuring chromosomal aberrations, sister chromatid exchange and micronucleus formation. Chromosomal aberrations induced in mammalian cells are characteristic of damage sustained in G_1 cells which are translated into breakage/exchange figures prior to chromosome replication. The aberrations, such as breaks, terminal and interstitial deletions, rings and dicentrics, can be detected in a wide range of mammalian cells. As a group chinese hamster cells in culture are probably the most well suited for such determinations, since they have short cell cycles and small numbers of large and varied chromosomes (Ishidate and Odashima, 1977; Mutsuoka *et al.*, 1979).

In addition to direct testing *in vitro* an *in vivo* approach can also be used to assess chromosomal effects. In the *in vivo* studies, cells, generally peripheral blood lymphocytes (Evans, 1976) or bone marrow cells (Cohen and Herrschhorn, 1972), are cultured after an *in vivo* exposure to the chemical under test. The subsequent techniques used for processing and analysis of the cells are then similar to those used in the direct *in vitro* method.

Sister chromatid exchange (Perry, 1980) involves symmetrical exchanges between sister chromatids and does not result in gross alteration in chromosome morphology. The exchange events between sister chromatids are visualized after the cells have been grown for two cycles in the thymidine analogue BUdR. Incorporation of the BUdR into DNA results in second division chromosomes having one chromatid unifilarly substituted and the other chromatid bifilarly substituted. After staining with a fluorescent dye and/or Giemsa, one chromatid appears dark and the other light. The test can be performed on cells in culture, cells from animals treated with the compound of interest, or in the intact animal. In the latter case, a sufficient level of BUdR must be maintained in order to obtain the differential staining of the chromatids in cells of the tissue to be evaluated.

Chromosomal bodies that are not incorporated in daughter nuclei at the time of cell division are known as micronuclei. These bodies can be formed from chromosomes as a result of the malfunction of the spindle apparatus or from chromosomal fragments and can be induced in mammalian cells both *in vivo* (Heddle, 1973; Matter and Schmid, 1971; Schmid, 1975) and *in vitro* (Heddle *et al.*, 1978). However, polychromatic erythrocytes from the bone marrow are most frequently used. Erythroblasts, precursor cells to erythrocytes, expel their nuclei after their last mitosis but retain their micronuclei. These then appear as densely-staining, small bodies in the bluish staining polychromatic erythrocytes. The most difficult problem encountered in scoring is not whether structures observed are micronuclei but whether the erythrocytes are polychromatic since there is a continual gradation from the polychromatic to the normochromatic staining characteristic as the cells develop.

A variety of techniques can be used to measure DNA damage and consequent DNA repair. Strand breakage can be assessed by either alkaline sucrose gradient centrifugation (Lett *et al.*, 1967; McGrath and Williams, 1966) or by alkaline elution from membrane filters (Kohn, 1979; Swenberg, *et al.*, 1976) However, care is required in interpreting the results of such assays, since dead or dying cells will display DNA fragmentation as a result of the action of degradative nucleases. Repair synthesis or unscheduled DNA synthesis can be measured either by autoradiography (Painter and Cleaver, 1969; Rasmussen and Painter, 1964) or by liquid scintillation counting (Evans and Norma, 1968; Stich and San, 1970). Only with autoradiography is it possible to unequivocally distinguish repair synthesis from replicative DNA synthesis, and this technique is preferred for screening. Among the cell types that have been used for repair studies are continuous cell lines such as WI-38 (San and Stich, 1975) and HeLa (Martin *et al.*, 1978). Cell lines require inhibition of replicative DNA synthesis, however, and such techniques as hydroxyurea supression or arginine deprivation are employed. Since the metabolic capabilities of the cells are limited, they also require addition of exogenous systems for metabolic activation. Both of these problems have been overcome with the development of a DNA assay in primary rat hepatocyte cultures (Williams, 1976, 1977). The freshly isolated non-dividing liver cells that are used have the capacity to metabolize carcinogens and respond with DNA repair. Studies to date have shown that this assay has substantial sensitivity and reliability with activation-dependent chemicals (Williams et al., 1982; Williams, 1980; Probst, 1980).

Although the morphological transformation of mammalian cells in culture is not a genetic endpoint, assays measuring the event are used in conjunction with mutagenesis assays in evaluating chemicals for carcinogenic potential. They contribute important information in the overall assessment of a chemical for genotoxic effects and thus should not be excluded from any discussion relating to the detection of carcinogens by short-term in vitro methods.

Both epithelial and fibroblastic cells can be used for studying transformation but the test systems now most commonly used for testing purposes all employ fibroblasts. The morphological change observed, whether as altered colonies or foci in a monolayer of normal cells, is generally characterized by piling up of the cells in an irregular criss-crossed pattern representing a loss of growth inhibition and cell-cell orientation. This is in contrast to the regular and orderly growth pattern of the non-transformed cells. With cell passage the transformed cells acquire other characteristics such as the ability to grow in semi-solid medium and the capacity to produce tumors after transplantation into syngeneic or immunosuppressed animals. Probably the transformation system which has been most extensively used, as determined by the number of chemicals tested (Heidelberger et al., 1983) is the Syrian hamster embryo clonal assay (Berwald and Sachs, 1963; DiPaolo et al., 1971; Pienta et al., 1977; Pienta, 1980). Primary or early passage cells are used as the target cell population and individual colonies are evaluated for the transformed phenotype. The cells are diploid and appear to have enzyme systems which allow metabolism of a fairly wide spectrum of chemicals to their active forms.

Continuous cell lines which can be used for transformation include BALB 3T3 (DiPaolo et al., 1972; Kakunaga, 1973, Sivak et al., 1980) C3H 10T 1/2 (Reznikoff, et al., 1973) and C3H mouse prostate, clone M2 (Marquardt, 1976). In assays with these cells, foci of morphologically transformed cells appear on a monolayer of normal cells. In contrast to hamster embryo cells, the mouse cell lines are aneuploid and appear to have more limited capacity to metabolize chemicals (Dunkel et al., 1981; Heidelberger et al., 1983).

C. TEST BATTERIES

Correlation studies in which mutagenicity/transformation test results are compared with those obtained in long-term carcinogenicity bioassays have been used to establish a foundation for the use of in vitro assays. Their purpose is to gain the necessary perspective for reasonable application of the methodology by providing a base of test information in terms of numbers of chemicals tested as well as the types of responses obtained with compounds in different chemical classes. Absolute precision in percent correlations cannot be expected since both biological and practical considerations have an impact on both the in vitro and in vivo evaluation of a chemical.

In general, a chemical is defined as a carcinogen if, in a well designed and conducted bioassay, it produces a statistically significant increase in the incidence of neoplasms in one or more target organs. The in vivo bioassay conducted according to the National Cancer Institute/National Toxicology Program (NCI/NTP) protocol (Sontag *et al.*, 1976) is itself a battery of four tests consisting of an assay with the male mouse, the female mouse, the male rat and the female rat. Although 50 animals are used per group, the bioassay is relatively insensitive since it is designed to detect levels of tumor incidences of 5-10 percent in the test groups as compared to none in the control (Chu, *et al.*, 1981). In addition there is well documented variability of response and assays for which no definite conclusion can be reached. Of 203 NCI carcinogenicity bioassays (data summarized in Chu, *et al.*, 1981) 67 gave no significant evidence for carcinogenicity and 15 were identified as inadequate for evaluation. The remaining 121 assays then fell into a number of different categories. In 20 assays (16.5%) there was positive evidence for carcinogenicity in both sexes of both species; in 23 assays (19.0%) there was positive evidence in at least one sex of both species; in 53 assays (43.8%) there was positive evidence in only one species and finally in 25 assays (20.6%) there was only suggestive evidence of a carcinogenic effect. Evaluation of in vivo bioassay data is difficult and requires a mix of toxicological, pathological and statistical interpretation. This is the standard (denominator) against which in vitro tests are measured—a standard with its own set of problems in data evaluation.

The numerator of the correlation equation contains the results from the various mutagenicity/transformation tests. An important factor here is the potential of any in vitro test to generate nonconcordant results which unfortunately have been referred to as false negative or false positives. A false-negative result is defined as one in which a short-term test gives a negative result for a known carcinogen, or more importantly, for carcinogens within a specific class of chemicals, and a false-positive result is one in which the test substance or related chemicals induce measurable responses in the in vitro test systems but have not induced tumors in carcinogenicity bioassys. It would be unrealistic to expect complete agreement between results obtained in vitro and those obtained in vivo, and there are some obvious explanations for this situation.

Nonconcordant responses could be related to the method used for biotransformation of particular substances to their ultimate reactive forms. Activating systems, either intact cells or liver S-9 fractions which are added to in vitro test systems, cannot duplicate the complex metabolic process of the whole animal and it can be expected that some procarcinogens may fail to show activity in certain short term test systems. On the other hand, the innate metabolic capabilities of the target cells must also be considered. The processing of certain classes of chemicals could possibly lead to the production of end products which would not be produced in vivo but which would have in vitro activity. Additionally, different substances may act through different mechanisms to induce tumors in the whole animal and in vitro tests may not be capable of mimicking such interactions. For example, some agents may act as promoters, simply enhancing the expression of cells which have already been initiated and such agents would not be detected by direct mutagenicity or transformation assays. With other substances, such as asbestos, the physical interaction with the affected tissue is important and such interactions cannot be duplicated in in vitro test systems. It can also be expected that sensitive in vitro tests may respond to the presence of impurities present at levels too low to be detected in whole animal carcinogenicity tests.

The use of a battery of in vitro tests for determining the carcinogenic potential of chemicals, in certain respects, parallels the application of a battery of tests (two sexes of two species of rodents) for long-term carcinogenicity bioassays. There is no expectation that one sex of one species of animal will provide the sought for information on carcinogenicity and it cannot be expected that any single in vitro test can reflect the species, strain, sex and organ specifities found in carcinogenicity bioassays. Since the somatic mutation theory of cancer forms a basis for the use of genetic endpoints, one might be tempted to conclude that any single endpoint could be sufficient for making a determination about a chemical. The information available, however, indicates that each test has its own range of detection and that there are nonconcordant results between microbial and mammalian cell systems, among the different mammalian cell systems and between a series of in vitro tests and the in vivo carcinogenicity results. Thus only a battery composed of assays using different target cells, measuring different endpoints, and using different sources of metabolic activation can be expected to provide the best approach for determining the carcinogenic potential of unknown chemicals.

The question which logically follows is what tests should be included in a battery. It has been stated (ICPEMC 1982) that there is no general agreement as to the most appropriate selection of tests and that certain factors contribute to the problem. These factors are : 1) few test systems have been adequately evaluated; 2) there is no definition of the ways in which the tests differ from each other; 3) there has been a failure to define the circumstances in which specific tests may be used; 4) there is inadequate consideration for the processes used to analyze the data, and finally, 5) there are strong personal preferences for specific tests. Although some of these factors may contribute to the selection of a test battery, evaluation of batteries proposed by individual investigators, regulatory agencies and other groups reveals that there is a fairly high degree of consistency in the assays (endpoints) included in testing schemes (Summarized in Grice, 1984). Although the number of specific in vitro tests within a battery varies, this tabulation shows that, in general, a basic core of assays is usually selected. Without exception, all schemes proposed include a mutation assay in prokaryotes. The other predominant assays include mutation in mammalian cells, a test for chromosomal aberrations and an assay for in vitro transformation. An interesting discrepancy exists with an assay for DNA repair synthesis. Among the batteries proposed by individual investigators relatively few (30%) include a test for DNA repair synthesis. In contrast, a major portion ($\sim$ 80%) of batteries devised by regulatory agencies or other organizations include a test for repair synthesis in mammalian cells. This difference could be attributed to the fairly recent development of the DNA repair test in primary rat hepatocytes and the fact that many of the batteries proposed by individual investigators preceded development and evaluation of this testing procedure.

Although there are a variety of applications for short-term tests, from use in product development to regulatory decisions, and many reasons could be set forth for the specific construction of a battery, it must be recognized that any combination of tests with genetic end points will not detect chemicals that act through non-genotoxic mechanisms. Nevertheless, based on the information currently available it would appear that a battery of in vitro tests consisting of an assay for mutation in bacteria and an assay for mutation in mammalian cells as well as assays for DNA repair synthesis and chromosomal aberrations covers the broadest spectrum of genetic damage and should give the most comprehensive evaluation of the activity of a chemical.

In view of the correspondence between in vivo carcinogenicity and transformation in vitro, inclusion of such an assay in a battery would be ideal. On a cellular level, in vitro transformation systems provide the simplest approach for studying various aspects of the carcinogenic process and can link chemical, biochemical and biological events which would be difficult to do in experimental animal systems. The major difficulty associated with the transformation assays, at this time, centers on metabolic activation. With the exception of a limited number of studies (Benedict et al., 1978; Poiley et al., 1979; McGlynn-Kraft et al., 1983), most chemicals have been tested in the various transformation assays without an exogenous source of metabolic activation. Since many of the cells used in these systems are deficient in the cytochrome P450 enzymes that metabolically activate many chemicals, it can be presumed that some of the negative responses obtained with carcinogens are the results of such enzyme deficiency. Until the difficulties associated with the use of exogenous metabolic activation systems have been satisfactorily resolved, transformation systems can only be considered of limited value in the testing of new chemicals of structural types for which there is little or no background on metabolism.

An example of how a battery of tests performs in the detection of chemical carcinogens is shown in Table 1. This data which is part of a larger set was developed by the In Vitro Carcinogenesis Program of the National Cancer Institute (NCI) (Dunkel, 1976). The chemicals were from among those tested for carcinogenicity in the NCI Bioassay Program and the same chemicals from the same batch used for the in vivo tests were used in the in vitro assays. According to the technical reports, six of the eleven chemicals were carcinogenic, one was judged suspect and four were reported as negative. The bioassay of two chemicals, 3-nitropropionic acid and N,N'-dicylohexythiourea were subsequently reclassified by Griesemer and Cueto (1980). The first showed sufficient evidence for carcinogenicity in one species and no evidence in a second based on an increased incidence, in the male rat, of heptocellular neoplasms which were primarily benign and of islet-cell adenomas of the pancreas. The second showed equivocal evidence of carcinogenicity based on an increased incidence of hyperplasia of the follicular cells of the thyroid.

The in vitro data for all the chemicals with definitive positive carcinogenicity bioassays, with the exception of nitrilotriacetic acid (NTA), is in overall agreement with the in vivo results. Although three chemicals, 4-4′-methylenebis (N′-N-dimethyl)benzenamine, 4-amino-2-nitrophenol and 3-chloromethylpyridine HC1, were not detected as positive, each in one in vitro test, the remaining test data are sufficient for a positive designation. The test conducted with 4,4′-methylenebis (N′N-dimethyl)benzenamine in the SHE transformation assay was without metabolic activation and it is possible that this might be a factor in the lack of a response with this chemical. All in vitro tests with NTA were negative. In the in vivo bioassay of this chemical, tumors of the urinary tract were observed at doses of 15,000 and 20,000 ppm and such high doses have been reported to be associated with crystalluria (Anderson and Kanorva, 1980). In addition, hydronephrosis and/or nephritis was observed in all animals treated with NTA (National Cancer Institute, 1977). The mechanisms through which tumor induction occurred is more than likely an important consideration with this chemical as it would appear that it may not be through direct interaction with DNA as evidenced by the lack of responses in the HPC/DNA repair, Salmonella and mouse lymphoma assays.

TABLE 1
In Vivo and In Vitro Results of Bioassay Chemicals

CHEMICAL[1]	CAR[2]	HPC/DNA[3]	SAL[4]	ML[5]	SHE[6]
2-Amino-5-nitrothiazole	+	+	+	+	+
4,4′-Bis(dimethylamino) benzophenone	+	+	+	ND	+
4,4′-Methylenebis (N′,N-dimethyl) benzenamine	+	W/+	W/+	+	–
Nitrilotriacetic acid (trisodium salt)	+	–	–	–	–
4-amino-2-nitrophenol	+	–	+	+	W/+
3-Chloromethylpyridine HC1	+	–	+	+	W/+
p-Chloroaniline	S	+	+	+	+
3-Nitropropionic acid	–	+	+	+	–
N,N′-Dicyclohexylthiourea	–	–	–	–	+
Anilizine	–	–	–	+	–
Lithocholic acid	–	–	–	+,-	–

[1]Chemicals tested for carcinogenicity and in the in vitro tests were all from the same lot; all chemicals were tested under codes.
[2]CAR, carcinogenicity; Data from NCI Technical Reports.
[3]HPC/DNA, Unscheduled DNA synthesis in primary rat hepatocytes; Data from Williams *et al.*, 1982.
[4]SAL, *Salmonella typhimurium* plate incorporation assay; Data from Dunkel and Simmon, 1980.
[5]ML, L5178Y Mouse lymphoma assay; results from two laboratories are combined when both were the same. Data from NTP Bulletin, 1983.
[6]SHE, Syrian hamster embryo transformation assay tests performed without metabolic activation; Data from Pienta, 1984.
[7]–, negative; +, positive; W/+, weak positive; S, suspect; ND, no data.

The bioassay with p-chloroaniline was judged to be suggestive of carcinogenicity based on the production of fibromas and sarcomas of the spleen (National Cancer Institute, 1979). This chemical was positive in all in vitro tests and thus may be a carcinogen which was not detected under the conditions of the bioassay. The National Toxicology Program is currently retesting this chemical and the outcome of this additional bioassay should clarify the situation with this chemical.

Interpretation of the bioassay results on 3-nitropropionic acid and N'N-dicyclohexylthiourea make it difficult to draw a conclusion on the comparison of the in vivo and in vitro data. The in vitro data on 3-nitropropionic acid indicate that this chemical is genotoxic and thus a potential carcinogen. This would be more in line with the classification by Griesemer and Cueto (1980) of this chemical as having sufficient evidence for carcinogenicity. On the other hand, if this chemical is not carcinogenic, the positive in vitro results could then be considered as false positives or the results could be attributed to a major impurity which was present in the test compound. This was identified as a dimeric ester of 3-hydroxypropionic acid, was present at a level of 5 percent (National Cancer Institute, 1978), and thus could have been detected in the in vitro tests while not being detected in the in vivo bioassay.

The remaining two chemicals, anilizine and lithocholic acid, were negative in the animal bioassay. If we assume the results in the SHE transformation assay are correct and would not change if an exogenous metabolic activation system was used, all data are negative except for the mouse lymphoma assay. In this assay the results in two laboratories were positive with anilizine and with lithocholic acid the results were positive in one lab and negative in the other lab. When all the data are considered for these two chemicals, it would appear that the results in the mouse lymphoma may be false negative responses.

Overall, these results show that in vitro assays can provide valuable information on the carcinogenic potential of chemicals. It is also obvious that no single assay can stand alone and must be coupled with other in vitro assays to obtain the most comprehensive evaluation of the potential activity of a chemical.

D. CONCLUSION

Significant advances have been made in the development and evaluation of short-term tests for use in determining the carcinogenic potential of chemicals. Although a number of aspects of carcinogenesis are inconsistent with the somatic mutation theory of cancer, it is nevertheless apparent that in vitro tests with genetic endpoints are of practical value in assessing the activity of chemicals. This area is still evolving and it can be expected, as we learn more about in vitro procedures, that there will be better definition and application of in vitro testing procedures.

REFERENCES

Abrahamson, S., Wurgler, F.E., DeJongh, C., and Meyer, H.U.: How many loci on the x-chromosome of *Drosophila melanogaster* can mutate to recessive lethals. Environ. Mutagen. **2**, 447–453 (1980).

Amacher, D.E., Paillet, S., Ray, V.A.: Point mutations at the thymidine kinase locus in L5178Y mouse lymphoma cells. I. Applications to genetic toxicological testing. Mutat. Res. **64**, 391–406 (1979).

Ames, B.N.: The Detection of Chemical Mutagens with Enteric Bacteria. In: Hollaender, A. (Ed.): Chemical Mutagens: Principles and Methods for their Detection. Vol. **1**, New York, N.Y., Plenum Press (1971).

Ames, B.N., McCann, J., Yamasaki, E.: Methods for detecting carcinogens and mutagens with the Salmonella/mammalian microsome mutagenicity test. Mutat. Res. **31**, 347–364 (1975).

Ames, B.N., Durston, W.E., Yamasaki, E., Lee, F.D.: Carcinogens are mutagens: A simple test system combining liver homogenates for activation and bacteria for detection. Proc. Natl. Acad. Sci. (USA) **70**, 2281–2285 (1973).

Anderson, R.L., Kanerva, R.L.: Hypercalcinuria and crystalluria during ingestion of dietary nitrilotriacetate. Food Cosmet. Toxicol. **16**, 569–574 (1978).

Auerbach, C., Robson, J.M.: Production of mutations by allyl isothiocyanate. Nature **154**, 81 (1944).

Auerbach, C., Robson, J.M.: Chemical production of mutations. Nature **157**, 302 (1946).

Barratt, R.W., Tatum, E.L.: An evaluation of some carcinogens as mutagens. Cancer Res. **11**, 234 (1951).

Benedict, W.F., Banerjee, A., Venkatesan, N.: Cyclophosphamide induced oncogenic transformation, chromosomal breaks and sister chromatid exchange following microsomal activation. Cancer Res. **38**, 2922–2924 (1978).

Berenblum, I.: Carcinogenesis as a Biological Problem, Amsterdam-Oxford: North-Holland Publishing Co. (1974).

Berenblum, I., Shubik, P.: An experimental study of the initiating stage of carcinogenesis and a re-examination of the somatic cell mutation theory of cancer. Brit. J. Cancer **3**, 109–118, (1949).

Berwald, Y., Sachs, L.: In vitro cell transformation with chemical carcinogens. Nature **200**, 1182–1184 (1963).

Bigger, C.A.H., Tomaszewski, J.E., Dipple, A., Lake, R.S.: Limitations of metabolic activation systems used with in vitro tests for carcinogens. Science **209**, 503–505 (1980).

Boveri, T.: The origin of malignant tumors (First published, Jena, 1914), Baltimore: Williams and Wilkins Co. (1929).

Boycott, A.E.: A discussion on experimental production of malignant tumors. Proc. Roy. Soc. London, s.B. **113**, 291–292 (1933).

Burdette, W.J.: The significance of mutation in relation to the origin of tumors. Cancer Res. **15**, 201–226 (1955).

Burdette, W.J., Haddox, Jr., C.H.H.: Mutation rate following treatment of Neurospora with 20-methylcholanthrene and 1,2,5,6-dibenzanthracene in tween-80. Cancer Res. **14**, 163–168 (1954).

Carr, J.G.: Production of mutations in mice by 1:2:5:6-dibenzanthracene. Brit. J. Cancer. **1**, 152–156 (1947).

Chu, E.H.Y., Malling, H.V.: Mammalian cell genetics. II. Chemical induction of specific locus mutations in Chinese hamster cells in vitro. Proc. Natl. Acad. Sci. U.S.A. **61**, 1306–1313 (1968).

Chu, K.S., Cueto Jr., C., Ward, J.M.: Factors in the evaluation of 200 National Cancer Institute Bioassays. J. Tox. and Environ. Health. **8**, 251–280 (1981).

Clive, D., Johnson, K.A., Spector, J.F.S., Spector, A.G., Brown, M.M.M.: Validation and characterization of the L5178Y/TK+/- mouse lymphoma mutagen assay system. Mutat. Res. **59**, 61–108 (1979).

Cohen, M.M., Hirschhorn, K.J.: Cytogenetic studies in animals. In: Hollaender, A. (Ed.): Chemical Mutagens: Principles and Methods for their Detection. Vol. **2**, New York, N.Y. (1972).

Cook, J.W., Duffy, E., Schoental, R.: Primary liver tumors in rats following feeding with alkaloids of *Senecio jacobae.* Brit. J. Cancer. **4**, 405–410 (1950).

Cook, J.W., Hervett, C.L., and Hieger, I.: The isolation of a cancer-producing hydrocarbon from coal tar. Parts I, II and III. J. Chem. Soc. 395–405 (1933).

Demerec, M.: Mutations induced by carcinogens. Brit. J. Cancer, **2**, 114–117 (1948).

de Serres, F.J., Malling, H.V.: Measurement of recessive lethal damage over the entire genome and at two specific loci in the ad-3 region of a two-component heterokaryon of *Neurospora crassa.* In: Hollaender, A. (Ed.): Chemical Mutagens: Principles and Methods for Their Detection, Vol. **2**, New York, N.Y., Plenum Press (1971).

DiPaolo, J.A., Nelson, R.L., Donovan, P.: In vitro transformation of Syrian hamster embryo cells by diverse chemical carcinogens. Nature **235**, 278–280 (1971).

DiPaolo, J.A., Takano, K., Papescu, N.C.: Quantitation of chemically induced neoplasic transformation of BALB/3T3 cloned cell lines. Cancer Res. **32**, 2686–2695 (1972).

Dunkel, V.C.: In Vitro carcinogenesis: A National Cancer Institute Coordinated Programme. In: Montesano, R., Bartsch, H., Tomatis, L. (Eds.): Screening Tests in Chemical Carcinogenesis. IARC Scientific Publications No. 12, Lyon (1976).

Dunkel, V.C., Simmon, V.F.: Mutagenic activity of chemicals previously tested for carcinogenicity in the National Cancer Institute Bioassay Program. In: Montesano, R., Bartsch, H., Tomatis, L. (Eds.): Molecular and Cellular Aspects of Carcinogen Screening Tests. IARC Scientific Publications No. 27, Lyon (1980).

Dunkel, V.C., Pienta, R.J., Sivak, A., Traul, K.: Comparative neoplastic transformation responses of BALB/3T3 cells, Syrian hamster embryo cells, and Rauscher murine leukemia virus-infected Fischer 344 rat embryo cells to chemical carcinogens. J. Natl. Cancer Inst. **67**, 1301–1315 (1981).

Dybing, E., Soderlund, E., Timm Haug, L., Thorgeirsson, S.S.: Metabolism and activation of 2-acetylaminofluorene in isolated rat hepatocytes. Cancer Res. **39**, 3268–3275 (1979).

Evans, H.J.: Cytological methods for detecting chemical mutagens. In: Hollaender, E. (Ed.): Chemical Mutagens: Principles and Methods for Their Detection, Vol. **4**, New York, N.Y. (1976).

Evans, R.G., Norma, A.: Radiation stimulated incorporation of thymidine into the DNA of human lymphocytes. Nature **216**, 455–456 (1968).

Gabridge, M., Legator, M: A host-mediated microbial assay for the detection of mutagenic compounds. Proc. Soc. Exp. Biol. Med. **130**: 831–834 (1969).

Grice, H.C. (Ed.): Use of short-term tests for mutagenicity and carcinogenicity in chemical hazard evaluation. In: Current Issues in Toxicology. Springer-Verlag. New York, In Press, 1984.

Griesemer, R.A., Cueto, Jr., C.: toward a classification scheme for degrees of experimental evidence for the carcinogenicity of chemicals for animals. In: Montesano, R., Bartsch, H., Tomatis, L. (Eds): Molecular and Cellular Aspects of Carcinogen Screening Tests. IARC Scientific Publications No. 27, Lyon (1980).

Geissler, E. Uber die werkung von Nitrosaminen auf Mikroorganismen. Naturwissenchaften **49**, 380–381 (1962).

Heddle, J.A.: A rapid in vivo test for chromosomal damage. Mutat. Res. **18**, 187–190 (1973).

Heddle, J.A., Benz, R.D., and Countryman, P.I.: Measurement of chromosomal breakage in cultured cells by the micronucleus technique. In: Evans, H.J., Lloyd, D.C. (Eds.): Mutagen-induced Chromosome Damage in Man. Edinburgh University Press (1978).

Heidelberger, C., Freeman, A.E., Pienta, R.J., Sivak, A., Bertram, J.S., Casto, B.C., Dunkel, V.C., Francis, M.W., Kakunaga, T., Little, J.B., Schechtman, L.M.: Cell transformation by chemical agents-a review and analysis of the literature. Mutat. Res. **114**, 283–385 (1983).

Heuper, W.C., Wiley, F.H., Wolfe, H.D.: Experimental production of bladder tumors in dogs by administration of beta-naphthylamine. J Ind. Hyg. Toxicol. **20**, 46–84 (1938).

Hsie, A.W., Couch, D.B., O'Neill, J.P., San Sebastian, J.R., Brimer, P.A., Machanoff, R., Riddle, J.C., Li, A.P., Fuscoe, J.C., Forbes, N., Hsie, M.H.: Utilization of a quantitative mammalian cell mutation system, CHO/HGPRT, in experimental mutagenesis and genetic toxicology. In: Butterworth, B.E. (Ed.): Strategies for Short-Term Testing for Mutagens/Carcinogens, CRC Press, West Palm Beach, Florida (1979).

Huberman, E., Sachs, L.: Cell mediated mutagenesis of mammalian cells with chemical carcinogens. Int. J. Cancer **13**, 326–333 (1974).

Huberman, E., Sachs, L.: Mutability of different genetic loci in mammalian cells by metabolically activated carcinogenic polycyclic hydrocarbons. Proc. Natl. Acad. Sci. U.S.A. (1976).

ICPEMC Committee 2 Final Report: Mutagenesis testing as an approach to carcinogenesis. Mutat. Res. **99**, 73–91 (1982).

Ishidate, M., Odashima, S.: Chromosome tests with 134 compounds on Chinese Hamster cells in vitro-a screening for chemical carcinogens. Mutat. Res. **48**, 337–354 (1977).

Kakunaga, T.: A quantitative system for assay of malignant transformation by chemical carcinogens using a clone derived from BALB/3T3. Int. J. Cancer **12**, 463–473 (1973).

Kohn, K.W.: DNA as a target in cancer chemotherapy: Measurement of macromolecular DNA damage produced in mammalian cells by anticancer agents and carcinogens. Methods Cancer Res. **16**, 291–345 (1979).

Kraybill, H.F., Skimkin, M.B.: Carcinogenesis related to foods contaminated by processing and fungal metabolites. Adv. Cancer Res. **8**, 191–248 (1964).

Kuroki, T.C., Drevon, C., Montesano, R.: Microsome-mediated mutagenesis in V79 Chinese hamster cells by various nitrosamines. Cancer Res. **37**, 1044–1050 (1977).

Langenbach, R., Freed, H.J., Huberman, E.: Liver cell-mediated mutagenesis of mammalian cells by liver carcinogens. Proc. Natl. Acad. Sci. U.S.A. **75**, 2863–2867 (1978).

Latarjet, R., Buu-Hoi, N.P., Elias, C.A.: Induction d'une mutation specifique chez une bacterie par des cancerigene hydrosolubles. Pubbl. Stas. Zool. Napoli **22**, 78–93 (1953).

Legator, M.S., Palmer, K.A., Adler, I.A.: A collaborative study of in vivo cytogenetic analysis. I. Interpretation of slide preparations. Toxicol. Appl. Pharmacol. **24**, 337–350 (1973).

Lett, J.T., Caldwell, I.R., Dean, C.J., Alexander, O.: Rejoining of x-ray induced breaks in the DNA of leukemia cells. Nature **214**, 790–792 (1967).

Lochart-Mummery, J.P.: The Origin of Tumors, London: John Bale, Sons & Danulson, Ltd. (1932).

Magee, P.N., Barnes, J.M.: The production of malignant primary hepatic tumors in the rat by feeding dimethylnitrosamine. Brit. J. Cancer. **10**, 114–122 (1955).

Malling, H.V.: Mutagenicity of two potent carcinogens dimethylnitrosamine and diethylnitrosamine in *Neurospora crassa.* Mutat. Res. 3, 537–540.

Malling, H.V.: Dimethylnitrosamine: Formation of mutagenic compounds by interaction with mouse liver microsomes. Mutat. Res. 13, 425–429 (1971).

Maron, D.M., Ames, B.N.: Revised methods for the Salmonella mutagenicity test. Mutat. Res. 113, 173–215 (1983).

Marquardt, H.: Malignant transformation in vitro: A model system to study mechanisms of action of chemical carcinogens and to evaluate the oncogenic potential of environmental chemicals. In: Montesano, R., Bartsch, H., Tomatis, L. (Eds.) Screening test for chemical carcinogens. IARC Scientific Publications No. 12, Lyon (1976).

Marquardt, H., Schwaier, R., Zimmerman, F.: Nicht-Mutagenitat von Nitrosaminene bei *Neurospora crassa.* Naturwissenschaften. 50, 135–136 (1963).

Marquardt, H., Zimmermann, F.K., Schwaier, R.: Die Werkung krebsauslosender Nitrosamin und Nitrosamide auf das Adenin-6-45-Ruckmutation system von *Saccharomyces crevisiae.* Z. Verebungl. 95, 82–96 (1964).

Martin, D.N., McDermid, A.C., Garner, R.C.: Testing of unknown carcinogens and non-carcinogens for their ability to induce unscheduled DNA synthesis in the HeLa cells. Cancer Res. 38, 2621–2627 (1978).

Matter, B. and Schmid, W.: Trenimon-induced chromosomal damage in bone marrow cells of six mammalian species, evaluated by the micronucleus test. Mutat. Res. 12, 417–425 (1971).

McCann, J., Choi, E., Yamasaki, E., Ames, B.N.: Detection of carcinogens as mutagens in the Salmonella/microsome test. Assay of 300 chemicals. Proc. Natl. Acad. Sci. USA 72, 5135–5139 (1975).

McGlynn-Kreft, A., Scribner, H.E., McCarthy, K.L.: An exogenous metabolic activation system for the C3H 10T1/2 cell Transformation assay. Mutat. Res. 5 (1983).

McGrath, R.A., Williams, R.W.: Reconstruction in vivo of irradiated *Escherichia coli* deoxyribonucleic acid, the rejoining of broken pieces. Nature 212, 534–535 (1966).

Mohn, G.R., Ellenberger, J., Van Bladeren, P.J.: Evaluation and relevance of *Escherichia coli* test systems for detecting and for characterizing chemical carcinogens and mutagens. In: Williams, G.M., Kroes, R., Waaijers, H.W., van de Poll, K.W. (Eds.): Applied Methods in Oncology., Vol. 3, Amsterdam: Elsevier/North-Holland Biomedical Press (1980).

Murray, J.A.: A discussion on experimental production of malignant tumors. Proc. Roy. Soc. London. s.B. 113, 268–273 (1933).

Mutsuoka, A., Hayashi, N., Ishidate Jr., M.: Chromosomal aberration tests on 29 chemicals combined with S9 mix in vitro. Mutat. Res. 66, 277–290 (1979).

National Cancer Institute: Bioassays of Nitrolotriacetic Acid (NTA) and Nitrolotriacetic Acid, Trisodium Salt, Monohydrate ($Na_3NTA \cdot H_2O$) for Possible Carcinogenicity. Technical Report Series No. 6. DHEW Publication No. (NIH) 77-806 (1977).

National Cancer Institute: Bioassay of 3-Nitropropionic Acid for Possible Carcinogenicity. Technical Report Series No. 52. DHEW Publication No. (NIH) 78-1302 (1978).

National Cancer Institute: Bioassay of p-Chloroaniline for Possible Carcinogenicity. Technical Report Series No. 189. DHEW Publication No. (NIH) 79-1745 (1979).

National Toxicology Program: NTP Technical Bulletin No. 9 (1983).

Nettleship, A., Henshaw, P.S.: Induction of pulmonary tumors in mice with ethyl carbamate (urethane). J. Natl. Cancer Inst. 4, 309–319 (1943).

Painter, R.B., Cleaver, J.E.: Repair replication, unscheduled DNA synthesis and the repair of mammalian DNA. Radiat. Res. 37, 4151–4166 (1969).

Pasternak, L.: Mutagene wirkung von dimethylnitrosamine bei *Drosophila melanogaster.* Naturwissenschaften 49, 381 (1962).

Perry, P.E.: Chemical mutagens and sister chromatid exchange. In: de Serres, F.J., Hollaender, A. (Eds.): Chemical Mutagens: Principles and Methods for Their Detection. Vol. **6**, New York, N.Y., Plenum Press (1980).

Pienta, R.J., Poiley, J.A., Lebherz, W.B.: III. Morphological transformation of early passage golden Syrian hamster embryo cells derived from cryopreserved primary cultures as a reliable in vitro bioassay for identifying diverse carcinogens. Int. J. Cancer **1**, 642–655 (1977).

Pienta, R.J.: A transformation bioassay employing cryopreserved hamster embryo cells. In: Mishra, N., Dunkel, V.C., Mehlman, M. (Eds.): Mammalian Cell Transformation by Chemical Carcinogens, Advances in Environmental Toxicology, Vol. **1**, Princeton Junction, N.J., Senate Press, Inc. (1980).

Pienta, R.J.: Personal Communication (1984).

Poiley, J.A., Rainier, R., Pienta, R.J.: Use of hamster hepatocytes to metabolize carcinogens in an in vitro bioassay. J. Natl. Cancer Inst. **61**, 519–523 (1979).

Probst, G.S., Hill, L.E., Bewsey, B.: Comparison of three in vitro assays for carcinogen-induced DNA damage. J. Toxicol. Environ. Health **6**, 33–49 (1980).

Rasmussen, R.E., Painter, R.B.: Evidence for repair of ultraviolet damaged deoxyribonucleic acid in cultured mammalian cells. Nature **203**, 1360–1362 (1964).

Reznikoff, C.A., Bertram, J.S., Brankow, D.N., Heidelberger, C.: Quantitative and qualitative studies of chemical transformation of cloned C3H mouse embryo cells sensitive to postconfluence inhibition of cell division. Cancer Res. **33**, 3239–3249 (1973).

San, R.H.C., Stich, H.F.: DNA repair synthesis of cultured human cells as a rapid bioassay for chemical carcinogens. Int. J. Cancer **16**, 284–291 (1975).

Schmeltz, I., Tosk, J. Williams, G.M.: Comparison of the metabolic profiles of benzo(a)pyrene obtained from primary cell cultures and subcellular fractions derived from normal and methylcholanthrene-induced rat liver. Cancer Lett. **5**, 81–89 (1978).

Schmid, W.: The micronucleus test. Mutat. Res. **31**, 9–15 (1975).

Selkirk, J.K.: Divergence of metabolic activation systems for short-term mutagenesis assays. Nature **270**, 604–605 (1977).

Sivak, A., Charest, M.C., Rudenko, L., Silveira, D.M., Simons, I., Wood, A.M.: BALB/c-3T3 cells as target cells for chemically induced neoplastic transformation. In: Mishra, M., Dunkel, V.C., Mehlman, M. (Eds.): Mammalian Cell Transformation by Chemical Carcinogens. Advances in Environmental Toxicology, Vol. **1**, Princeton Junction, N.J., Senate Press, Inc. (1980).

Smith, D.W.E.: Mutagenicity of cycasin aglycone (methylazoxymethanol), a naturally occurring carcinogen. Science. **192**, 1273–1274 (1966).

Sontag, J.A., Page, N.P., Saffiotti, U.: Guidelines for carcinogen bioassay in small rodents. Carcinogenesis Tech. Rep. Ser. 1, DHEW Publ. NIH 76–81 (1976).

Stich, H.F., San, R.H.C.: DNA repair and chromatid anomalies in mammalian cells exposed to 4-nitroquinoline 1-oxide. Mutat. Res. **10**, 389–404 (1970).

Strong, L.C.: The induction of mutations by a carcinogen. Brit. J. Cancer. **3**, 97–108 (1949).

Swenberg, J.A., Petzold, G.L., Harback, P.R.: In vitro DNA damage/alkaline elution assay for predicting carcinogenic potential. Biochem. Biophys. Res. Commun. **72**, 732–738 (1976).

Vogel, E.: Recent advancements with Drosophila as an assay system for carcinogens. In: Stich, H.F., San, R.H.C. (Eds.): Short-term Tests for Chemical Carcinogens. New York, N.Y. Springer-Verlag (1981).

Williams, G.M.: Carcinogen-induced DNA repair in primary rat liver cell cultures; a possible screen for chemical carcinogens. Cancer Lett. **1**, 231–236 (1976).

Williams, G.M.: The detection of chemical carcinogens by unscheduled DNA synthesis in rat liver primary cell cultures. Cancer Res. **37**, 1845–1851 (1977).

Williams, G.M.: The predictive value of DNA damage and repair assays for carcinogenicity. In: Williams, G.M., Kroes, R., Waaijers, H.W., van de Poll, K.W. (Eds.): Applied Methods in Oncology, Vol. **3**, Amsterdam, Elsevier/North-Holland Biomedical Press (1980).

Williams, G.M., Laspia, M.F., Dunkel, V.C.: Reliability of the hepatocyte primary culture/DNA repair test in testing of coded carcinogens and noncarcinogens. Mutat. Res. **97**, 359–370 (1982).

Wilson, R.H., De Eds, F., and Cox, Jr., A.J.: Toxicity and carcinogenic activity of 2-acetaminofluorene. Cancer Res. **1**, 595–608 (1941).

Yamagiwa, K., Ichikawa, K.: Experimentelle Studie uber die Pathogenese der Epithelialgeschwulste. Mitteilungen Med. Facultat Kaiserl. Univ. Tokyo. **15**, 295–344 (1915).

Yoshida, T.: Uber die serienweise verfolgung der veranderungen der leber der experimentellen hepatomerseugung durch o-aminoazotoluol. Trans. Japan Pathol. Soc. **23**, 636–638 (1933).

Zimmerman, H.K.: Detection of genetically active chemicals using various yeast systems. In: Hollaender, A. (Ed.): Chemical Mutagens: Principles and Methods for their Detection, Vol. **3**, New York, N.Y., Plenum Press (1973).

CHAPTER IV

METABOLIC ACTIVATION

Edward Bresnick
The Eppley Institute for Research in Cancer
University of Nebraska Medical Center
Omaha, Nebraska

A. INTRODUCTION

A number of potentially-reactive agents occur in a form which requires metabolic activation while some can elicit their toxic or mutagenic effects without such enzymatic action. The latter are referred to as '*direct-acting*' mutagens, toxins, etc., while the former fall into the category of '*indirect-acting*'. The fates of these two classes of agents are depicted in Figure 1.

Through metabolic activation of procarcinogens or promutagens or through spontaneous reaction of direct-acting carcinogens or mutagens, electrophilic substances are formed which may interact in covalent fashion with nucleophilic regions of macromolecular components (or smaller molecular weight intracellular materials). Such interaction may lead to the formation of alkylated protein, RNA or DNA. These "lesions" contribute in some manner to the toxic, mutagenic or carcinogenic event(s). The alkylation of DNA in a number of instances will trigger a repair process which could occur prior to cell division, i.e., *prereplication repair*, or during replication in preparation for cell division, i.e., *replication repair*. Were repair to occur prior to replication, the alkylated DNA could be restored to its original structure, i.e., 'normal' DNA, or inappropriate bases could be inserted as a result of lack of conformance to Watson-Crick base-pairing rules. The latter mechanism is known as *error-prone repair* and has been demonstrated in some bacterial systems. Furthermore, alkylated DNA could be partially repaired during the replication mechanism again resulting in either complete restoration of the original structure, i.e., 'normal' DNA, or in a DNA molecule which contains aberrant or inappropriate bases. Examples of each will be provided in a later section.

Not all monooxygenases that function in biotransformation contain cytochrome P450. Thus, as reviewed by Ziegler (1980), the microsomes contain a flavin-dependent monooxygenase which catalyzes the oxygenation of imidazole mercaptans, e.g., methimazole, to imidazole sulfenic acids, of sulfides to sulfoxides and sulfones and of thioamides and thiocarbonates to sulfoxides and sulfenes, respectively. In addition, this enzyme catalyzes the production of

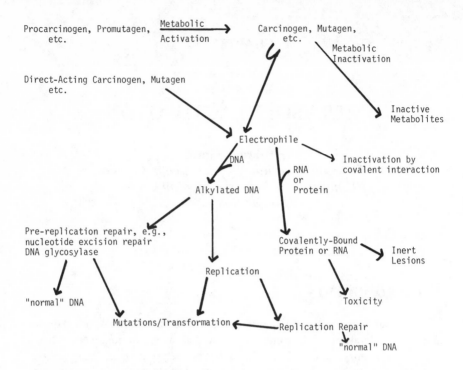

FIGURE 1: Activation of Prodrugs and Interaction with Macromolecules.

amine oxides from tertiary amines, of hydroxylamines from secondary amines and of reactive, not completely identified species from 1,1-disubstituted hydrazines and N-substituted aziridines.

In addition to the oxidative reactions catalyzed by the enzymes of biotransformation, reductions also proceed within the sphere of cytochrome P450. These reductive reactions are tabulated in Table II.

TABLE I
Monooxygenase-Catalyzed Drug Biotransformations

Involving a Carbon Moiety
    Hydroxylation of an aromatic ring → phenol
    Side-chain oxidation → sec alcohol
    Epoxidation → Epoxide
Involving a Nitrogen Moiety
    N-Dealkylation → sec or primary amine
    N-Oxidation of tertiary amines → N-oxide
    Oxidation deamination → ketones
Involving an Oxygen or Sulfur Moiety
    O or S-Dealkylation of ethers or thioether → alcohols or mercaptans
    S-Oxidation of ring-sulfur or thiono-sulfur compounds → S-oxides
    Oxidative desulfuration of sulfides → oxygen substitution
Involving a Phosphorous Moiety
    Phosphothionate oxidation → cleavage of bond

TABLE II
Reductions Catalyzed by Cytochrome P450-Dependent Enzymes

Affecting a Nitrogen Moiety
   Nitrogroup reduction → Amines
   Azo-bond reductive cleavage → 2 amine functions
   N-Dehydroxylation of hydroxylamines → amines
Affecting an Oxygen Moiety
   Epoxide reduction → aromatic or olefinic group
Affecting a Halogen Group
   Dehalogenation → replacement by a hydrogen

I. Other Enzymes Involved in the Biotransformation of Drugs, Particularly Those Which Lead to Activation or Inactivation

A number of particulate-bound and cytosolic enzymes function in either the activation of prodrugs or the inactivation of drugs. Epoxide hydrolase, an enzyme which is located within the endoplasmic reticulum (Oesch, 1973) or in the nucleus (Thomas, et al, 1979), catalyzes the hydration of epoxides to yield *trans* dihydrodiols (Figure 3). No co-factors are required for this reaction. Epoxide hydrolase is an interesting enzyme in view of its participation as a component of the activating mechanism leading to the formation of ultimate carcinogenic forms of polycyclic hydrocarbons, e.g., benzo(a)pyrene, or as a component in the inactivation of the biological reactive species, the 2,3-oxide of aflatoxin B_1.

Glucoronidation is an important reaction of detoxification which is catalyzed by a family of microsomal UDP-glucuronyltransferases (Figure 4). The enzymes and their actions have been reviewed by Sutton and Burchell (1977). The net effect of this chemical reaction is to increase the hydrophilicity of the acceptor molecule prior to secretion from the liver to the circulation. Substrates for this enzyme family include hydroxyl-bearing compounds such as bilirubin or morphine; phenols such as p-nitrophenol or hydroxylated benzo(a)pyrenes; amines such as aniline; mercaptans such as thiophenol; and carboxyl-containing substances such as benzoic acid.

Conjugation of appropriate acceptors with glutathione is another mechanism of detoxification (Figure 5). This reaction is catalyzed by a family of isozymes which are located in the cytosolic compartment of a number of tissues, in particular, liver (Jakoby and Habig, 1980). At least 7 glutathione transferases have been isolated from rat liver. Each has a broad but overlapping specificity in regard to substrates. Included amongst the substrates are oxides, and mono- and dihalogenated di- and mono-nitrobenzenes. The major form present in rat liver cytosol, glutathione S-transferase B, is identical with ligandin or the Y-protein (reviewed in Jakoby and Habig, 1980) which is purported to shuttle bilirubin (or certain carcinogens) from the hepatocyte plasma membrane to the endoplasmic reticulum.

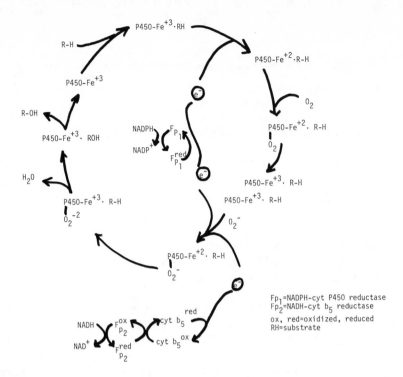

FIGURE 2: Hydroxylation of Substrates by Cytochrome P450-Dependent Monooxygenases.

The cytosolic enzyme, N-acetyltransferase, catalyzes a major pathway for the metabolism of arylamines and arylhydrazides (Figure 6). The reaction generally leads to the detoxification of active amine-containing moieties, e.g., sulfanilamide, although, in the case of the insecticide, aminofluorene, the acetylation step is requisite for the formation of penultimate carcinogens.

Phenolic or hydroxyl groups are generally detoxified by the formation of sulfate esters as catalyzed by the cytosolic sulfotransferases (Jakoby, et al, 1980). The reactions are indicated in Figure 7. The sulfotransferases are another example of isozymes, each member of which has overlapping substrate specificity. Although the sulfation reaction is generally considered to represent a detoxification, the sulfate ester of N-hydroxy-2-acetylaminofluorene appears to more readily form a reactive electrophile than the sulfated N-hydroxy compound. Therefore, this reaction would more truly represent an activation mechanism.

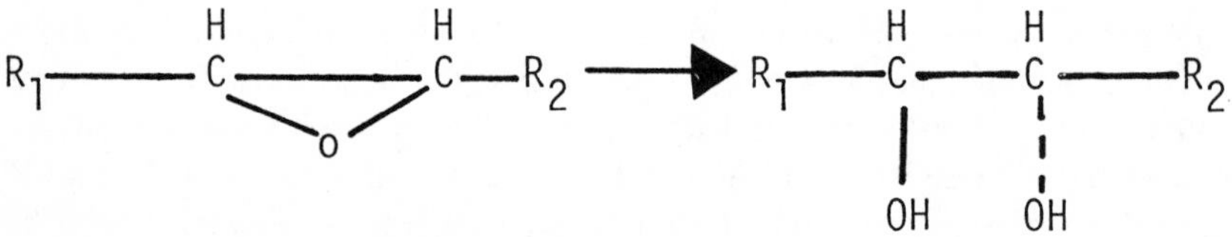

FIGURE 3: Epoxide Hydrolase.

UDP-Glucuronide + Acceptor $\longrightarrow$ Acceptor-Glucuronide
$$+$$
$$UDP$$

FIGURE 4: UDP-Glucuronyl Transferase Activity.

G-SH + Acceptor $\longrightarrow$ Acceptor-S-G + H^+

Reduced Glutathione, G-SH

FIGURE 5: Glutathione S-Transferase Activity.

$$CH_3-\overset{O}{\overset{\|}{C}}-Coenzyme\ A + Acceptor \longrightarrow Coenzyme\ A + CH_3-\overset{O}{\overset{\|}{C}}-Acceptor$$

FIGURE 6: N-Acetyltransferase Activity.

ATP + $SO_4^=$ $\xrightarrow{\text{sulfurylase}}$ adenosine-5'-phosphosulfate (APS)

APS + ATP $\xrightarrow{\text{APS Kinase}}$ 3'-phospho-5'-adenosine phosphosulfate (PAPS)

PAPS + Acceptor-OH $\xrightarrow{\text{sulfotransferase}}$ Acceptor-O-sulfate + adenosine-
$$3',5'-diphosphate$$

FIGURE 7: Sulfate Ester Formation.

II. Multiplicity of Cytochrome P450's

The initial observation suggesting the multiplicity of cytochrome P450's within a specific mammalian host was made by Conney, et al (1959). These investigators reported that the administration of benzo(a)pyrene to rats effected a dramatic increase in the microsomal metabolism of a number of substrates, e.g., zoxazolamine; the metabolism of others such as mepiridine was decreased, while the metabolism of chlorpromazine was unaffected.

The effects of a number of inducers of varying chemical structure have also contributed to the multiplicity problem. In this regard, Richardson and Cunningham (1951) reported in 1951 that the incidence of azo dye-induced hepatocellular carcinoma was markedly reduced by the coadministration of the polycyclic hydrocarbon, 3-methylcholanthrene (3MC). Subsequently, Conney and the Millers (1956) demonstrated the induction of the liver cytochrome

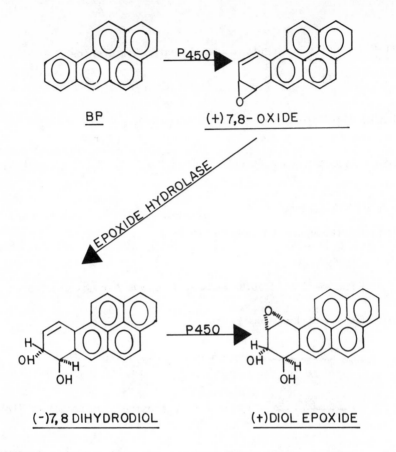

FIGURE 8: Activation of Benzo(a)pyrene (BP). P450 = Cytochrome P450.

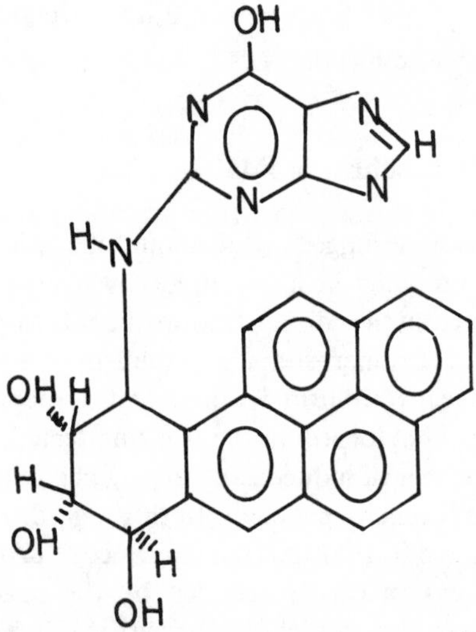

FIGURE 9: Benzo(a)pyrene Guanine Adduct.

P450-dependent enzyme, N-demethylase, and the resultant decrease in carcinogenicity of the azo dye upon injection of rats with 3-methylcholanthrene. The polycyclic hydrocarbon-induced cytochrome P450 exhibited an altered difference spectrum from control microsomal preparations (reviewed in Lu and West, 1979). The responsible hemoprotein was named the 3MC-inducible cytochrome P450, cytochrome P_{448}, cytochrome P_1-450 or cytochrome P450c.

In addition to 3MC, phenobarbital administration also resulted in elevated liver cytochrome P450 levels. This cytochrome has been termed cytochrome P450b and LM_2 in rat and rabbit, respectively (see Lu, 1978). The polychlorinated biphenyl mixture, Aroclor 1254, also induces hepatic cytochrome P450 in rats. Ryan, et al (1979) have shown that Aroclor 1254 is a mixed inducer, i.e., causes an elevation in both cytochromes P450b and P450c. Since Aroclor 1254 administration does lead to increases in multiple cytochrome P450's and since activation of different procarcinogens or promutagens often requires different hemoproteins, S9 fractions from livers of polychlorinated biphenyl-treated rats are employed as the activating system in the Ames *Salmonella* mutagenesis assay. Finally, the administration to rodents of pregnenolone-16 α-carbonitrile, a steroid analog, results in the induction of a unique cytochrome P450 (Elshourbagy and Guzelian, 1980).

D. FACTORS WHICH INFLUENCE MONOOXYGENASE ACTIVITY

In addition to induction of the cytochrome P450's elicited by a number of xenobiotics (see above), total monooxygenase activity is altered by physiological factors such as age, genetics and the hormonal milieu and by pathological factors such as neoplasia.

Previous work with rodents has shown that biotransformation of drugs takes place at a much reduced rate in fetal and neonatal tissues but increases dramatically shortly after birth (Fouts and Adamson, 1959; Conney, 1967). In contrast, human fetuses have greater drug metabolic activity during early gestation (Pelkonen, et al, 1971). In addition to the monooxygenases, epoxide hydrolase and the conjugating enzymes undergo ontogenetic changes in activity. With 3MC-11, 12-oxide as substrate, hepatic epoxide hydrolase was barely detectable in rat fetuses and in 1 day old neonates (Stoming and Bresnick, 1974). Enzyme activity rose rapidly to adult values by 3 weeks of age.

Glutathione S-epoxide transferase activity exhibited a somewhat similar ontogenetic pattern in rat liver and lung (Mukhtar and Bresnick, 1976). Enzyme activity in 18 day old fetal liver or lung was approximately 20% of that observed in the respective adult tissue; adult values were reached by 3 weeks of age.

UDP glucuronyltransferase activity in rat liver changes in a complex manner as a result of development (Henderson, 1971; Lucier and McDaniel, 1977). Enzyme activity is undetectable in rat liver prior to 5 days before birth; it rises rapidly reaching a maximum shortly after birth. Glucuronyltransferase then falls to a nadir at weaning. In contrast to the above examples, N-acetyltransferase is present in fetal and neonatal rodents (Sonawane and Lucier, 1975). The type of developmental pattern was a reflection of the tissue and the species.

Although monooxygenase and related enzyme activities are diminished in fetal liver, induction by a variety of agents can take place. Thus, addition of 3MC or β-naphthoflavone to fetal liver organ cultures resulted in a profound increase in the monooxygenase, aryl hydrocarbon hydroxylase (Burke, et al, 1973a). The magnitude of the induction was dependent upon the age of the fetus from which the liver was extirpated; older fetuses yielded higher induction of this enzyme. Similar type studies have been conducted under *in vivo* conditions. The administration of the potent inducer of aryl hydrocarbon hydroxylase, 2,3,7,8-tetrachlorodibenzo-p-dioxin (TCDD), to pregnant rats at 10 days of gestation resulted in a marked increase in fetal enzyme (Lucier, et al, 1975; Berry, et al, 1976). Transplacental induction of the monooxygenase had obviously occurred.

As mentioned in a previous section, the cytochrome P450-dependent monooxygenases are located in the nucleus as well as in the endoplasmic reticulum. Studies from our laboratory have addressed the question of the ontogenetic changes of nuclear aryl hydrocarbon hydroxylase in rat liver (Nunnick, et al, 1978). The nuclear activity was detectable in fetal liver, increased approximately 30-fold by 1 day after birth and rose an additional 4-fold by the time the rats were 2 weeks old. Furthermore, administration of 3MC to the rat dams effected an 8-fold increase in fetal nuclear aryl hydrocarbon hydroxylase. The most "inducible" in regard to nuclear enzyme activity was the 4 week old rat. Parenthetically, it should be mentioned that in recent studies from out laboratory (Bresnick, et al, 1979; 1980), 3MC-inducible aryl hydrocarbon hydroxylase has been demonstrated in 2 morphologically-distinct forms within rat liver nuclei, a) a fibrillar form which resembles the nucleo-cytoplasmic skeleton and b) a macrodeposit which was established as nucleoli. What the function of this monooxygenase is within nucleoli is not known. Within nuclei, the monooxygenase may serve as a second means for disposing of lipid-soluble components. Unfortunately, during the transition of the latter to more hydrophilic components, toxic ingredients may be produced. This is exemplified by the nuclear activation of benzo(a)pyrene (Bresnick, et al, 1977).

It is well known that in certain species sex plays a very prominent role in determining the extent of basal activity of the enzymes of drug metabolism. The adult female rat has a much less active liver monooxygenase system than the adult male (reviewed in Conney, 1967). In regard to rat liver aryl hydrocarbon hydroxylase, during normal ontogeny, the specific activity in the male rose to 6-fold that present in the female. The increased enzymatic activity in the male is a reflection of the sensitivity to carcinogenesis as a result of exposure to aflatoxin B_1 (Purchase and Steyn, 1969). The level of the microsomal mono-oxygenase in the female can be increased upon administration of androgens; the activity in the male can be reduced upon castration (Conney, 1967).

It is of interest that the sex effect discussed for the rat is opposite to that portrayed in the mouse. As reported previously (Burki, et al, 1973b), the activity of aryl hydrocarbon hydroxylase in the livers obtained from female mice of several strains was 2-fold higher than that observed in the male. This increased activity in the female coincided with the increased metabolic products obtained after incubation of 3MC with mouse microsomes.

The contribution of genetics to metabolic activation is discussed in another chapter and accordingly, will not be treated in this section.

E. SPECIFIC EXAMPLES OF METABOLIC ACTIVATION

In this section, the metabolic activation of certain specific protoxins, promutagens and procarcinogens will be discussed. In particular, the polycyclic hydrocarbons, aflatoxins, dimethylnitrosamine, acetylaminofluorene and acetaminophen will be employed as examples.

I. Polycyclic hydrocarbons

Most environmental polycyclic hydrocarbons are biologically inert and therefore require metabolic activation, presumably in the target cell destined for mutagenesis or carcinogenesis. During the more recent years, a key to unlocking the mechanism of action of these substances was provided by Borgen, et al (1973) who noted that microsomal metabolites of benzo(a)pyrene, (BP)-7,8-dihydrodiol covalently bound to DNA to a greater extent than did the parent compound or other metabolites. This observation was quickly followed by the report of Sims, et al (1974) in which BP-7,8-dihydrodiol-9,10-epoxide was suggested as the reactive metabolite which contributed to the binding of DNA. The reactions by which the reactive intermediates are generated are interesting in that the enzymes exhibit a considerable amount of selectivity. These enzymes include the cytochrome P450-dependent monooxygenases and epoxide hydrolase. We are indebted to the studies of Yang, et al (1976), and Thakker, et al (1976; 1977) for the details of the stereospecific enzymatic reactions.

In animal tissues, BP is metabolized by the monooxygenases to form primarily the (+) 7,8-oxide of BP (Figure 8). The latter is hydrated as a result of the action of epoxide hydrolase to yield the (−) 7,8-dihydrodiol of BP which then undergoes a secondary round of metabolism via the cytochrome P450-dependent monooxygenases. The product is primarily r-7,t-8-dihydroxy-t-9,10-oxy-7,8,9,10-tetrahydro BP, diol epoxide 2 or the *anti* diol epoxide. Diol epoxide 2 is a very reactive substance which easily generates an electrophile that is capable of covalently interacting with nucleophilic centers of a variety of macromolecules, including DNA. The most prevalent, although not *de facto* the most important, adduct with DNA is the N2-substituted guanine moiety (Figure 9). As indicated previously, the entire sequence of activation is present within nuclei (Bresnick et al, 1977).

The presence of a unique structural feature in the diol epoxides of BP formed the nidus of the bay region theory of carcinogenesis postulated by Jerina and his colleagues (see Jerina and Daly, 1976). The epoxide of a saturated, angular benzo-ring forms a segment of the bay region of polycyclic hydrocarbons

(Figure 10). The metabolic formation of dihydrodiol derivatives at the 2 most distal carbon atoms from the sterically-hindered bay region should provide very reactive diol epoxides which exhibit carcinogenic and mutagenic properties. Jerina and his colleagues were able to calculate the ease of carbonium ion formation using quantum mechanics and have observed a good correlation between the relative carcinogenicity of the bay region diol epoxides of a number of polycyclic hydrocarbons and this computation.

Several additional pathways have been proposed for the metabolic activation of polycyclic hydrocarbons such as BP. Lorentzen, et al (1975) have proposed that oxidation of BP at the 6 position which would take place by a mechanism which does not involve prior epoxidation. Such a reaction could lead to the generation of a free radical at the 6-position of BP and the subsequent bond formation with an appropriate macromolecule. The actual contribution of this pathway to the metabolism of BP, its covalent binding to nucleic acids and protein or its relationship to carcinogenesis has not been fully evaluated, although the current belief is that this reaction plays only a minor role.

Of perhaps greater importance to the activation of BP is the peroxidative oxidation of this polycyclic hydrocarbon in concert with prostaglandin biosynthesis (Marnett and Reed, 1979). Prostaglandin synthesis is depicted in Figure 11. During the microsomal conversion of arachidonate to PGH_2, BP is oxidized to quinones or other metabolites. Sivarajah, et al (1978) have reported that during this prostaglandin synthetase (sum total of endoperoxide synthetase and cyclooxygenase)—dependent oxidation of BP, covalent attachment of the latter occurs to DNA. Furthermore, Marnett, et al (1978) have demonstrated the formation of derivatives that are strongly mutagenic to *Salmonella typhimurium* TA 98 during the prostaglandin synthetase-dependent cooxygenation of BP-7,8-dihydrodiol. This mechanism would represent a very viable alternative

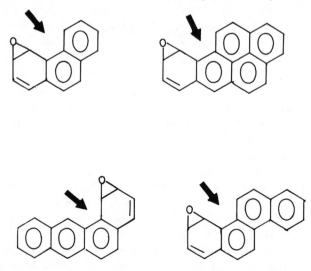

FIGURE 10: Bay Region of Polycyclic Hydrocarbons. The *arrow* indicates the Bay Region.

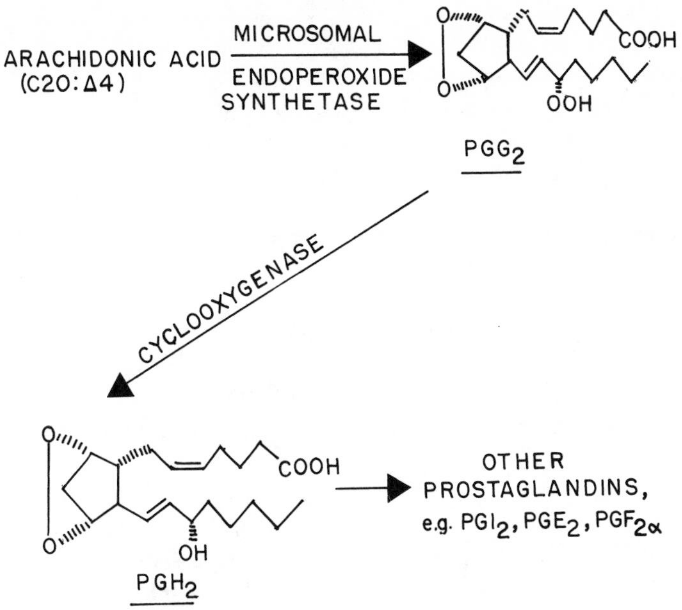

FIGURE 11: Prostaglandin Synthesis.

for tissues with active prostaglandin synthesis to the monooxygenase-epoxide hydrolase system for the activation of polycyclic hydrocarbons.

II. Some Naturally-Occurring Mutagens and Carcinogens

It has long been known that mutagens and carcinogens occur naturally in our foodstuffs. In this regard, cycasin that occurs in the cycad tree which provides food for some natives in tropical and subtropical countries and aflatoxin B_1, a heterocyclic compound elaborated by a mold that contaminates grains and nuts, are prime examples. Both chemicals share the property of hepato-carcinogenesis.

Cycasin (Figure 12) is partially hydrolyzed in the gastrointestinal lumen by our resident bacteria yielding methylazoxymethanol. The latter substance via either the catalytic action of certain dehydrogenases or the spontaneous decomposition of some of the reactive intermediates, eventually gives rise to the CH_3^+ electrophile. It is the latter agent which is purported to be the ultimate mutagen and carcinogen. This pathway is particularly important because it demonstrates the contributory role of the gut bacterial flora to the problem of metabolic activation and subsequently, to carcinogenesis.

Aflatoxin B_1 (Figure 13) is formed within and secreted by certain strains of *Aspergillus flavus*. It is apparently activated by the cytochrome P450-dependent monooxygenases to form the very reactive ultimate mutagen or carcinogen, the 2,3-oxide of aflatoxin B_1 (Swenson, et al, 1973) (Figure 13). This reactive substance which has not been isolated to date immediately interacts

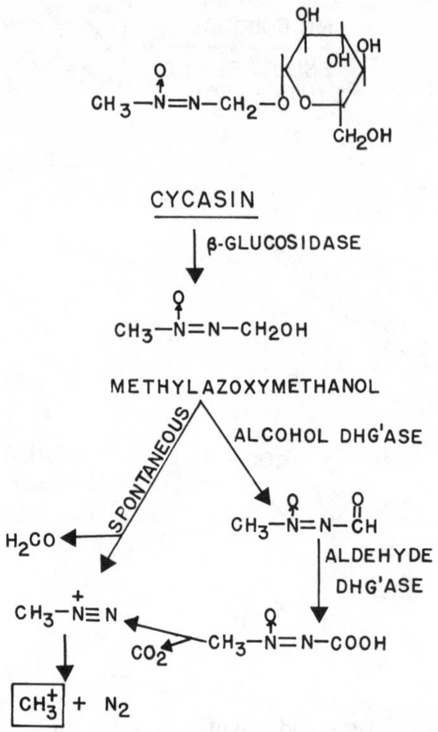

FIGURE 12: Activation of Cycasin. β-glucosidase is a bacterial enzyme. DHG'ase = dehydrogenase.

with nucleophiles such as the guanine moiety of DNA resulting in the formation of the N-7 derivative at the C2 of aflatoxin B_1). It should be mentioned that epoxide hydrolase would serve in a protective capacity by hydrating the 2,3-oxide to inactive dihydrodiols.

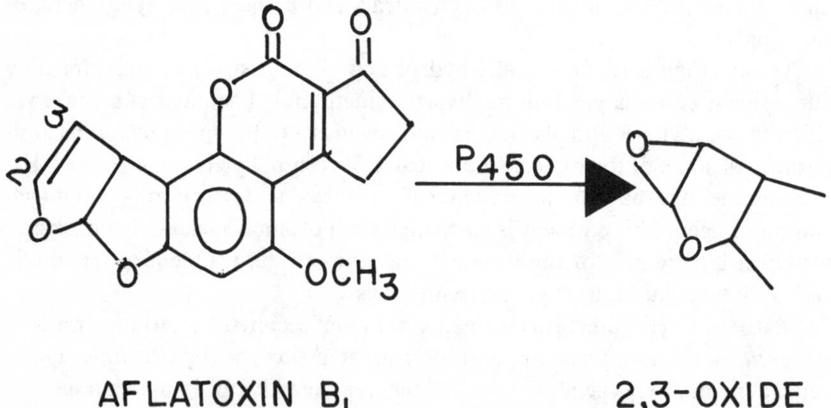

FIGURE 13: Activation of Aflatoxin B_1.

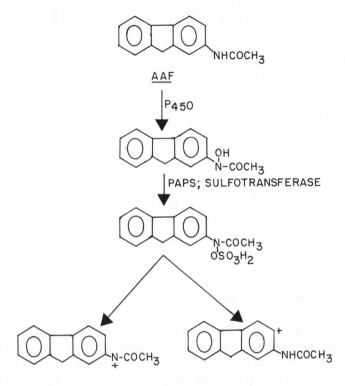

FIGURE 14: Activation of Acetylaminofluorene (AAF).

III. Aromatic Amines

2-Acetylaminofluorene (AAF) (Figure 14) is one of the first carcinogens which was demonstrated to require metabolic activation (reviewed in Miller and Miller, 1969). AAF undergoes a cytochrome P450-dependent monooxygenase catalyzed N-hydroxylation leading to the formation of the proximate carcinogen, N-hydroxy AAF. It is of interest that the guinea pig is unable to carry out the N-hydroxylation reaction and accordingly, is resistant to AAF-induced carcinogenesis. The N-hydroxy AAF subsequently is either sulfated (as shown in the Figure), glucuronidated, or acetylated. These reactions are then followed by the removal of sulfate, glucuronide of acetyl group, generating several electrophile possibilities. The electrophiles interact with the guanine moiety at the C-8 position and to a much less extent at the N-2 position.

AAF is carcinogenic for rat mammary tissue which unfortunately (for the proposed mechanism) does not appear to contain any sulfotransferase. King, et al (1979) have proposed an additional mechanism of activation utilizing the catalytic activity of a N-O-acyltransferase, which is present in mammary tissue. This enzyme transfers the N-acetyl moiety of N-hydroxyarylamides to the oxygen of the N-hydroxy group forming an N-O-acyl derivative which is very reactive and which loses the O-acyl group, yielding an electrophile.

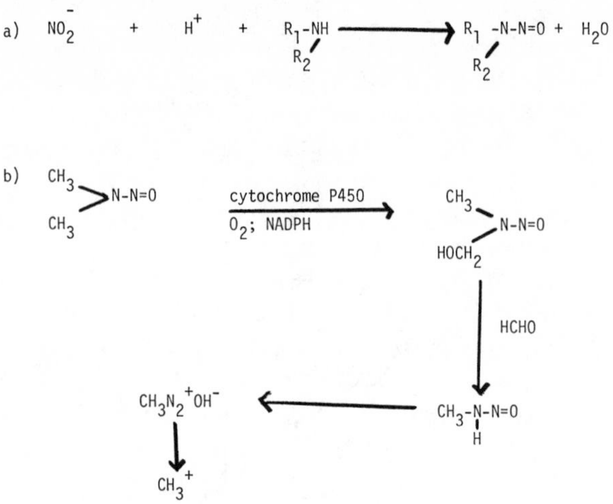

a) $NO_2^- + H^+ + R_1-NH \longrightarrow R_1 -N-N=O + H_2O$
R_2 R_2

b)
$$\begin{array}{c} CH_3 \\ CH_3 \end{array} > N-N=O \xrightarrow[O_2; NADPH]{cytochrome\ P450} \begin{array}{c} CH_3 \\ HOCH_2 \end{array} > N-N=O$$

$CH_3N_2^+OH^- \longleftarrow CH_3-N-N=O$
$\downarrow$ H
CH_3^+

$\downarrow HCHO$

FIGURE 15: The Nitrosation Reaction and Activation of Nitrosamines.

IV. Nitrite and Nitrosamine Formation

The nitrosamines are very potent carcinogens affecting a wide spectrum of species and in many cases, exhibiting considerable tissue specificity. Since many of the tumors that result from application of some of the nitrosamines are often seen in the human species, the induction of these cancers has been employed as biological models for the human disease.

The two nitrosamines can form non-enzymatically from nitrite and the appropriate amine under acid conditions (see Sander, 1972). Accordingly, the formation of the nitrosamines can occur in the stomach, their absorption may

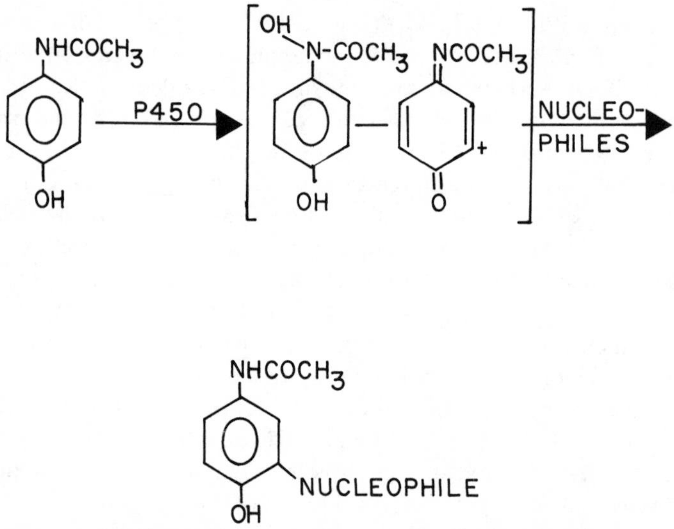

FIGURE 16: Acetaminophen Activation.

take place through the gastrointestinal tract and subsequently, they may be distributed to target tissues. The nitrosation reaction is shown in Figure 15.

The secondary amines which contribute to the nitrosation reaction, e.g., dimethylamine, are found in nature as the result of bacterial decomposition of N-containing foodstuffs. Some secondary amines are formed in the cooking process and the pyrolysis of tobacco. Nitrite may be contributed from nitrite-yielding drugs, from food additives in for example packaged meat products, or from well water. Furthermore, our own symbiotic bacterial flora generates considerable nitrite.

The metabolic activation of dimethylnitrosamine formed from the nitrosation of dimethylamine is indicated in Figure 15. The monooxygenase system catalyzes the C-hydroxylation and subsequent removal of one of the methyl groups (oxidative demethylation). The monomethylnitrosamine is reacted further to ultimately yield the methyl electrophile. It is the latter which is purported to be the ultimate mutagen or carcinogen.

V. Acetaminophen

Although acetaminophen is *not* mutagenic or carcinogenic, it does result in a certain amount of toxicity which is due to some interesting mechanisms of metabolic activation. The proposed metabolic scheme by which this drug is rendered toxic is depicted in Figure 16. Other aromatic amines, e.g., benzidine, may behave in a similar metabolic manner.

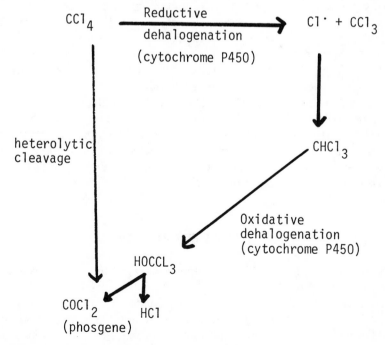

FIGURE 17: Metabolism of Carbon Tetrachloride.

VI. Halogenated Hydrocarbons

The halogenated hydrocarbons are volatile solvents that have been extensively used commercially in industrial laboratories and as anesthetics. Furthermore, these substances are formed from organic wastes under the conditions of chlorination in water purification plants and therefore, they may be present in substantial concentration in potable water, posing a peculiar health hazard. The halogenated hydrocarbons require metabolic activation generating both reactive free radicals and toxic metabolites. The metabolic scheme is exemplified in Figure 17 with carbon tetrachloride although other chlorinated hydrocarbons would be activated in a similar fashion. In this regard, it is germane to point out to the reader the idiosyncratic hepatotoxicity observed upon repeated exposures to the halogenated anesthetic, halothane, 2-bromo-2-chloro-1,1,1-trifluorethane. The latter also undergoes a reductive dehalogenation (VanDyke and Gandolfi, 1976) yielding a halogen free radical which may contribute to the toxic reaction.

F. CONCLUSIONS

In this report, we have considered some of the mechanisms by which certain xenobiotics are metabolically activated to carcinogenic, mutagenic or toxic ingredients. Such mechanisms often implicate the cytochrome P450-dependent monooxygenases but not exclusively so. Indeed, many enzymes which in the past had been considered to be components of a detoxification system are really involved in the toxicity event. For example, epoxide hydrolase, sulfotransferase, or N-acetyl transferase all played vital roles in the activation pathway for specific prodrugs. This lesson should teach us not to label reactions in a general sense but to consider the individual possibilities.

We have also discussed some of the factors which modulate the activation or inactivation mechanisms. In this regard, the often exquisite sensitivity of the fetus to a number of drugs is at least in part due to a reduction in the capacity of this organism to detoxify toxic xenobiotics. Finally, the contributions of free radical generating mechanisms and cooxygenation reactions to the generation of toxic metabolites have been briefly discussed.

ACKNOWLEDGMENTS

The author's research studies were supported by a grant from the National Cancer Institute (CA 20711).

It is a pleasure to acknowledge the assistance and the intellectual stimulation of Drs. W. Bornstein, K. Burki, A.H.L. Chuang, H. Mukhtar, and T. Stoming. In addition, Drs. Wayne Levin and Paul Thomas have proven to be super collaborators.

REFERENCES

Berry, D.L., Zachariah, P.K., Namking, M.J., and Juchau, M.R. Transplacental induction of carcinogen-hydroxylating systems with 2,3,7,8-tetrachlorodibenzo-p-dioxin. Toxicol. Appl. Pharmacol. **36**: 569–84 (1976).

Borgen, A., Darvey, H., Castagnoli, N., Crocker, T.J., Rasmussen, R.E., and Wang, I.Y. Metabolic conversion of benzo(a)pyrene by Syrian hamster liver microsomes and binding of metabolites to deoxyribonucleic acid. J. Med. Chem. **16**: 502–6 (1973).

Bresnick, E., Boraker, D., Levin, W., Hassuk, B., and Thomas, A. Intranuclear localization of hepatic cytochrome P448 by an immunochemical method. Molecular Pharmacology **16**: 324–31 (1979).

Bresnick, E., Hassuk, B., Levin, W., and Thomas, P.E. Nucleolar cytochrome P450. Molecular Pharmacology **18**: 550–2 (1980).

Bresnick, E., Stoming, T.A., Vaught, J.B., Thakker, D.R., and Jerina, D.M. Nuclear metabolites of benzo(a)pyrene and of (+ / −)-trans-7-8-dihydroxy-7-8,-dihydro-benzo(a)pyrene; Comparative chromatographic analysis of alkylated DNA. Arch. Biochem. Biophys. **183**: 31–7 (1977).

Brodie, B.B., Axelrod, J., Cooper, J.R., Gaudette, L., LaDue, B.N., Mitoma, C., and Udenfriend, S. Detoxification of Drugs and Other Foreign Compounds by Liver Microsomes. Science **121**: 603–4 (1955).

Burki, K., Liebelt, A.G., and Bresnick, E. Expression of aryl hydrocarbon hydroxylase induction in mouse tissues in vivo and in organ culture. Arch. Biochem. Biophys. **158**:641–9 (1973a).

Burki, K., Liebelt, A.G., and Bresnick, E. Induction of aryl hydrocarbon hydroxylase in mouse tissues from a high and low cancer strain and their F1 hybrids. J. Natl. Cancer Inst. **50**: 369–80 (1973b).

Conney, A.H., Gillette, J.R., Inscoe, J.K., Trams, E.R., and Posner, H.S. Induced Synthesis of Liver Microsomal Enzymes Which Metabolize Foreign Compounds. Science **130**: 1478–9 (1959).

Conney, A.H., Miller, E.C., and Miller, J.A. The Metabolism of Methylated Aminoazo Dyes V. Evidence for Induction of Enzyme Synthesis in the Rat by 3-Methylcholanthrene. Cancer Res. **16**: 450–9 (1956).

Conney, A.H. Pharmacological implications of microsomal enzyme induction. Pharmacol Rev. **19**: 317–66 (1967).

Elshourbagy, N.A., and Guzelian, P.S. Separation, purification, and characterization of a novel form of hepatic cytochrome P-450 from rats treated with pregnenolone-16 alpha-carbonitrile. J. Biol. Chem. **255**: 1279–85 (1980).

Fouts, J.R., and Adamson, R.H. Drug Metabolism in the Newborn Rabbit. Science **129**: 897–8 (1959).

Gander, J.E., and Mannering, G.J. Kinetics of hepatic cytochrome P-450-dependent mono-oxygenases systems. Pharmacol. Therap. **10**: 191–221 (1980).

Hayaishi, O., Katgiri, M., and Rothberg, S. Mechanism of the Pyrocatechase Reaction. J. Am. Chem. Soc. **77**: 5450–51 (1955).

Hayaishi, O. in *Oxygenases* Ed. O. Hayaishi. Academic Press, NY, pp. 1–29 (1962).

Henderson, P.T. Metabolism of drugs in rat liver during the perinatal period. Biochem. Pharmacol. **20**: 1225–32 (1971).

Jakoby, W.B., and Habig, W.H. Glutathione Transferases, Enzymatic Basis of Detoxification. **2**: 63–94 (1980).

Jakoby, W.B., Sekura, R.D., Lyon, E.S., Marcus, C.J., and Wang, J.L. Sulfotransferases, Enzymatic Basis of Detoxification. **2**: 199–228 (1980).

Jerina, D.M., and Daly, J.W. Oxidation of Carbon, in Drug Metabolism, Eds. D.V. Parke and R.L. Smith, Taylor and Francis Ltd., London, 15–33 (1977).

King, C.M., Traub, N.R., Lortz, Z.M., and Thissen, M.R. Metabolic activation of arylhydroxamic acids by N-O-acyltransferase of rat mammary gland. Cancer Res. **39**: 3369–71 (1979).

Klingenberg, M. Pigments of Rat Liver Microsomes. Arch. Biochem. Biophys. **75**: 376 (1958).

Lorentzen, R.J., Caspary, W.J., Lesko, S.A., and Ts'o, P.O. The autoxidation of 6-hydroxybenzo(a)pyrene and 6-oxobenzo(a)-pyrene radical, reactive metabolites of benzo(a)pyrene. Biochemistry **14**: 3970–77 (1975).

Lu, A.Y.H., and West, S.B. Multiplicity of Mammalian Microsomal Cytochromes P-450. Pharmacol. Rev. **31**: 277–95 (1979).

Lu, A.Y.H. Multiplicity of Liver Drug Metabolizing Enzymes. Drug Metabolism Rev. **10**: 187–208 (1978).

Lucier, G.W., and McDaniel, O.S. Steroid and non-steroid UDP glucuronyltransferase: glucuronidation of synthetic estrogens as steroids. J. Ster. Biochem. **8**: 867–72 (1977).

Lucier, G.W., Sonawane, B.R., McDaniel, O.S., and Hook, G.E.R. Postnatal stimulation of hepatic microsomal enzymes following administration of TCDD to pregnant rats. Chem.-Biol. Interactions **11**: 15–26 (1975).

Lucier, G.W. Perinatal development of conjugative enzyme systems. Environ. Health Perspect. **18**: 25–34 (1976).

Mannering, G.J. Hepatic Cytochrome P-450-Linked Drug-Metabolizing Systems, in Concepts in Drug Metabolism, part B, Eds. P. Jenner and B. Testa. Mercel Dekker, NY 53–166 (in press).

Marnett, L.J., and Reed, G.A. Peroxidatic oxidation of benzo(a)pyrene and prostaglandin biosynthesis. Biochemistry **18**: 2923–29 (1979).

Marnett, L.J., Reed, J.A., and Dennison, D.J. Prostaglandin synthetase dependent activation of 7,8-dihydro-7,8-dihydroxy-geno (a) pyrene to mutagenic derivatives. Biochem. Biophys. Res. Communs. **82**: 210–16 (1978).

Mason, H.S., Fowlks, W.L., and Peterson, E. Oxygen Transfer and Electron Transport by the Phenolase Complex. J. Am. Chem. Soc. **77**: 2914–15 (1955).

Mason, H.S. Mechanisms of Oxygen Metabolism. Science **25**: 1185–88 (1957).

Miller, J.A., and Miller, E.C. The metabolic activation of carcinogenic aromatic amines and amides. Prog. Exp. Tumor Res. **11**: 273–301 (1969).

Mueller, G.C., and Miller, J.A. The Reductive Cleavage of 4-Dimethyl-aminoazobenzene by Rat Liver: The Intracellular Distribution of the Enzyme System and its Requirement for Triphosphopyridine Nucleotide. J. Biol. Chem. **180**: 1125–26 (1949).

Mueller, G.C., and Miller, J.A. The Metabolism of Methylated Aminoazo Dyes. J. Biol. Chem. **202**: 579–87 (1953).

Mikhtar, H., and Bresnick, E. Glutathione-S-epoxide transferase activity during development and the effect of partial hepatectomy. Cancer Res. **36**: 937–40 (1976).

Nunnick, J.C., Chuang, A.H.L., and Bresnick, E. The Ontogeny of Nuclear Aryl Hydrocarbon Hydroxylase. Chem.-Biol. Interactions **22**: 225–30 (1978).

Oesch, F. Mammalian epoxide hydrases: inducible enzymes catalysing the inactivation of carcinogenic and cytotoxic metabolites derived from aromatic and olefinic compounds. Xenobiotica **3**: 305–40 (1973).

Omura, T., and Sato, R. A new cytochrome in liver microsomes. J. Biol. Chem. **237**: 1375-6 (1962).

Pelkonen, O., Arvela, P., and Karki, N.T. 3,4-Benzpyrene and N-methyl-aniline and metabolizing enzyme in the immature human foetus and placenta. Acta Pharmacol. Toxicol. **30**: 385–95 (1971).

Purchase, I.F.H., and Steyn, M. The metabolism of aflatoxin B_1 in rats. Brit. J. Cancer **23**: 800–5 (1969).

Richardson, H.L., and Cunningham, L. The Inhibitory Action of Methylcholanthrene on Rats Fed the Azo Dye 3'-Methyl-4-Dimethyl-Aminoazo-benzene. Cancer Res. **11**: 274 (1951).

Ryan, D.E., Lu, A.Y.H., Korzeniowski, D., and Levin, W. Separation and characterization of highly purified forms of liver microsomal cytochrome P-450 from rats treated with polychlorinated biphenyls, phenobarbital, and 3-methylcholanthrene. J. Biol. Chem. **254**: 1365–74 (1979).

Sander, J. Formation of Carcinogenic Compounds Under Biological Conditions, in Environment and Cancer. The University of Texas at Houston, M.D. Anderson Hospital and Tumor Inst. Williams and Wilkins Co. 109–117 (1972).

Sims, P., Grover, P.L., Swaisland, A., Pal, K., and Hewer, A. Metabolic activation of benzo(a)pyrene proceeds by a diol-epoxide. Nature **252**: 326–8 (1974).

Sivarajah, K., Anderson, M.W., and Eling, T. Metabolism of benzo(a)pyrene to reactive intermediate(s) via prostaglandin biosynthesis. Life Sci. **23**: 2571–8 (1978).

Sonowane, B.R., and Lucier, G.W. Hepatic and extrahepatic N-acetyl-transferase. Perinatal development using a new radioassay. Biochem. Biophys. Aca. **411**: 97–105 (1975).

Stoming T.A., and Bresnick, E. Hepatic epoxide hydrase in neonatal and partially hepatectomized rats. Cancer Res. **34**: 2810–13 (1974).

Sutton, G.J., and Burchell, B. Newer Aspects of Glucuronidation, in Progress in Drug Metabolism. **2**: 1–70. Eds. J.W. Bridges and L.F. Chasseaud. Wiley, London (1977).

Swenson, D.H., Miller, J.A., and Miller, E.C. 2,2-Dihydro-2,3-dihydroxy-aflatoxin B_1: an acid hydrolysis product of an RNA-aflatoxin B_1 adduct formed by hamster and rat liver microsomes in vitro. Biochem. Biophys. Res. Commons. **53**: 1260–7 (1973).

Thakker, D.R., Yagi, H., Lu, A.Y.H., Levin, W., Conney, A.H., and Jerina, D.M. Metabolism of benzo(a)pyrene: conversion of $(+ \ / \ -)$-trans-7,8-dihydroxy-7,8-dihydrobenzo(a)pyrene to highly mutagenic 7,8-diol-9,10-epoxides. Proc. Natl. Acad. Sci. **73**: 3381–5 (1976).

Thakker, D.R., Yagi, H., Akagi, H., Koreeda, M., Lu, A.Y.H, Levin, W., Wood, A.W., Conney, A.H., and Jerina, D.M. Metabolism of benzo(a)pyrene, VI, Stereoselective metabolism of benzo(a)pyrene and benzo(a)pyrene 7,8-dihydrodiol to diol epoxides. Chem.-Biol. Interactions **16**: 281–300 (1977).

Thomas, P.E., Korzeniowski, D., Bresnick, E., Bornstein, W.A., Kasper, C.B., Fahl, W.E., Jefcoate, C.R., and Levin, W. Hepatic cytochrome P-448 and epoxide hydrase: enzymes of nuclear origin are immunochemically identical with those of microsomal origin. Arch. Biochem. Biophys. **192**: 22–26 (1979).

VanDyke, R.A., and Gandolfi, A.J. Anaerobic Release of Fluoride from Halothane, Relationship to the Binding of Halothene Metabolites to Hepatic Cellular Constituents. Drug Metabl. Dispos. **4**: 40–44 (1976).

Yang, S.K., McCourt, D.W., Roller, P.P., and Gelboin, H.V. Enzymatic conversion of benzo(a)pyrene leading predominantly to the diol-epoxide r-7,t-8-dihydroxy-t-9,10-oxy-7,8,9,10-tetrahydrobenzo(a)pyrene through a single enantiomer of r-7,t-8-dihydroxy-7,8-dihydrobenzo(a)pyrene. Proc. Natl. Acad. Sci. **73**: 2594–8 (1976).

Ziegler, D.M. Microsomal Flavin-Containing Monooxygenases: Oxygenation of Nucleophilic Nitrogen and Sulfur Compounds, Enzymatic Basis of Detoxication. **1**: 201–27 (1980).

CHAPTER V

MEASUREMENTS OF CHEMICAL INTERACTIONS WITH DNA

Matthews O. Bradley,[1] **Joseph F. Sina**[1]
Leonard C. Erickson[2]
[1]*Merck Institute for Therapeutic Research,*
West Point, PA 19486
[2]*Laboratory of Molecular Pharmacology,*
National Cancer Institute, National Institutes of Health,
Bethesda, MD 20205

A. INTRODUCTION

One of the major canons of modern biology is that the genotype of a cell resides in its DNA and that the sequence and regulation of this DNA determines a cell's phenotype within a particular environment. Malignant cells certainly vary from normal ones in some aspect of their phenotype, and therefore, in some aspect of their DNA. This reasoning leads one to consider DNA as a most critical target for chemical and physical carcinogens.

We have known for years that many mutagens and carcinogens damage DNA either directly by covalent binding or indirectly by intercalation, by chromosomal protein binding, or by alterations in DNA precursors. The somatic mutation model for carcinogenesis (reviewed in Chapter 2) states that the mutation of one or more genes is necessary for the initiation of malignant change within a cell. The accumulating evidence that many carcinogens are mutagens lends a great deal of support to this model. Nevertheless, we should keep in mind that other events besides mutation occur after a chemical reacts with DNA and that these may be critical for carcinogenesis. For instance, the critical events induced by chemicals may be equivalent to the sort of differential gene expression that occurs during embryonic development and may not depend on structural gene mutations at all. These theories are often called epigenetic, to distinguish them from mutagenic theories. No matter what DNA mediated event is found to be critical, alterations in gene number, mutation, structure, sequence, expression, or function will undoubtedly form the basis for understanding chemical carcinogenesis and the cancer phenotype.

This review will concentrate on 1) methods for measuring the interaction of chemicals with DNA, 2) the types of modification made by chemicals in DNA, and 3) the biological consequences of such modifications.

B. TYPES OF INTERACTIONS WITH DNA

I. Covalent Binding of Adducts to DNA

1. General:

Carcinogenic compounds often bind to cellular protein and nucleic acids. Such covalent binding interferes with the biochemical and biological integrity of the cell. However, most work has focused on DNA because it transfers genetic information from one cell generation to the next. The binding of either large or small adducts to DNA can produce distortions of the molecule that result in base mispairing during DNA synthesis, strand breakage, loss of bases, and errors of repair. Any of these lesions may lead to cytotoxicity, mutagenesis, or carcinogenesis.

Miller, et al (1966, 1971) showed that esters of aromatic animes and amides react non-enzymatically with nucleic acids and hypothesized that many ultimate carcinogens are electrophiles capable of interacting covalently with DNA through Sn1 and Sn2 reactions. The Sn1 reactions involve the relatively slow ionization of a compound to form a carbonium ion (CH_3^+), then an almost immediate interaction with a nucleophile. The Sn2 reaction occurs in one-step where the nucleophile and compound combine to form an unstable complex which breaks down, leaving a chemical group bound to the nucleophile. If the xenobiotic-DNA interaction persists for a long enough time, the chemical is no longer required for the continuation of the carcinogenic or mutagenic process (Miller and Miller, 1971). This finding suggests that the lesion(s) induced in DNA by covalently bound adducts initiate both mutagenesis and carcinogenesis.

Though most carcinogens can interact with DNA, chemical reactivity is not always a good measure of biological activity. Dipple *et al.* (1981) found that alkylating agents of intermediate reactivity were most likely to form tumors in rats. They postulated that some compounds react so quickly in solution and others react so slowly that in neither case is DNA damaged.

Studies with isolated DNA have shown that every nucleoside is a potential site for covalent binding of xenobiotics (Singer, 1975). The site of alkylation *in situ*, however, is quite variable. Some adducts of guanine and adenine are unstable and not detectable under physiological conditions, while uracil and thymine are only significantly alkylated by some agents. In addition, the site of covalent interaction determines the ultimate biological effect. Alkylation of cytosine, adenine, and guanine amino groups has little effect on base pairing, while alkylation of base oxygens and ring nitrogens causes extensive base mispairing (Singer and Kroger, 1979). Specificity in the binding of adducts to DNA may also determine the biological effect. For instance, Winkle and Krugh

(1981) have demonstrated that N-hydroxy-AAF and 4-nitroquinoline oxide, two potent carcinogens, have relatively few binding sites on phage DNA. In addition, the sites seem to overlap and cluster, which may be comparable to mutational hot spots in bacteria (Coulondre and Miller, 1977). On the other hand, Slor *et al.* (1981) have observed by immunochemical methods that benzo(a)pyrene diol-epoxide 1 binds randomly to purified Col El DNA. Further study of the random and non-random binding of other carcinogens to DNA is of great importance.

In the sections to follow, we will describe in detail the mechanism of covalent interaction and the potential biological consequences of DNA binding by two representative classes of compounds—alkylating agents and polycyclic aromatic hydrocarbons. For specific details on other classes of xenobiotics see the following reviews: Irving, 1973 and Kriek and Westra, 1979.

2. Alkylating Agents:

Alkylating agents generally interact with DNA to form a relatively small DNA adduct, a bound alkyl group. While many DNA sites may be alkylated, some occur more often and cause greater cell damage. Substitutions at the N-1 position of adenosine, N-7 and O^6 of guanosine, N-3, O^2, O^4 of uridine, and N-3 and O^2 of cytidine give rise to mutagenic lesions (Singer and Kroger, 1979). Depurination occurs rapidly at 7-alkyl guanosine and 3-alkyladenosine; this may result in breaks in the DNA backbone (Singer, 1975). Phosphotriester adducts may also result in DNA strand breaks (Singer, 1975).

Although some studies have shown that the extent of DNA binding by alkylating agents correlates well with tumor initiating ability (Colburn and Boutwell, 1968), other studies suggest that the site of alkylation is of more importance (Frei and Lawley, 1975; Lawley, 1980; and Margison and O'Connor, 1979). For example, early studies showed that the N7 position of guanine was a major site of DNA alkylation (Brookes and Lawley, 1961; Magee and Farber, 1962; Montesano, 1980; Roberts, 1980) by mono- and difunctional alkylating agents such as MMS, EMS, DMN, ENU, and mustard compounds. But these studies did not find a consistent correlation between N7 alkylation and biological effect (Lawley, 1976a,b; Margison and O'Connor, 1979). The amount of N7 binding is equal with both weak and strong alkylating agents (Pegg and Nicoll, 1976). The adduct does not stimulate DNA repair (Kirtikar and Goldthwart, 1974; Margison and O'Connor, 1979). Additionally, N7 alkyl guanine did not cause mutations in bacteria nor base mispairing in DNA *in vitro* (Lawley, 1976a; Loveless, 1969; Pegg and Nicoll, 1976). The extent of N7 alkylation, however, is a useful quantitative estimate of the initial amount of DNA binding and can be used as an internal standard against which the quantity and persistence of other DNA alkylations can be measured.

Loveless (1969) found that methylnitrosourea reacted with deoxyguanosine to form an 06-methylated derivative and suggested that this lesion had more biological significance than the N-7 lesion. Subsequent studies led to the conclusion that the more potent carcinogenic alkylating agents extensively modified most of the oxygen atoms of nucleic acids (Margison and O'Connor, 1979; Roberts, 1980; Singer, 1976). Alkylation of guanine at the 06 position causes GC → AT transition mutations (Coulondre and Miller, 1977; Lawley, 1980), presumably because the adduct interferes with hydrogen bonding between bases (Deutsch et al., 1981). 06-Methylguanine may also cause most mutations induced by methylating agents in mammalian cells (Newbold, et al., 1980). Furthermore, Frei *et al.* (1978) demonstrated that the extent of 06-alkylation of guanine correlated well with thymoma formation in mice.

What are the biological consequences of the covalent binding of alkyl groups to cellular DNA? Depending upon the site of alkylation, these consequences include cytotoxicity, mutagenicity, and carcinogenicity. For instance, alkylation decreases the stability of the N-glycosidic bond in DNA leading to depurination (Margison and O'Connor, 1979; O'Connor, 1981) and subsequent DNA strand breakage (Kuebler and Goldthwart, 1977; Ljungquist and Lindahl, 1974). If these breaks are not repaired they may be lethal (Margison and O'Connor, 1979). In addition, the alkylation lesion may interfere with new DNA synthesis preventing cell replication. Some lesions (06-methylguanine, and 03-methyladenine, but not N7-methylguanine) are enzymatically removed from the DNA of *E. coli* (Kirtikar and Goldthwart, 1974) and higher organisms (Pegg, 1978). In the case of alkylated *E. coli* DNA, this enzyme activity results in double strand breaks in DNA (Kirtikar and Goldthwart, 1974), which may be lethal. And, as discussed above, the 06-alkylation of guanine may be mutagenic (Lawley, 1980; Newbold et al., 1980) and carcinogenic (Frei et al., 1978). In fact, it has been estimated (Lawley, 1980) that one alkylation/10^6 DNA bases can result in tumors.

However, the level of 06-alkylation of guanine does not always correlate well with the *site* of tumor occurrence (O'Connor, 1981; Pegg and Nicoll, 1976). For instance, after rats are exposed to ethylnitrosourea, 06-alkylation is found to the same extent in DNA from liver and brain tissues, while tumors are found only in the brain (Goth and Rajewsky, 1974). The removal of the lesion in brain, however, is significantly slower (T1/2 = 220 hr) than in liver (T1/2 = 30 hr), implying that the persistence of the lesion may be more important for tumorigenicity. Other studies (Jerino et al. 1977; and Nicoll et al., 1975) have also found a slower repair of alkylation damage in target tissues than in non-target tissues. But, some recent work does not support this conclusion (Buecheler and Kleihues, 1977; Nicoll et al., 1977; Margison et al., 1977; Rogers and Pegg, 1977). Thus, other unknown factors besides the type and persistence of DNA binding may play a role in tumorigenicity induced by alkylating agents.

3. Polycyclic Aromatic Hydrocarbons:

Polycyclic aromatic hydrocarbons, in contrast to direct-acting alkylating agents, need to be metabolically activated to a form which binds to DNA (Archer and Eng, 1981). The overall binding of the hydrocarbon, however, does not always correlate well with carcinogenicity. The quantitative binding of methylcholanthrene, benzo(a)pyrene, and dimethylbenzanthracene to the DNA of mouse skin, for example, does not show a good correlation with species variations in susceptibility to tumorigenesis (Phillips *et al.*, 1978). The non-carcinogen dibenz(a,c)anthracene and the carcinogen dibenz(a,h)anthracene react equally well with DNA (Kuroki and Heidelberger, 1971) and the non-carcinogenic K-region phenol of dibenz(a,h)anthracene is more reactive than the carcinogenic K-region epoxide (Kuroki et al., 1971). Nonetheless, the fact that most carcinogens do bind to DNA (Miller and Miller, 1971) suggests that we simply have not determined the *specific* binding product of importance.

Recent evidence indicates that the ultimate reactive intermediates of hydrocarbons are the bay-region diol epoxides (Jerina et al., 1977). For instance, bay-region diol epoxides of hexacyclic hydrocarbons have been shown to be mutagenic (Wood et al., 1981). And for the carcinogen benzo(a)pyrene, 7,8-dihydroxy-9,10-epoxy benzapyrene, a bay-region diol epoxide appears to be the biologically active form (Buening et al., 1978; Cooper et al., 1980; Newbold and Brookes, 1976; Sims et al., 1974). Other forms may also be important. For instance, MacNicoll *et al.* (1979) have shown that non-bay region diol epoxides may be involved in benz(a)anthracene binding to DNA.

The nature of the diol epoxide-DNA interaction is also controversial. The site of critical adduct formation by the diol epoxides in DNA may be the N-2 position of guanine (Ivanovic et al., 1978). But DiGiovanni *et al.* (1979) have found a better correlation between mouse skin tumorigenicity and benz(a)pyrene binding to adenine than to guanine. Frenkel *et al.* (1978) have suggested that once the benzpyrene diol epoxide covalently binds to guanine, the complex rotates into the DNA helix, forming a stacking-type intercalation with the neighboring bases. However, recent work (Geacintov et al., 1981) suggests that the initial diol epoxide-DNA interaction is originally a non-covalent intercalation which then rearranges to form a covalently bound adduct.

What are the physical consequences of adduct formation and their biological significance? In contrast to the alkylating agents, which generally induce a base mispairing lesion, hydrocarbons produce bulky lesions which physically distort the DNA. Structural studies (Jerina *et al.*, 1977) indicate that when the benzpyrene diol epoxide adduct is formed at the N-2 position of guanine, the DNA helix is bent and several base pairs are unwound. It has been suggested (Deutsch et al., 1981) that the size of hydrophobic nature of this adduct blocks the polymerases from synthesizing DNA (Moore and Strauss, 1979). It has also been shown (Gamper et al., 1980) that 1 percent of the benzpyrene diol epoxide adduct sites in DNA cleave at neutral pH, possibly through a depurination or depyrmidination mechanism. Thus, the bulky hydrocarbon lesions appear to physically inhibit base pairing and chain elongation, which inhibits DNA synthesis, repair, and transcription (Deutsch et al., 1981; Moore and Strauss, 1979). Bulky lesions usually cause frameshift mutations in bacteria (Grunberger and Weinstein, 1979), while the smaller alkylation lesions predominantly cause miscoding mutations. However, both lesions are carcinogenic suggesting that whatever change in DNA is critical to carcinogenisis is made by both types of lesions.

II. Non-Covalent Interactions of Chemicals with DNA

1. Intercalation:

Although most current work focuses on the covalent binding of carcinogens and mutagens to DNA, we should not overlook the potential importance to mutagenesis and carcinogenisis of non-covalent chemical interaction. The clearest example of such interaction is the intercalation of planar molecules such as acridines and phenanthridines between the base pairs of DNA that cause the helix to uncoil because the sugar-phosphate chain is extended in normal B-form DNA (Waring, 1970 and 1981). The easiest way to measure intercalation is by the decrease in supercoiling of the closed circular DNA of phage ϕX174. Since supercoiled circles are more compact than open circles, they sediment more rapidly. Measurements with ϕX174 have shown that a number of mutagens and carcinogens intercalate into DNA including actinomycin D, adriamycin, and the acridines proflavin, ethidium bromide, duanomycin, and propidium (Waring, 1970). No one knows whether the structural alterations in DNA caused by intercalators lead directly to genotoxic changes or whether other alterations occur. There are, however, certain hints. Sirover and Loeb (1980) have shown that intercalators such as adriamycin and duanomycin, as well as several steroids, all decrease the fidelity of *in vitro* DNA synthesis. Their assay measures the frequency with which [^{3}H]dGTP is incorporated into a polynucleotide synthesized *in vitro* by avian myeloblastosis virus DNA polymerase from a template of poly [d(A–T)]. The fact that non-covalent interactions of the sort made by the intercalators and steroids decreases the fidelity of DNA synthesis suggests that base-pair substitution mutations, and perhaps malignant transformation, could result by this mechanism.

Intercalators form other sorts of DNA alterations that may be related to their genotoxic potential. For instance, Ross and Bradley (1981) have shown that adriamycin, ellipticine, and actinomycin D make both DNA single and double strand breaks in L1210 cells. Previous work (Ross *et al.*, 1979) had shown that the single strand breaks are associated with protein. Double strand breaks are repaired in mammalian cells (Bradley and Kohn, 1979), but if unrepaired (Bradley and Taylor, 1981), they might be potent genotoxic lesions.

2. Precursor pool imbalances:

Hydroxyurea kills cells primarily by inactivating ribonucleotide reductase which is required for the reduction of ribonucleotides to deoxyribonucleotides. The pools of these DNA precursors fall to levels low enough to cause cytotoxic but non-mutagenic DNA damage during DNA synthesis (Bradley and Sharkey, 1978). High exogenous levels of thymidine ($>$ 1 mm) also kill actively proliferating cells, but, unlike hydroxyurea, produce large numbers of mutations at the hypoxanthine-guanine phosphoribosyl transferase locus (Bradley and Sharkey, 1978).

3. DNA breakdown associated with cell death:

Little is known about the events that accompany cell death. A few reports have indicated that DNA breakdown may occur during cell autolysis by treatments such as hypotonic shock that do not damage DNA directly (Williams, 1974). Presumably, lysosomal DNA hydrolases are released in dying cells and digest the cells' DNA (Allison, 1969), although little is known about the overall process.

We have recently begun to study the relationship between non-DNA based toxicity and DNA damage. In one study we have found that some carcinogens make DNA single strand breaks (SSBs) in rat hepatocytes only at toxic doses. Without toxicity the compounds induce no DNA SSBs (Sina *et al.*, 1983). If DNA is a necessary target for carcinogens, then some of these compounds may be carcinogenic because of lysosome-based DNA hydrolases rather than because of direct attack on DNA by the compounds or their metabolites.

Dead cells cannot become malignant, so one necessary condition for a lysosomal hydrolase or other nuclease model of malignancy is that the enzymes are released before the cell is irretrievably dead. The model demands that a certain fraction of cells could repair toxic damage and survive even though nucleases have begun to digest the DNA. We have recently shown that hypotonic shock produces DNA SSBs in mouse L1210 cells and that these breaks are repaired if the cells are returned to isotonicity (Bradley, 1982, unpublished). Perhaps this rejoining process is error-prone and leads to mutation or transformation.

C. MEASUREMENTS OF CHEMICAL INTERACTION WITH DNA

This section is divided into indirect and direct methods for measuring chemical interactions with DNA. The indirect methods include neutral and alkaline sucrose gradient sedimentation, neutral and alkaline filter elution, alkaline unwinding as measured by S-1 nuclease, viscoelastometry, and nucleoid sedimentation. These techniques provide sensitive measurements of chemical attack on DNA that result in single strand breaks, double strand breaks, DNA-DNA crosslinks, DNA-protein crosslinks, single stranded regions in DNA, and excision repair.

The direct methods measure the covalent binding of chemical adducts to DNA at specific sites. The methods involve hydrolyzing the DNA, separating the products, and then identifying them by some chemical method such as thin layer chromatography, high pressure liquid chromatography, fluorescence spectroscopy, nuclear magnetic resonance, or mass spectroscopy. A new approach utilizes modified radioimmunoassays to measure specific DNA adducts down to pico- and femtomole sensitivity.

I. Indirect Methods for Measurement of Chemical Interaction with DNA

1. Alkaline Filter Elution:

Kohn and Ewig (1973) first described the alkaline elution techique in 1973. Since then the methodology and sensitivity of the technique have improved dramatically, and it now detects a varity of DNA lesions including DNA single strand breaks (SSB), DNA-protein crosslinks (DNP), DNA interstrand crosslinks (ISC), and alkali labile sites (ALS). In the alkaline procedure, cells are deposited on a membrane filter using mild suction, and lysed with a detergent solution. Virtually all of the cellular components are washed through the filter with only the DNA being retained. Following lysis an optional deproteinizing step can be included, depending upon the lesion being studied. A denaturing solvent, usually tetrapropylammonium hydroxide and 0.02 M EDTA at pH 12.1, is then pumped through a filter at approximately 2 ml/hr. Elution of DNA from the filter is a function of the molecular weight of the DNA with low molecular weight DNA eluting early, and higher molecular weight DNA eluting later. Fractions are collected and processed for either liquid scintillation counting or fluorometric measurements of the amount of DNA. A number of alkaline elution studies have shown that many known carcinogens produce DNA damage in cells exposed to these agents. Table I lists selected references showing the lesions and suspected genotoxic agents studied by alkaline elution.

In addition to these studies, Sina et al. (1983) have recently developed a technique for routinely screening large numbers of compounds for their ability to induce DNA SSBs in freshly isolated rat hepatocytes without radioactively labeling the cells. Cell viability was also simultaneously determined. Three people working half time were able to screen 91 compounds in 10 weeks with an overall accuracy of about 90 percent. These results are summarized in Table II.

2. Neutral Filter Elution:

Bradley and Kohn (1979) described a neutral filter elution method for measuring DNA double strand breaks in mammalian cells after X-ray. The method differs from alkaline elution in that it uses polycarbonate filters that do not adsorb protein and DNA-associated protein must be stringently removed by 2 percent sodium dodecyl sulfate and proteinase K. Otherwise, DNA associated protein slows the elution of double stranded DNA. The assay is done at pH values between 7.0 and 10.0 which do not denature DNA. Table I lists the agents that have been studied by neutral elution.

3. Alkaline Sucrose Sedimentation:

Comprehensive reviews by Cleaver (1975) and Kohn (1979) should be consulted for the details and theory of alkaline sedimentation. There are probably as many variations in the technique of alkaline sedimentation as there are laboratories performing this analysis. Obvious variations include choice of rotor, rpm, length of spin, and w^2t. In addition to these variations, changes are made in sucrose concentration, the degree of alkalinity, sodium concentration, and cell lysis conditions. In some cases, cells are lysed on top of the gradient, with or without detergent, and the centrifuge started after an appropriate incubation period. An alternative method described by Dingman and Kakunaga (1976) involves lysis in a test tube, followed by deproteinization with proteinase K, and gentle layering of the DNA lysate onto the preformed sucrose gradient. Using this method we have reproducibly measured DNA breaks from X-ray doses as low as 250 Rads (Bradley *et al.*, 1976), and drug treatments producing DNA strand break frequencies in 100–200 Rad range (Erickson *et al.*, 1978). Table I lists selected references of genotoxic agents studied by alkaline sucrose sedimentation.

4. *Alkaline Unwinding of DNA:*

The alkaline unwinding method described by Rydberg (1975) was developed as an extension of the observations of Ahnstrom and Erixon (1973) that the unwinding of DNA on top of a gradient could be accelerated by irradiating the cells with 50 or more rads of X-ray. Using this observation as a basis Rydberg developed an assay in which irradiated cells are injected into denaturing solvents, and after appropriate incubation times quickly neutralized to renature non-separated DNA strands. The neutralized sample is then chromatographed on hydroxyapatite columns and the fraction of single strand and double strand DNA determined. The sensitivity of this technique is in the range of 10–20 Rads of X-irradiation and is thus comparable to the sensitivity of alkaline elution. Although alkaline unwinding has not been widely used to detect carcinogen induced DNA damage Table I lists references using this technique, or a variation of the method.

5. *Viscoelastometry:*

The technique for viscoelastometry has been used in several studies of carcinogenic agents. The apparatus consists of a rotating inner cylinder, a rotor submersed in the DNA lysate which is contained in a concentric outer cylinder. Torque is applied to the rotor using an electro-magnet. The rotor is moved through an angular displacement, the torque is removed, and the rotor turns back towards its original position. The recoil opposite the torque is produced by the stretched DNA molecules in the solution. The recoil is mathematically described as an exponential decay of the angular position of the rotor with time, and T^c, the retardation time, is a function of the molecular weight of the DNA. In addition to the effects of radiation, several other genotoxic agents have been studied with this method and are listed in Table I.

107

6. Nucleoid Sedimentation:

The sedimentation of nucleoids was first described by Cook and Brazell (1975). Nuclei, isolated from cells using non-ionic detergent, are layered over neutral sucrose gradients containing high salt (2 M NaCl). This treatment strips the histone and non-histone proteins from the DNA, and leaves a residual nuclear structure called a "nucleoid." Supercoiling of the DNA keeps the DNA within the nucleoid, but if DNA breaks are present which disrupts the supercoiling, the nucleoid expands and sediments more slowly. Thus agents which change the supercoiling of the DNA (i.e. ethidium), and agents producing DNA strand breaks, can be studied using this method (Cook and Brazell, 1976). Listed in Table I are representative references.

C. MEASUREMENTS OF CHEMICAL INTERACTION WITH DNA (Cont'd)

II. Direct Methods for Measurement of Chemical Interaction With DNA

1. Binding:

One can examine the interaction of xenobiotics with DNA at a gross level, i.e., total binding of compound, or at the molecular level, i.e., the specific reaction products formed. For total binding studies, the approach is relatively straightforward although subject to many errors. The target cells, *in vivo* or *in vitro*, are exposed to a radiolabelled compound, the DNA is extracted, and total radioactivity is measured by scintillation counting. The amount of label is expressed as a percentage of the total DNA as determined chemically.

An alternative to DNA extraction is the equilibrium dialysis method of Sun and Dent (1980). In this technique. the total covalent interaction of a radiolabelled compound with cellular macromolecules is measured after removal of unbound isotope by dialysis. The method is rapid and non-destructive, leaving a sample which can be further analyzed. One drawback to this method is that, although it appears to be somewhat more sensitive for determination of *total* binding than are assays requiring the extraction of macromolecules, the method lacks specificity because labeled compound may be bound to other macromolecules besides DNA.

Total binding assays, however, are subject to certain errors. For instance, many carcinogens also bind to RNA and protein (Miller and Miller, 1971) which often contaminate a DNA preparation. Label may be lost from the compound either spontaneously or during DNA repair. And, Baird and Brookes (1973) have found that radiolabel can be incorporated into normal DNA presumably by a non-specific release of the label from the compound and reincorporation into DNA precursors. These, and other factors would lead to over or underestimation of the total binding (see Baird, 1979 for further discussion).

The specific identification of xenobiotic-DNA reaction products is a more accurate method. The general approach is, again, to expose the target cells to a labelled compound and to isolate the DNA. The DNA is degraded to nucleosides or bases, and bound adducts are separated by some form of chromatography (see Baird, 1979 for review). In some of the early studies, alkylation of the N7 position of guanine was examined by hydrolysing the DNA in acid and by separating the products with paper chromatography or ion exchange on Dowex 50 (Brookes and Lawley, 1961; Magee and Farber, 1962). However, as the chemistry of carcinogen-nucleic acid interactions developed, it became apparent that these methods were unsatisfactory for some reaction products. Loveless (1969) found that a major alkylation product, 06-alkyguanine, was labile in acid. Lawley and Shah (1972) re-examined the separation techniques used in studying alkylating agent-nucleic acid interactions. They found that many acid-labile reaction products (06-methylguanine, N7-methylguanine) were better analyzed after enzymatic degradation. Various resins were also found more suitable for some applications than others. For example, Dowex 50 (NH_4^+ form) separated nucleosides, while other resins separated bases.

Other classes of xenobiotics required different conditions. For instance, Kriek (1968) isolated AAF-deoxynucleoside adducts by using Sephadex G-25 and eluting with urea. Later he found (Kriek, 1969) that by using Sephadex LH20, which is compatible with organic solvents, the urea could be omitted. Polycyclic aromatic hydrocarbon metabolism and binding has also been analyzed by chromatography on LH20 columns. Baird and Brookes (1973) developed a technique whereby DNA reacted with 7-methylbenz(a)anthracene was degraded by DNAse I, phosphodiesterase, and alkaline phosphatase, then applied to LH20 columns. Adducts could be eluted from the column with a water:methanol (7:3) to methanol gradient. For DNA that had been reacted with benzo(a)pyrene, a useful modification is elution with a borate-containing buffer. This technique better resolves the 2 isomers of benzpyrene-7, 8-diol-9,10-epoxide (King, et al., 1976). Usually the amount of adduct recovered from column chromatography is too small for chemical identification, so synthetic markers are run and their position is determined by UV absorption.

One limitation of chromatography is that although an LH20 column can accept a fairly large DNA sample, resolution is limited. However, this can be overcome by collecting the fractions from the column and analyzing them further by HPLC, which offers better resolution (though sample size is limited). This method has been applied, for instance, to DNA reacted with 7,12-dimethylbenzanthracene (Jeffrey, et al., 1976), benzo(a)pyrene (Baird, et al., 1981), and various alkylating agents (Frei, et al., 1978).

HPLC is probably the best tool at present for resolving reaction products of closely related structure due to its large number of theoretical plates, reproducibility, rapidity, and gradient elution capabilities (Selkirk, 1978). Further refinements such as HPLC recycling (Selkirk, 1978) add to the resolving power and utility of this technique.

One potential problem with these analyses is that the DNA must be isolated and degraded. One must, therefore, be aware that the adducts may be labile.

TABLE I
**DNA Lesions Induced by Genotoxic Agents Measured by Alkaline Elution,
Neutral Elution, Alkaline Sedimentation, Alkaline Unwinding,
Viscoelastometry, and Nucleoid Sedimentation.
Most references selected from a computer search of 1981–1976.**

Alkaline Elution

DNA Lesion Detected	Genotoxic Agent	Reference
SSB	64 carcinogens 27 non-carcinogens	Sina, et al., 1983
SSB	6-N-nitroso compounds	Brambilla, et al., 1981a
SSB	7,12-Dimethyl Benzo-(A) anthracene and Benzo-(A)-pyrene	Parodi et al., 1981c
SSB	X-irradiation, H_2O_2	Bradley and Erickson, 1981
ISC	8-methoxy psoralen	Kraemer, et al., 1981
DNP	Chromate	Fornace et al., 1981
ISC, DNP	4-sulfido-cyclophosphamide	Ramonas et al., 1981
SSB, DNP	Nickel carbonate	Ciccarelli et al., 1981
SSB	Near-U.V. light and gamma irradiation	Hirschi et al., 1981
DNP	Chromate	Tsapakos et al., 1981
SSB	16 hydrazine derivatives	Parodi et al., 1981b
SSB	Procarbazine	Brambilla et al., 1981b
SSB	Azaserine	Zurlo et al., 1981
ISC	Trimethyl psoralen	Cohen et al., 1980
SSB, DNP	Adriamycin	Levin et al., 1981
ISC, DNP	Cis-diamminedichloro-platinum II and melphalen	Zwelling et al., 1981
SSB	N-trifluoro acetyl Adriamycin 14 valerate	Brox et al., 1980a
SSB, ISC	Phosphoramide mustard and Acrolein	Erickson et al., 1980c
SSB	X-irradiation	Suzuki et al., 1980
SSB	Lithocholic acid	Kulkarni et al., 1980
SSB	X-irradiation	Fornace and Little, 1980
SSB	2-acetylaminofluorene 2-aminofluorene and N-hydroxy-2-acetylamino-fluorene	Staiano et al., 1980
SSB	Nitrite and Aminopyrine	Parodi et al., 1980
ISC	L-phenylalanine mustard	Brox et al., 1980b
ISC, DNP	Cis-diamminedichloro-platinum II	Meyn et al., 1980
SSB	2-acetylaminofluorene	Stout and Becker, 1980
SSB, ISC, DNP	Chloroethylnitrosoureas	Erickson et al., 1980a
SSB	Chloroethylnitrosoureas	Kann et al., 1980
DNP	Fluorescent Light	Gannt et al., 1979

TABLE I (Con'td).

Alkaline Elution

DNA Lesion Detected	Genotoxic Agent	Reference
SSB	X-irradiation	Bolognesi et al., 1979
SSB	Bleomycin	Sognier and Hittleman, 1979
SSB	U.V. Light	Netrawali and Cerutti, 1979
SSB, DNP	Adriamycin and Ellipticine	Ross et al., 1979
DNP	trans-diamminedichloroplatinum II	Kohn and Ewig, 1979
DNP	DMBA, N-acetylaminofluorene	Fornace and Little, 1979
SSB, DNP, ISC	trans and cis-PtII diammine dichloride; fluorescent and near U.V. light, H_2O_2	Bradley et al., 1979
SSB	Methylmethanesulfonate	Eastman and Bresneck, 1978
SSB, ISC, DNP	Haloethylnitrosoureas	Ewig and Kohn, 1978
SSB	Visible Light	Bradley et al., 1978
SSB	MeCCNU	Thomas et al., 1978
SSB	1,2 dimethyl hydrazine	Brambilla et al., 1978
SSB	Multiple carcinogens	Petzold et al., 1978
SSB	Benzo(A)pyrene diol epoxides I and II	Cerruti et al., 1978
ISC, DNP	Melphalan and nitrogen mustard	Ross et al., 1978
SSB	Multiple carcinogens	Petzold and Swenberg, 1978
DNP, SSB	X-irradiation	Fornace and Little, 1977
SSB	Multiple carcinogens	Swenberg et al., 1976
SSB	Bleomycin	Kohn and Ewig, 1976
SSB	Bleomycin	Iqbal et al., 1976
SSB, ISC	X-irradiation, nitrogen mustard	Bradley et al., 1976

Neutral Elution

DNA Lesion Detected	Genotoxic Agent	Reference
DSB, SSB	4-nitroquinoline oxide methylnitrosourea, I^{125}	Bradley, unpublished
DSB	U.V. Light	Bradley and Taylor, 1981
DSB, SSB, DNP	Adriamycin, Ellipticine, Actinomycin D	Ross and Bradley, 1981
DSB, SSB, DNP	m-AMSA	Zwelling et al., 1981
DSB	X-irradiation	Bradley and Kohn, 1979

Alkaline Sedimentation

DNA Lesion Detected	Genotoxic Agent	Reference
SSB	Ethylnitrosourea	Heyting et al., 1980
SSB	N-butyl-N3-carboxypropyl nitrosamine	Miyata et al., 1980
SSB	MNNG	Koropatnick and Stich, 1980

TABLE I (Con'td).

Alkaline Elution

DNA Lesion Detected	Genotoxic Agent	Reference
SSB	Rhodamine 6G and B	Nestmann et al., 1979
SSB	Chromate	Whiting et al., 1979
SSB	Ethyl and methyl nitrosamine	Floot et al., 1979
SSB	Dimethyl nitrosamine	Abanobi et al., 1979
SSB	Dimethyl nitrosamine Diethyl nitrosamine	Engelese & Philippus, 1978
SSB	N-Diazoacetyl glycine amide	Parodi et al., 1977
SSB	Azaserine	Lilja et al., 1977
SSB/ALS	1,3,bis-2-chloroethyl nitrosourea	Erickson et al., 1977
SSB	N-methyl nitrosourea, U.V. light	Cox and Irving, 1976
SSB	X-irradiation	Dingman & Kakunaga, 1976; Bradley et al., 1976 Erickson et al., 1978

Alkaline Unwinding

SSB	10 Anthracycline derivatives	Kantner & Swartz, 1979b
SSB	Adriamycin, duanorubicin and related compounds	Kantner & Swartz, 1979a
SSB	Gamma irradiation	Sheridan and Huang, 1977
SSB	X-irradiation	Ryberg, 1975

VISCOELEASTOMETRY
Lesion Detected

SB	X-irradiation	Shafer et al., 1981
SSB	methyl nitrosamine	Parodi et al., 1981a
SSB, ISC	BCNU, Nitrogen mustard	Shafer and Chase, 1980
SSB	X-irradiation	Chase and Shafer, 1979

NUCLEOID SEDIMENTATION

SSB	Lithocholic acid	Kulkarni et al., 1980
SSB	Ionizing radiation	Weniger, 1979
SSB	U.V. Light	Kulkarni and Yielding, 1978
SSB	Ionizing radiation	Cook and Brazell, 1976

Autrup (1979) has developed a technique whereby water-soluble BP conjugates are analyzed by HPLC without prior organic extraction, thereby giving a more reliable measurement of conjugated vs free metabolites. The problem of preserving DNA adducts during isolation has been the subject of extensive reviews and will not be further discussed here. For a discussion of conditions of DNA isolation which preserve different adducts see Irving (1973). Excellent discussions of various DNA degradation procedures have been published by Lawley (1976) and Margison and O'Connor (1979).

2. Colorimetric Methods

Other methods of analyzing DNA interactions are also available. For instance, the extent of DNA alkylation can be determined colorimetrically. 4-(p-nitrobenzyl)pyridine (PNBP) reacts with alkylating agents to yield a colored product which can be quantitated (Archer and Eng, 1981). The ability of compounds to react with PNBP is, thus, a quantitative measure of the alkylating potential of unknowns; but this technique does not measure specific types of interactions.

3. Nuclear Magnetic Resonance

NMR spectroscopy has been applied to the study of DNA methylation at various base sites (Krepinsky, et al., 1979). This technique offers the advantage that isolation of the adducts is not required. However, in this study $(^{13}C)H_3$ enriched methylating agents were required. NMR spectroscopy has also been utilized to study alkylation products without specially labelled alkylating agents (Hemminki, et al., 1980), but purified deoxyribonucleosides were required.

4. Electric Dichroism

Conformational studies of DNA adducts can also be useful. Electric linear dichroism studies have been used to determine the relative orientation of DNA adduct and base (Kadlubar, et al., 1981). This data can predict the amount of DNA distortion expected, and whether the damage is likely to be recognized by repair enzymes or persist into replication. The technique is limited to cases where the adduct of interest is relatively abundant. In addition, DNA has to be isolated and degraded.

5. X-Ray Crystallography

X-ray crystallography can also be used to show the conformation of the adduct and base, and how this will interact with the rest of the DNA. For instance, Carrell et al. (1981) showed by x-ray crystallography that N-6(12-methylbenz(a)anthracene-7-methyl) deoxyadenine is in a conformation which would distort base stacking and which would account for its ability to induce enzymatic repair. The limitation to this technique is that a crystalline base-adduct structure must be prepared.

6. Radioimmunoassays for DNA Adducts

Radioimmunoassay (RIA) has greatly increased our ability to detect small quantities of biological molecules such as hormones, drugs, protein, and micro-organisms (Wisdom, 1976; Yalow, 1978). These assays determine the concentration of an unknown, unlabelled antigen by comparing its inhibitory effect on

TABLE II

Summary of the Response of 91 Compounds Tested in the Alkaline Elution/Rat Hepatocyte Assay

Chemical Classification	Category 1 — DNA Single Strand Breaks (SSB's) < 30% Toxicity	Category 2 — No DNA SSB's < 30% Toxicity	Category 3 — DNA SSB's > 30% Toxicity	Category 4 — No DNA SSB's > 30% Toxicity
Cyanamide		Cyanamid		
Diazo	Azaserine			
Azo	Azobenzene			
Hydrazine	Hydrazine 1,2-dimethylhydrazine 1,1-dimethylhydrazine	Methylhydrazine Isoiazid (C)		
N-nitroso	MNNG Methylnitrosourea 1-nitrosopiperidine Diphenylnitrosamine Dimethylnitrosamine	Piperidine		
Carbamyl, thiocarbayml	Thiourea	Acetamide (C) Urea	Thioacetamide	
Aromatic amine	2-AAF Auramine 4-aminobiphenyl 2-aminonaphthalene 2-aminoanthracene 2-aminofluorene	2,4-diaminotoluene (C)	2-aminobiphenyl 1-aminonaphthalene	Tetramethyl benzidine
Nitroaromatic	Metronidazole 4-nitrobiphenyl		2-nitrobiphenyl (NC) 2,4-dinitrotoluene	

114

Category			
Phenyl	4-nitroquinoline oxide 2,3-dinitrotoluene 2,6-dinitrotoluene 3,4-dinitrotoluene	Benzene Phenobarbital	
Benzodioxole	Aroclor 1254		Safrole
Substituted diphenylethane		p,p'-DDT	p,p'-DDE
Stilbenediol	DES		
Polycyclic Aromatic	7,12-DMBA 3-methylcholanthrene B(a)P	B(e)P Pyrene	Anthracene
Oxirane, thiirane	Propylene oxide Epichlorhydrin		
Dioxane			1,4-dioxane
Anhydride		Succinic anhydride (C)	
Heteroaromatic	Quinoline Actinomycin D Aflatoxin B_1		
Halomethane, haloethane	1,2-dibromoethane Nitrogen mustard		CCl_4
Chloroethylene	Lindane Aldrin		
Sulfate, Sulfonate sultone	Dimethyl sulfate MMS EMS		
Sulfanilamide Phosphate	Sulfanilamide Trimethylphosphate		

TABLE II (Cont'd).

Chemical Classification	DNA Single Strand Breaks (SSB's) Category 1 < 30% Toxicity	Category 2 No DNA SSB's < 30% Toxicity	Category 3 DNA SSB's > 30% Toxicity	Category 4 No DNA SSB's > 30% Toxicity
Steroid	Testosterone propionate	Estradiol		
Inorganic	Na dichromate cadmium sulfate	Arsenic pentoxide	Nickel sulfide Cupric sulfate (NC) Phenanthrene (NC)	
Miscellaneous	Styrene oxide Saccharin Mitomycin C Adriamycin	Chloroform (C) 1% ethanol 1% acetone 1% DMSO Acetaldehyde TPA	Styrene Toluene Urethane	Naphthalene Fluorene
Total Number of Compounds	51	21	16	3
Carcinogenic Activity	All compounds carcinogenic	16 non-carcinogens 5 carcinogens	4 non-carcinogens 12 carcinogens	3 non-carcinogens

Legend to Table II: DNA single strand break induction was considered significant when the elution slope was 3 times greater than the control elution slope. Cytotoxicity was measured by trypan blue exclusion or release of glutamate-axaloacetate transaminase activity into the medium. Cytotoxicity greater than 30% was considered biologically significant.

C — reported to be carcinogenic

NC — Non-carcinogenic

the binding of a known radioactively labelled antigen to a specific antibody (against the antigen) with the inhibitory effect of known standards. Recent studies have used RIA to measure DNA adducts formed by benzo(a)pyrene (Poirier, et al., 1980) and N-acetoxy-acetylaminofluorene (N-Ac-AAF) (Poirier, et al., 1977).

The sensitivity of RIA is generally high but is limited by the specific activity of the isotopes. In practice, this has meant a detection level in the picomole range for DNA adducts. Two recent methodological developments have increased the limits of sensitivity beyond that of standard RIA: the first is ELISA, enzyme-linked immunosorbent assay (Yolken, et al., 1978), and the second is USERIA, ultrasensitive enzymatic radioimmunoassay (Harris, et al., 1979). Both methods are similar to solid-phase RIA except they do not use gamma emitting isotopes. Because a single enzyme molecule (bound to the antibody) reacts with a large number of substrate molecules, the final sensitivity is increased. ELISA and USERIA both use alkaline phosphatase conjugated to IgG (usually goat anti-rabbit IgG) in combination with a rabbit antibody directed against a specific DNA-carcinogen adduct. ELISA uses a para-nitrophenolphosphate as a substrate, measuring the formation of the reaction product para-nitrophenol with a spectrophotometer at 405 nm. USERIA uses purified $[^3H]$ adenosine-5'-monophosphate as substrate; the reaction product, adenosine, is measured by separating the $[^3H]$ adenosine from the $[^3H]$ adenosine-5'-monophosphate by DEAE-Sephadex A-25 chromatography. Alkaline phosphatase is stable and its reaction rate is constant for about 6 to 10 hr. The relative sensitivities of these methods were first shown for cholera toxin and rotavirus (Harris, et al., 1979). USERIA was the most sensitive assay, detecting 10^{-16}g of cholera toxin (i.e., 6×10^2 molecules) after a 1000 min reaction, while ELISA detected 10^{-13}g (i.e., 6×10^5 molecules) after 1000 min of reaction. For measuring rotavirus, USERIA was 100-fold more sensitive than ELISA and 1000-fold more sensitive than RIA.

Recently, both USERIA and ELISA have been used for detecting certain DNA-carcinogen adducts. Hsu, et al. (1980) measured acetylated and deacetylated C-8 adducts of acetylaminofluorene (AAF) with deoxyguanosine, n-(deoxyguanosin-8-yl)-acetylamino fluorene (dG-8-aAAF) and n-(deoxyguanosin-8-yl) aminofluorene (dG-8-AF). A competitive USERIA assay detected less than 3 fmol of the specific adduct, n-(deoxyguanosin-8-yl)-AAF. USERIA was 60 and 10-fold more sensitive for these DNA adducts than either RIA or ELISA, respectively. Hsu et al. (1981) also measured 3 fmol of B(a)P-DNA adducts bound to DNA by non-competitive USERIA and 10 fmol of adducts in 25 ug of DNA in a competitive assay (approximately 1 DNA adduct/7×10^6 nucleotides). For the B(a)P adduct, USERIA was 500-fold more sensitive than RIA and 5-fold more sensitive than ELISA. Hangen et al. (1981) prepared a monoclonal antibody to aflatoxin-B₁ modified DNA which was used in a USERIA assay.

The main disadvantage of these methods is that many DNA-carcinogen adducts are weakly immunogenic (for instance, methylated and ethylated bases), a property which limits the sensitivity and usefulness of these procedures. Nevertheless, for those DNA-adducts that are strongly immunogenic, these methods will allow us to study DNA damage and repair, human environmental exposure, organ specific carcinogenesis, and other instances of human exposure to non-radioactive drugs and environmental chemicals.

REFERENCES

Abanobi, S.E., Farber, E., Sarma, D.S.R.: Persistence of DNA damage during development of liver angiosarcoma in rats fed dimethylnitrosamine. Cancer Res. **39**, 1592–1596 (1979).

Ahnstrom, G., Exixon, K.: Radiation-induced strand breakage in DNA from mammalian cells. Strand separation in alkaline solution. Int. J. Radiat. Biol. **23**, 285–289 (1973).

Allison, A.C.: Lysosomes and cancer. In: Lysosomes in Biology and Pathology, Amsterdam: North-Holland Publishing Co., 1969.

Archer, M.D., Eng, V.W.S.: Quantitative determination of carcinogens and mutagens as alkylating agents following chemical activation. Chem. Biol. Interact. **33**, 207–214 (1981).

Autrup, H.: Separation of water-soluble metabolites of benzo(a)pyrene formed by cultured human colon. Biochem. Pharmacol **28**, 1727–1730 (1979).

Baird, W.M.: The use of radioactive carcinogens to detect DNA modifications. In: Chemical Carcinogens and DNA, vol. 1. Boca Raton, Fla.: CRC Press, Inc. 1979.

Baird, W.M., Brookes, P.: Isolation of the hydrocarbon-deoxyribonucleoside products from the DNA of mouse embryo cells treated in culture with 7-methyl-benz(a)anthracene-^{3}H. Cancer Res. **33**, 2378–2385 (1973).

Baird, W.M., Diamond, L.: The nature of benzo(a)pyrene-DNA adducts formed in hamster embryo cells depends on the length of time of exposure to benzo(a)pyrene. BBRC **77**, 162–167 (1977).

Baird, W.M., O'Brien, T.G., Diamond, L.: Comparison of the metabolism of benzo(a)pyrene and its activation to biologically active metabolites by low-passage hamster and rat embryo cells. Carcinog. **2**, 81–88 (1981).

Bolognesi, C., Cesarone, C.F., Santi, L.: Standardization of the alkaline elution procedure using x-ray damaged nuclear DNA. Tumori **65**, 511–516 (1979).

Bradley, M.O., Erickson, L.C.: Comparison of the effects of hydrogen peroxide and x-ray irradiation on toxicity, mutation, and DNA damage/repair in mammalian cells (V-79). Biochim. Biophys. Acta. **654**, 135–141 (1981).

Bradley, M.O., Erickson, L.C., Kohn, K.W.: Normal DNA strand rejoining and absence of DNA crosslinking in progeronal and aging human cells. Mut. Res. **37**, 279–292 (1976).

Bradley, M.O., Erickson, L.C., Kohn, K.W.: Non-enzymatic DNA strand breaks induced in mammalian cells by fluorescent light. Biochim. Biophys. Acta. **520**, 11–20 (1978).

Bradley, M.O., Hsu, I.C., Harris, C.C.: Relationships between sister chromatid exchange and mutagenicity, toxicity, and DNA damage. Nature **282**, 318–320 (1979).

Bradley, M.O., Kohn, K.W.: X-ray induced DNA double strand break production and repair in mammalian cells and measured by neutral filter elution. Nuc. Acids Res. **7**, 793–804 (1979).

Bradley, M.O., Sharkey, N.A.: Mutagenicity of thymidine to cultured Chinese hamster cells. Nature **274**, 607–608 (1978).

Bradley, M.O., Taylor, V.I.: DNA double-strand breaks induced in normal human cells during the repair of ultraviolet light damage. Proc. Natl. Acad. Sci. USA **78**, 3619–3623 (1981).

Brambilla, G., Cavanna, M., Parodi, S., Sciaba, L., Pino, A., Robbiano, L.: DNA damage in liver, colon, stomach, lung and kidney of BALB-C mice treated with 1,2-dimethylhydrazine. Int. J. Cancer **22**, 174–180 (1978).

Brambilla, G., Cavanna, M., Pino, A., Robbiano, L.: Quantitative correlation among DNA damaging potency of 6′N-nitroso compounds and their potency in inducing tumor growth and bacterial mutations. Carcinogenesis **2**, 425–430 (1981a).

Brambilla, G., Cavanna, M., Pino, A., Robbiano, L.: DNA damage and repair in mouse tissues following procarbazine administration. Pharmacol. Res. Commun. **13**, 213–222 (1981b).

Brent, T.P.: Purification and characterization of human endonucleases specific for damaged DNA. Analysis of lesions induced by ultraviolet or x-radiation. BBA **454**, 172–183 (1976).

Brookes, P., Lawley, P.D.: The reaction of mono- and di-functional alkylating agents with nucleic acids. Biochem. J. **80**, 496–503 (1961).

Brox, L., Gowans, B., Belch, A.: N-tri-fluoroacetyl adriamycin 14 valerate and adriamycin induced DNA damage in the RPMI-6410 human lymphoblastoid cell line. Can. J. Biochem. **58**, 720–725 (1980a).

Brox, L.W., Gowans, B., Belch, A.: L-phenyl alanine mustard melphalan uptake and cross linking in the RPMI-6410 human lymphoblastoid cell line. Cancer Res. **40**, 1169–1172 (1980b).

Beucheler, J., Kleihues, P.: Excision of 06-methylguanine from DNA of various mouse tissues following a single injection of N-methyl-N-nitrosourea. Chem-Biol. Interact. **16**, 325–333 (1977).

Buening, M.K., Wislocki, P.G., Levin, W., Yogi, H., Thakkei, D.R., Akagi, H., Koreeda, M.L., Jerina, D.M., Conney, A.H.: Tumorigenicity of the optical enantiomers of the diostereomeric benzo(a)pyrene 7,8-diol-9,10-epoxides in newborn mice: Exceptional activity of (+)−7B,8a-dihydroxy-9a,10a-epoxy-7,8,9,10-tetrahydrobenzo(a)pyrene. PNAS **75**, 5358–5356 (1978).

Carrell, H.L., Glusker, J.P., Moschel, R.C., Hudgins, W.R., Dipple, A.: Crystal structure of a carcinogen: nucleoside adduct. Cancer Res. **41**, 2230–2234 (1981).

Cerutti, P.A., Sessions, F., Hariharan, P.V., Lusby, A.: Repair of DNA damage induced by benzo(a)pyrene diol epoxides I and II in human alveolar tumor cells. Cancer Res. **38**, 2118–2124 (1978).

Chase, E.S., Shafer, R.H.: Viscoelastic behavior of mammalian DNA. Biophys. J. **28**, 93–106 (1979).

Ciccarelli, R.B., Hampton, T.H., Jennette, K.W.: Nickel carbonate induces DNA protein cross links and DNA strand breaks in rat kidney. Cancer Lett. **12**, 349–354 (1981).

Cleaver, J.E.: Methods for studying repair of DNA damaged by physical and chemical carcinogens. In: Methods Cancer Res, **11**, New York: Academic Press, 1975.

Cohen, L.F., Ewig, R.A.G., Kohn, K.W., Glaubiger, D.: Inter strand DNA cross linking by 4,5′8-trimethylpsoralen plus monochromatic UV light studies by alkaline elution in mouse L-1210 leukemia cells. Biochim. Biophys. Acta. **610**, 56–63 (1980).

Colburn, N.H., Boutwell, R.K.: The binding of β-propiolactone and some related alkylating agents to DNA, RNA, and protein of mouse skin; relation betwen tumor-initiating power of alkylating agents and their binding to DNA. Cancer Res. **28**, 653–660 (1968).

119

Cook, P.R., Brazell, J.A.: Supercoils in human DNA. J. Cell Sci. **19**, 261–279 (1975).

Cook, P.R., Brazell, J.A.: Detection and repair of single strand breaks in nuclear DNA. Nature **263**, 679–682 (1976).

Cooper, C.S., Ribeiro, O., Farmer, P.B., Hewer, A., Walsh, C., Pal, K., Grover, P.L., Sims, P.: The metabolic activation of benzo(a)anthracene in hamster embryo cells: evidence that diol-epoxides react with guanogene, deoxyguanogene and adenogene in nucleic acids. Chem-Biol. Interact. **32**, 209–231 (1980).

Coulondre, C., Miller, J.H.: Genetic studies of the lac repressor. IV. Mutagenic specificity in the lac I gene of *Escherichia coli*. J. Mol. Biol. **117**, 577–606 (1977).

Cox, R., Irving, C.C.: Effect of N-methyl-N-nitrosourea on the DNA of rat bladder epithelium. Cancer Res. **36**, 4114–4118 (1976).

Deutsch, J., Cavalieri, L.F., Rosenberg, B.H.: Effects of ethylating agents on DNA synthesis *in vitro*: implications for the mechanism of carcinogenesis. Carcinog. **2**, 363–371 (1981).

Di Giovanni, J., Romson, J.R., Linville, D., Juchau, M.R.: Covalent binding of polycyclic aromatic hydrocarbons to adenine correlates with tumorigenesis in mouse skin. Cancer Lett. **7**, 39–43 (1979).

Dingman, C.W., Kakanuga, T.: DNA strand breaking and rejoining in response to ultraviolet light in normal human and *Xeroderma pigmentosum* cells. Int. J. Rad. Biol. **30**, 55–66 (1976).

Dipple, A., Levy, L.S., Lawley, P.D.: Comparative carcinogenicity of alkylating agents: comparisons of a series of alkyl and aralkyl bromides of differing chemical reactivities as inducers of sarcoma at the site of a single injection in the rat. Carcinog. **2**, 103–107 (1981).

Eastman, A., Bresnick, E.: A technique for the measurement of breakage and repair of DNA alkylated in vivo. Chem-Biol. Interact. **23**, 369–378 (1978).

Engelse, L.D., Philippus, E.J.: In vivo repair of rat liver DNA damaged by dimethylnitrosamine or diethylnitrosamine. Chem-Biol. Interact. **19**, 111–124 (1977).

Erickson, L.C., Bradley, M.O., Ducore, J.M., Ewig, R.A.G., Kohn, K.W.: DNA cross linking and cytotoxicity in normal and transformed human cells treated with anti-tumor nitrosoureas. Proc. Natl. Acad. Sci. USA **77**, 467–471 (1980a).

Erickson, L.C., Bradley, M.O., Kohn, K.W.: Strand breaks in DNA from normal and transformed human cells treated with 1,3-bis(2-chloroethyl)-1-nitrosourea. Cancer Res. **37**, 3744–3750 (1977).

Erickson, L.C., Bradley, M.O., Kohn, K.W.: Differential inhibition of the rejoining of x-ray induced DNA strand breaks in normal and transformed human fibroblasts treated with 1,3-bis(2-chloroethyl)-1-nitrosourea *in vitro*. Cancer Res. **38**, 672–677 (1978).

Erickson, L.C., Dsieka, R., Sharkey, N.A., Kohn, K.W.: Measurement of DNA damage in unlabeled cells by alkaline elution and a flurometric DNA assay. Anal. Biochem. **106**, 169–174 (1980b).

Erickson, L.C., Ramonas, L.M., Zaharko, D.S., Kohn, K.: Cytotoxicity and DNA cross linking activity of 4 sulfido cyclophosphamides in mouse leukemia cells in vitro. Cancer Res. **40**, 4216–4220 (1980c).

Ewig, R.A.G., Kohn, K.W.: DNA protein cross linking and DNA inter strand cross linking by haloethylnitrosoureas in L-1210 cells. Cancer Res. **38**, 3197–3203 (1978).

Floot, B.G.J., Philippus, E.J., Hart, A.A.M., Den Engelse, L.: Persistence and accumulation of potential single strand breaks in liver DNA of rats treated with diethylnitrosamine or dimethylnitrosamine correlation with hepatocarcinogenicity. Chem.-Biol. Interact. **25**, 229–242 (1979).

Fornace, A.J., Jr., Little, J.B.: DNA cross linking induced by x-rays and chemical agents. Biochem. Biophys. Acta **477**, 343–355 (1977).

Fornace, A.J., Jr., Little, J.B.: DNA cross linking by chemical carcinogens in mammalian cells. Cancer Res. **39**, 704–710 (1979).

Fornace, A.J., Jr., Little, J.B.: Normal repair of DNA single strand breaks in patients with ataxia telangiectasia. Biochim. Biophys. Acta **607**, 432–437 (1980).

Fornace, A.J., Seres, D.S., Lechner, J.F., Harris, C.C.: DNA protein cross linking by chromium salts. Chem.-Biol. Interactions **36**, 345–354 (1981).

Frei, J.V., Lawley, P.D.: Methylation of DNA in various organs of C57BL mice by a carcinogenic dose of N-methyl-N-nitrosourea and stability of some methylation products up to 18 hours. Chem.-Biol. Interact. **10**, 413–427 (1975).

Frei, J.V., Swenson, D.H., Warren, W., Lawley, P.D.: Alkylation of deoxyribonucleic acid *in vivo* in various organs of C57BL mice by the carcinogens N-methyl-N-nitrosourea, N-ethyl-N-nitrosourea and ethyl methanesulfonate in relation to induction of thymic lymphoma. Biochem. J. **174**, 1031–1044 (1978).

Frenkel, K., Greenberger, D., Boublik, M., Weinstein, I.B.: Conformation of denucleoside monophosphates modified with benzo(a)pyrene-7,8-dehydrodiol 9,10-oxide as measured by circular dichroism. Biochem. **17**, 1278–1282 (1978).

Gamper, H.B., Bartholomew, J.C., Calvin, M.: Mechanism of benzo(a)pyrene diol epoxide induced deoxyribonucleic acid strand scission. Biochem. **19**, 3948–3956 (1980).

Gantt, R., Jones, G.M., Stephens, E.V., Baeck, A.E., Sanford, K.K.: Visible light induced DNA cross links in cultured mouse and human cells. Biochim. Biophys. Acta **565**, 231–240 (1979).

Garner, R.C., Martin, C.N., Smith, J.R.L., Coles, B.F., Tolson, M.R.: Comparison of aflatoxin B_1 and aflatoxin G_1 binding to cellular macromolecules *in vitro*, *in vivo*, and after peracid oxidation; characterization of the major nucleic acid adducts. Chem.-Biol. Interact. **26**, 57–73 (1979).

Geacintov, N.E., Yoshida, H., Ibanez, V., Harvey, R.G.: Non-covalent intercalative binding of 7,8-dihydroxy-9,10-epoxybenzo(a)pyrene to DNA. BBRC **100**, 1569–1577 (1981).

Goth, R., Rajewsky, M.F.: Persistence of 06-ethylguanine in rat-brain DNA: correlation with nervous system-specific carcinogenesis by ethylnitrosourea. PNAS **71**, 639–643 (1974).

Grunberger, D., Weinstein, I.B.: Biochemical effects of the modification of nucleic acids by certain polycyclic aromatic carcinogens. Prog. Nucl. Acid Res. Mol. Biol. **23**, 105–149 (1979).

Harris, C.C., Yolken, R.H., Hsu, I.-C.: Ultrasensitive enzymatic radioimmunoassay: Application to detection of cholera toxin and rotavirus. Proc. Natl. Acad. Sci. USA **76**, 5336–5339 (1979).

Haugen, A., Groupman, J.P., Hsu, I.-C., Goodrich, G.R., Wogan, G.N., Harris, C.C.: Monoclonal antibody to aflatoxin B_1-modified DNA detected by enzyme immunoassay. Proc. Natl. Acad. Sci. USA **78**, 4124–4217 (1981).

Hemminki, K., Paasivirta, J., Kurkirinne, T., Virkki, L.: Alkylation products of DNA bases by simple epoxides. Chem-Biol. Interact. **30**, 259–270 (1980).

Heyting, C., Huigen, A., Engelse, L.D.: Repair of ethylnitrosourea induced DNA damage in the newborn rat. Alkali labile lesions and in-situ breaks. Carcinogenesis **1**, 769–778 (1980).

Hirschi, M., Netrawali, M.S., Remsen, J.F., Cerutti, P.A.: Formation of DNA single strand breaks by near UV and gamma-rays in normal and Blooms syndrome skin fibroblasts. Cancer Res. **41**, 2003–2007 (1981).

Hogan, M.E., Dattagupta, N., Whitlock, J.P.: Carcinogen-induced alteration of DNA structure. J. Biol. Chem. **256**, 4504–4513 (1981).

Hsu, I.-C., Poirier, M.C., Yuspa, S.H., Grunenberger, D., Weinstein, I.B., Yolken, R.H., Harris, C.C.: Measurement of benzo(a)pyrene-DNA adducts by enzyme immunoassays and radioimmunoassay. Cancer Res. **41**, 1091–1095 (1981).

Hsu, I.-C., Poirier, M.C., Yuspa, S.H., Yolken, R.H., Harris, C.C.: Ultrasensitive enzymatic radioimmunoassay (USERIA) detects femtomoles of acetylaminofluorene-DNA adducts. Carcinogen. **1**, 455–458 (1980).

Iqbal, Z.M., Kohn, K.W., Ewig, R.A.G., Fornace, A.J., Jr.: Single strand scission and repair of DNA in mammalian cells by bleomycin. Cancer Res. **36**, 3834–3838 (1976).

Irving, C.C.: Interaction of chemical carcinogens with DNA. In: Methods in Cancer Research, vol. VII, New York, Academic Press: 1973.

Ivanovic, V., Geacintov, N.E., Yamasaki, H., Weinstein, I.B.: DNA and RNA adducts formed in hamster embryo cell cultures exposed to benzo(a)pyrene. Biochem. **17**, 1597–1603 (1978).

Jeffrey, A.M., Blobstein, S.H., Weinstein, I.B., Harvey, R.G.: High pressure liquid chromatography of carcinogen-nucleoside conjugates: separation of 7,12-dimethylbenzanthracene derivatives. Anal. Biochem. **73**, 378–385 (1976).

Jerina, D.M., Lehr, R., Schaefer-Ridder, M., Yogi, H., Karle, J.M., Thakkei, D.R., Wood, A.W., Lu, A.Y.H., Ryan, D., West, S., Levin, W., Conney, A.H.: Bay-region epoxides of dihydrodiols: A concept explaining the mutagenic and carcinogenic activity of benzo(a)pyrene and benzo(a)anthracene. In: Origins of Human Cancer, Book C, Cold Spring Harbor Press: 1977.

Kadlubar, F.F., Melchior, W.B., Flammang, T.J., Gagliano, A.G., Yoshida, H., Geacintov, N.E.: Structural consequences of modification of the oxygen atom of guanine in DNA by the carcinogen N-hydroxy-1-naphthylamine. Cancer Res. **41**, 2168–2174 (1981).

Kann, H.E., Jr., Schott, M.A., Petkas, A.: Effects of structure and chemical activity on the ability of nitrosoureas to inhibit DNA repair. Cancer Res. **40**, 50–55 (1980).

Kanter, P.M., Schwartz, H.S.: Effects of N'trifluoroacetyl adriamycin 14 valerate and related agents on DNA strand damage and thymidine incorporation in CCRF-CEM cells. Cancer Res. **39**, 448–451 (1979a).

Kanter, P.M., Schwartz, H.S.: Quantitative models for growth inhibition of human leukemia cells by antitumor anthracycline derivatives. Cancer Res. **39**, 3661–3671 (1979b).

King, H.W.S., Obsorne, M.R., Beland, F.A., Harvey, R.G., Brookes, P.: (±)-7a,8B-dihydroxy-9B,10B-epoxy-7,8,9,10-tetrahydrobenzo(a)pyrene is an intermediate in the metabolism and binding to DNA benzo(a)pyrene. PNAS **73**, 2679–2681 (1976).

Kirtikar, D.M., Cathcart, G.R., Goldthwart, D.A.: Endonuclease II, apurinic acid endonuclease, and exonuclease III. PNAS **73**, 4324–4328 (1976).

Kirtikar, D.M., Goldthwart, D.A.: The enzymatic release of 06-methylguanine and 3-methyladenine from DNA reacted with carcinogen N-methyl-N-nitrosourea. PNAS **71**, 2022–2026 (1974).

Kleihues, P., Margison, G.P.: Carcinogenicity of N-methyl-N-nitrosourea: possible role of excision repair of 06-methylguanine from DNA. JNCI **53**, 1839–1841 (1974).

Kohn, K.W.: DNA as a target in cancer chemotherapy: measurement of macromolecular DNA damage produced in mammalian cells by anticancer agents and carcinogens. In: Methods. Cancer Res. **14**, New York: Academic Press, 1979.

Kohn, K.W., Erickson, L.C., Ewig, R.A.G., Friedman, C.A.: Fractionation of DNA from mammalian cells by alkaline elution biochemistry **15**, 4629–4637 (1976).

Kohn, K.W., Ewig, R.A.G.: Alkaline elution analysis, a new approach to the study of DNA single-strand interruptions in cells. Cancer Res. **33**, 1849–1853 (1973).

Kohn, K.W., Ewig, R.A.G.: Effect of pH on the bleomycin induced DNA single strand scission in L-1210 cells and the relation to cell survival. Cancer Res. **36**, 3839–3841 (1976).

Kohn, K.W., Ewig, R.A.G.: DNA protein cross linking by trans platinum II di ammine di chloride in mammalian cells: a new method of analysis. Biochim. Biophy. Acta **562**, 32–40 (1979).

Kohn, K.W., Ewig, R.A.G., Erickson, L.C., Zwelling, L.A.: Measurements of strand breaks and cross links by alkaline elution. In: DNA Repair—A Laboratory Manual of Research Procedures, vol. I, Part B. New York: Marcel Dekker, Inc. 1981.

Koropatnick, D.J., Stich, H.F.: The modifying effect of sodium ascorbate on DNA damage and repair after N-methyl-N'-nitro-N-nitrosoguanidine treatment in vivo. Biochem. Biophys. Res. Commun. **92**, 292–298 (1980).

Kraemer, K.H., Waters, H.L., Cohen, L.F., Popescu, N.C., Amsbaugh, S.C., DiPaolo, J.A., Glaubiger, D., Ellingson, O.L., Tarone, R.E.: Effects of 8 methoxypsoralen and UV radiation on human lymphoid cells in-vitro. J. Invest. Dermatol. **76**, 80–87 (1981).

Krepinsky, J., Carver, J.P., Rajalakshmi, S., Rao, P.M., Sarma, D.S.R.: Detection by nuclear magnetic resonance of methylation sites on rat liver DNA utilizing magneti- cally labelled N-methyl-N-nitrosourea and methyl methane sulfonate. Chem.-Biol. Interact. **27**, 381–386 (1979).

Kriek, E.: Difference in binding 2-acetylaminofluorene to rat liver deoxyribonucleic acid and ribosomal ribonucleic acid *in vivo*. BBA **161**, 273–275 (1968).

Kriek, E.: On the mechanism of action of carcinogenic aromatic amines. I. Binding of 2-AAF and N-hydroxy-2-AAF to rat liver nucleic acids *in vivo*. Chem.-Biol. Interact. **1**, 3–17 (1969).

Kriek, E., Westra, J.G.: Metabolic activation of aromatic amines and amides and interactions with nucleic acids. In: Chemical Carcinogens and DNA, vol. II. Boca Raton: CRC Press, Inc. 1979.

Kuebler, J.P., Goldthwart, D.A.: An endonuclease from calf liver specific for apurinic sites in DNA. Biochem. **16**, 1370–1377 (1977).

Kuroki, T., Heidelberger, C.: The binding of polycyclic aromatic hydrocarbons to the DNA, RNA and proteins of transformable cells in culture. Cancer Res. **31**, 2168–2176 (1971).

Kuroki, T., Huberman, E., Marquardt, H., Selkirk, J.K., Heidelberger, C., Grover, P.L., Sims, P.: Binding of K-region epoxides and other derivatives of benzo(a)an- thracene and dibenz(a,b)anthracene to DNA, RNA and proteins of transformable cells. Chem.-Biol. Interact. **4**, 389–397 (1971).

Kulkarni, M.S., Heidepreim, P.M., Yielding, K.L.: Production by lithocholic acid of DNA strand breaks in L-1210 cells. Cancer Res. **40**, 2666–2669 (1980).

Kulkarni, M.S., Yielding, K.L.: Inhibition of UV induced DNA repair at different steps by quinacrine and anthralin. Biochem. Biophys. Res. Commun. **83**, 1531–1537 (1978).

Lang, M.C.E., Freund, A.M., de Murcia, G., Fuchs, R.P.P., Daune, M.P.: Unwinding of supercoiled Col E_1-DNA after covalent binding of the ultimate carcinogen N- acetoxy-N-2-acetylaminofluorene and its 7-iodo derivative. Chem.-Biol. Interact. **28**, 171–180 (1979).

Lawley, P.D.: a. Carcinogenesis by alkylating agents. In: Chemical Carcinogens. Washington, D.D.: American Chemical Society, 1976.

Lawley, P.D.: b. Methylation of DNA by carcinogens: some applications of chemical analytical methods. In: Screening Tests in Chemical Carcinogenesis. Lyon: IARC 1976.

Lawley, P.D.: DNA as a target of alkylating techniques. Br. Med. Bull. **36**, 19–24 (1980).

Lawley, P.D., Shah, S.A.: Methylation of ribonucleic acid by the carcinogens dimethyl sulphate, N-methyl-N-nitrosourea and N-methyl-N'-nitro-N-nitrosoguanidine. Biochem. J. **128**, 117–132 (1972).

Levin, M., Silber, R., Israel, M., Goldfeder, A., Khetarpal, V.K., Potmesil, M.: Protein associated DNA breaks and DNA protein cross links caused by DNA nonbinding derivatives of adriamycin in L-1210 cells. Cancer Res. **41**, 1006–1010 (1981).

Lilja, H.S., Hyde, E., Longnecker, D.S., Yager, J.D., Jr.: DNA damage and repair in rat tissues following administration of azaserine. Cancer Res. **37**, 3925–3931 (1977).

Ljungquist, S., Lindahl, T.: A mammalian endonuclease specific for apurinic sites in double-stranded deoxyribonucleic acid. J. Biol. Chem. **249**, 1530–1535 (1974).

Loveless, A.: Possible relevance of 0-6 alkylation of deoxyguanosine to the mutagenicity and carcinogenicity of nitrosamines and nitrosamides. Nature **223**, 206–207 (1969).

Mac Nicoll, A.D., Cooper, C.S., Ribeizo, O., Gervasi, P.G., Hewer, A., Walsh, C., Grover, P.L., Sims, P.: The involvement of a non 'bay-region' diol-epoxide in the formation of benzo(a)anthracene-DNA adducts in a rat liver microsomal system. BBRC **91**, 490–497 (1979).

Magee, P.N., Farber, E.: Toxic liver injury and carcinogenesis. Methylation of rat liver nucleic acids by dimethylnitrosamine *in vivo*. Biochem. J. **83**, 114–124 (1962).

Margison, G.P., Margison, J.M., Montesano, R.: Accumulation of 06-methylguanine in non-target tissue deoxyribonucleic acid during chronic administration of dimethyl-nitrosamine. Biochem. J. **165**, 463–468 (1977).

Margison, G.P., O'Connor, P.J.: Nucleic acid modification by N-nitroso compounds. In: Chemical Carcinogens and DNA, vol. I. Boca Raton: CRC Press, Inc. 1979.

Marquardt, H.: DNA—The critical cellular target in chemical carcinogenesis? In: Chemical Carcinogens and DNA, vol. II. Boca Raton: CRC Press, Inc. 1979.

Meyn, R.E., Corry, P.M., Fletcher, S.E., Demetriades, M.: Thermal enhancement of DNA damage in mammalian cells treated with cis diammine dichloro platinum II. Cancer Res. **40**, 1136–1139 (1980).

Mhaskar, D.N., Chang, M.J.W., Hart, R.W., D'Ambrosio, S.M.: Analysis of alkylated sites at N-3 and N-7 positions of purines as an indicator of chemical carcinogens. Cancer Res. **41**, 223–229 (1981).

Miller, E.C., Juhl, U., Miller, J.A.: Nucleic acid guanine: reaction with the carcinogen N-acetyl-2-acetylaminofluorene. Science **153**, 1125–1127 (1966).

Miller, J.A., Miller, E.C.: Chemical carcinogenesis: mechanism and approaches to its control. JNCI **47**, 5–14 (1971).

Miyata, Y., Hagiwara, A., Nakatsuka, T., Murasaki, G., Arai, M., Ito, N.: Effects of caffeine and saccharin on DNA in the bladder epithelium of rats treated with N-butyl-N-3-carboxypropyl nitrosamine. Chem.-Biol. Interact. **29**, 291–302 (1980).

Montesano, R., Pegg, A.E., Margioon, G.P.: Alkylation of DNA and carcinogenicity of N-nitroso compounds. J. Toxicol. Environ. H. **6**, 1001–1008 (1980).

Moore, P., Strauss, B.: Site of inhibition of *in vitro* DNA synthesis in carcinogen and UV treated ϕX174 DNA. Nature **278**, 664–666 (1979).

Nestmann, E.R., Douglas, G.R., Matula, T.I., Grant, C.E., Kowbel, D.J.: Mutagenic activity of rhodamine dyes and their impurities as detected by mutation induction in Salmonella typhimurium and DNA damage in Chinese hamster ovary cells. Cancer Res. **39**, 4412–4417 (1979).

Netrawali, M.S., Cerutti, P.A.: Increased near UV induced DNA fragmentation in Xeroderma pigmentosum variants. Biochem. Biophys. Res. Commun. **87**, 802–810 (1979).

Newbold, R.F., Brookes, P.: Exceptional mutagenicity of a benzo(a)pyrene diol epoxide in cultured mammalian cells. Nature **261**, 52–54 (1976).

Newbold, R.F., Warren, W., Medcalf, A.S.C., Amos, J.: Mutagenicity of carcinogenic methylating agents is associated with a specific DNA modification. Nature **283**, 596–599 (1980).

Nicoll, J.W., Swann, P.F., Pegg, A.E.: Effect of dimethylnitrosamine on persistence of methylated guanines in rat liver and kidney DNA. Nature **254**, 261–262 (1975).

Nicoll, J.W., Swann, P.F., Pegg, A.E.: The accumulation of 06-methylguanine in the liver and kidney DNA of rats treated with dimethylnitrosamine for a short or a long period. Chem.-Biol. Interact. **16**, 301–308 (1977).

O'Connor, P.J.: Interaction of chemical carcinogens with macromolecules. J. Cancer Res. Clin. Oncol. **99**, 167–186 (1981).

Panthananickal, A., Marnett, L.J.: Comparison of commercial reversed-phase high performance liquid chromatographic columns for the separation of benzo(a)pyrene diolepoxide-nucleic acid adducts. J.Chromatog. **206**, 253–265 (1981).

Parodi, S., Bolognesi, O., Cavanna, M., Pollack, R.L., Santi, L., Brambilla, G.: Damage and repair of DNA in cultured mammalian cells with N-di-azo acetyl glycine amide. Cancer Res. **37**, 4460–4466 (1977).

Parodi, S., Carlo, P., Martelli, A., Taningher, M., Finollo, R., Pala, M., Giaretti, W.: A circular channel crucible oscillating viscometer detection of DNA damage induced in-vivo by exceedingly small doses of dimethylnitrosamine. J. Mol. Biol. **147**, 501–522 (1981a).

Parodi, S., Deflora, S., Cavanna, M., Pino, A., Robbiano, L., Bennecelli, C., Brambilla, G.: DNA damaging activity in-vivo and bacterial mutagenicity of 16 hydrazine derivatives as related quantitatively to their carcinogenicity. Cancer Res. **41**, 1469–1482 (1981b).

Parodi, S., Pala, M.T.M., Brambilla, G., Cavanna, M., Tanningher, M.: Detection by alkaline elution of rat liver DNA damage induced by simultaneous subacute administration of nitrite and aminopyrine. J. Toxicol. Environ. Health **6**, 167–174 (1980).

Parodi, S., Taningher, M., Pala, M., Santi, L.: Alkaline DNA fragmentation in-vivo borderline or negative results obtained respectively with 7,12-dimethyl-benzo(a)-anthracene and benzo(a)pyrene. Tumori. **67**, 87–94 (1981c).

Pegg, A.E.: Enzymatic removal of 06-methylguanine from DNA by mammalian cell extracts. BBRC **84**, 166–173 (1978).

Pegg, A.E., Nicoll, J.W.: Nitrosamine carcinogenesis: the importance of the persistence in DNA of alkylated bases in the organotropism of tumor induction. In: Screening Tests in Chemical Carcinogenesis. Lyon: IARC (1976).

Petzold, G., Harbach, P., Bedell, M., Swenberg, J.A.: In-vitro DNA damage alkaline elution assay for predicting carcinogenic potential. Mutat. Res. **53**, 110 (1978).

Petzold, G., Swenberg, J.A.: Detection of DNA damage induced in-vivo following exposure of rats to carcinogens. Cancer Res. **38**, 1589–1594 (1978).

Phillips, D.H., Grover, P.L., Sims, P.: The covalent binding of polycyclic hydrocarbons to DNA in the skin of mice of different strains. Int. J. Cancer **22**, 487–494 (1978).

Poirer, M.C., Santella, R., Weinstein, I.B., Greenberger, D., Yuspa, S.H.: Quantitation of benzo(a)pyrene-deoxyguanosine adducts by radioimmunoassay. Cancer Res. **40**, 412–416 (1980).

Poirer, M.C., Yuspa, S.H., Weinstein, I.B., Blobstein, S.: Detection of carcinogen-DNA adducts by radioimmunoassay. Nature **270**, 186–188 (1977).

125

Prakash, L., Strauss, B.: Repair of alkylation damage: stability of methyl groups in *Bacillus subtilis* treated with methyl methanesulfonate. J. Bact. **102**, 760–766.

Ramonas, L.M., Erickson, L.C., Klesse, W., Kohn, K.W., Zaharko, D.S.: Differential cytotoxicity and DNA cross linking produced by polymeric and monomeric activated analogs of cyclophosphamide in mouse L-1210 leukemia cells. Mol. Pharmacol. **19**, 331–336 (1981).

Roberts, J.J.: Cellular responses to carcinogen-induced DNA damage and the role of DNA repair. Br. Med. Bull. **36**, 25–31 (1980).

Rogers, K.J., Pegg, A.E.: Formation of 06-methylguanine by alkylation of rat liver, colon, and kidney DNA following administration of 1,2-dimethylhydrazine. Cancer Res. **37**, 4082–4087 (1977).

Ross, W.E., Bradley, M.O.: DNA double-strand breaks in mammalian cells after exposure to intercalating agents. Biochim. Biophys. Acta **654**, 129–134 (1981).

Ross, W.E., Ewig, R.A.G., Kohn, K.W.: Differences between melphalan and nitrogen mustard in the formation and removal of DNA cross links. Cancer Res. **38**, 1502–1506 (1978).

Ross, W.E., Glaubiger, D., Kohn, K.W.: Qualitative and quantitative aspects of intercalator induced DNA strand breaks. Biochim. Biophys. Acta **562**, 41–50 (1979).

Rydberg, B.: The rate of strand separation in alkali of DNA of irradiated mammalian cells. Radiat. Res. **61**, 274–287 (1975).

Selkirk, J.K.: Analysis of benzo(a)pyrene metabolism by high pressure liquid chromatography. Adv. Chromatog. **16**, 1–36 (1978).

Shafer, A.H., Chase, E.S.: DNA damage in rat 92 cells treated with nitrogen mustard and 1,3-bis(2-chloroethyl)-1-nitrosourea assayed by visco-elastometry and 51 nuclease. Cancer Res. **40**, 3186–3193 (1980).

Shafer, A.H., Chase, E.S. Eisenach, J.: Slow repair of x-ray induced DNA damage in rat 92 cells *in vitro* analyzed by viscoelastometry. Radiat. Res. **85**, 47–56 (1981).

Sheridan, R.B., Huang, P.C.: Single strand breakage and repair in eukaryotic DNA as assayed by S1 nuclease. Nuc. Acids Res. **4**, 299–318 (1977).

Shinohara, K., Cerutti, P.A.: Excision repair of benzo(a)pyrenedeoxyguanosine adducts in baby hamster kidney 21/C13 cells and in secondary mouse embryo fibroblasts C57BL/6J. PNAS **74**, 979–983 (1977).

Shooter, K.V., Merrifield, R.K.: An assay for phosphotriester formation in the reaction of alkylating agents with deoxyribonucleic acid *in vitro* and *in vivo*. Chem.-Biol. Interact. **13**, 223–236 (1976).

Sims, P., Grover, P.L., Swaisland, A., Pal., A., Hewer, A.: Metabolic activation of benzo(a)pyrene proceeds by a diol-epoxide. Nature **252**, 326–328 (1974).

Sina, J.F., Bean, C.L., Dysart, G.R., Taylor, V.I., Bradley, M.O.: Evaluation of the alkaline elution/rat hepatocyte assay as a predictor of carcinogenic/mutagenic potential. Mutation Res., **113**, 357–391 (1983).

Singer, B.: The chemical effects of nucleic acid alkylation and their relation to mutagenesis and carcinogenesis. Prog. Nucl. Acid Res. Mol. Biol. **15**, 219–284 (1975).

Singer, B.: All oxygens in nucleic acids react with carcinogenic ethylating agents. Nature **264**, 333–339 (1976).

Singer, B., Kroger, M.: Participation of modified nucleosides in translation and transcription. Prog. Nucl. Acid Res. Mol. Biol. **23**, 151–194 (1979).

Sirover, M.A., Loeb, L.A.: On the fidelity of DNA synthesis: Effects of steroids and intercalating agents. Chem.-Biol. Interact. **30**, 1–8 (1980).

Slor, H., Mizusawa, H., Neihart, N., Kakefunda, T., Day, R.S., Bustin, M.: Immunochemical visualization of binding of the chemical carcinogen benzo(a)pyrene diolepoxide 1 to the genome. Cancer Res. **41**, 3111–3117 (1981).

Snyder, R.D., Regan, J.D.: Quantitative estimation of the extent of alkylation of DNA following treatment of mammalian cells with non-radioactive alkylating agents. Mutat. Res. **91**, 307–314 (1981).

Sognier, M.A., Hittelman, W.N.: The repair of bleomycin induced DNA damage and its relationship to chromosome aberration repair. Mutat. Res. **62**, 517–528 (1979).

Staiano, N., Erickson, L.C., Thorgeirsson, S.S.: Bacterial mutagenesis and host cell DNA damage by chemical carcinogens in the Salmonella typhimurium hepatocyte system. Biochem. Biophys. Res. Commun. **94**, 837–842 (1980).

Stout, D.L., Becker, F.F.: Progressive DNA damage in hepatic nodules during 2 acetylamino fluorene carcinogenesis. Cancer Res. **40**, 1269–1273 (1980).

Sun, J.D., Dent, J.G.: A new method for measuring covalent binding of chemicals to cellular macromolecules. Chem.-Biol. Interact. **32**, 41–61 (1980).

Suzuki, F., Watanabe, E., Horikawa, M.: Repair of x-ray induced DNA damage in aging human diploid cells. Exp. Cell Res. **127**, 299–308 (1980).

Swenberg, J.A., Petzold, G.L., Harbach, P.R.: In vitro DNA damage alkaline elution assay for predicting carcinogenic potential. Biochem. Biophys. Res. Commun. **72**, 732–738 (1976).

Swenson, D.H., Farmer, P.B., Lawley, P.D.: Identification of the methylphospho-triester of thymidylyl (3'-5') thymidine as a product from reaction of DNA with the carcinogen N-methyl-N-nitrosourea. Chem.-Biol. Interact. **15**, 91–100 (1976).

Thomas, C.B., Osieka, R., Kohn, K.W.: Chloroethyl-3-4-methylcyclohexyl-1-nitroso-urea of sensitive and resistant human colon carcinoma xeno grafts in nude mice. Cancer Res. **38**, 2448–2454 (1978).

Tsapakos, M.J., Hampton, T.H., Jennette, K.W.: The carcinogen chromate induces DNA cross links in rat liver and kidney. J. Biol. Chem. **256**, 3623–3626 (1981).

Waring, M.J.: DNA modification and cancer. Ann. Rev. Biochem. **50**, 159–192 (1981).

Weniger, P.: An improved method to detect small amounts of radiation damage in DNA of eukaryotic cells. Int. J. Rad. Biol. **36**, 197–199 (1979).

Whiting, R.F., Stich, H.F., Koropatnick, D.J.: DNA damage and DNA repair in cultured human cells exposed to chromate. Chem.-Biol. Interact. **26**, 267–280 (1979).

Williams, J.R., Little, J.B., Shipley, W.U.: Association of mammalian cell death with a specific endonucleolytic degradation of DNA. Nature **252**, 754–755 (1974).

Winkle, S.A., Krugh, T.R.: Equilibrium binding of carcinogens and antitumor antibio-tics to DNA: site selectivity, cooperativity, allosterism. Nucl. Acids Res. **9**, 3175–3186 (1981).

Wisdom, G.B.: Enzyme immunoassay. Clin. Chem. **22**, 1243–1255 (1976).

Wood, A.W., Chang, R.L., Levin, W., Ryan, D.E., Thomas, P.E., Kehr, R.E., Kumas, S., Sardella, D.J., Boger, E., Yogi, H., Sayer, J.M., Jerina, D.M., Conney, A.H.: Mutagenicity of the bay-region diol-epoxides and other benzo-ring derivatives of dibenzo(a,h)pyrene and dibenzo(a,i)pyrene. Cancer Res. **41**, 2589–2597 (1981).

Yalow, R.S.: Radioimmunoassay: A probe for the fine structure of biologic systems. Science **200**, 1236–1245 (1978).

Zurlo, J., Longnecker, D.S., Cooney, D.A., Kuhlmann, E.T., Curphey, T.J.: Studies of pancreatic nodule induction and DNA damage by D-azaserine. Cancer Lett. **12**, 75–80 (1981).

Zwelling, L.A., Michaels, S., Erickson, L.C., Ungerleider, R.S., Nichols, M., Kohn, K.W.: Protein-associated deoxyribonucleic acid strand breaks in L-1210 cells treated with the deoxyribonucleic acid intercalating agents 4'-(9-acridinylamino)metha-nesulfon-m-anisidide and adriamycin. Biochemistry, in press (1982).

Zwelling, L.A., Michaels, S., Schwartz, H., Dobson, P.P., Kuhn, K.W.: DNA cross linking as an indicator of sensitivity and resistance of mouse L-1210 leukemia to cis di ammine dichloro platinum II and L-phenyl alanine mustard. Cancer Res. **41**, 640–649 (1981).

CHAPTER VI

MAMMALIAN CELL DNA REPAIR ASSAYS FOR CARCINOGENS

Charlene A. McQueen and Gary M. Williams
Naylor Dana Institute for Disease Prevention
American Health Foundation
1 Dana Road
Valhalla, New York 10595

A. INTRODUCTION

Two principal characteristics determine the usefulness of an *in vitro* short-term test: the nature of the biotransformation processes that are provided and the test end point that is measured. An ideal *in vitro* test for chemical carcinogens would be one that preserved *in vivo* parameters of xenobiotic metabolism and offered an end point that measures the critical action of chemicals that underlies their carcinogenicity.

Evaluation of the relevance of test end points must consider the likelihood that carcinogens operate by different mechanisms of action (Williams, 1979a,b). This concept is reflected in a classification of carcinogens in which carcinogens are divided into two major categories, DNA reactive (genotoxic) and epigenetic (Table 1). DNA reactive carcinogens are defined as those that are capable of damaging DNA through covalent interactions, while epigenetic carcinogens are designated as those that lack this property and produce another biological effect that could underlie their carcinogenicity (Weisburger and Williams, 1980; 1982). Short-term tests that measure genetic effects of chemicals are potentially capable of detecting genotoxic carcinogens, but will not respond to epigenetic carcinogens. Approaches to defining epigenetic agents have been discussed elsewhere (Williams, 1979a; 1980b; 1983).

A number of observations indicate that DNA is a critical target for the action of chemical carcinogens (Table 2). Therefore, tests for genotoxicity very likely measure, for one category of carcinogens, an action that is responsible for their carcinogenicity (Dunkel and Williams, 1981).

The genotoxic effects of chemicals can be detected by measuring their DNA interactions or determining the biochemical or biologic consequences of interaction such as DNA damage, inhibition of DNA synthesis, DNA repair, chromosomal effects, and mutagenesis. Only DNA damage tests actually measure the chemical effect that may initiate the neoplastic process. The techniques by which DNA damage can be detected have been reviewed (IARC, 1980; Larsen *et al.,* 1982). Those which have been applied to chemical screening include DNA fragmentation (Kohn, 1979), inhibition of DNA synthesis (Painter, 1978) and DNA repair (Stitch *et al.,* 1971; Flamm, 1973; Williams, 1976a). The three major types of DNA damage caused by chemical carcinogens, base damage, strand breakage and cross-linkage, all elicit DNA repair and therefore repair is an end point with a broad sensitivity for detecting genotoxic chemicals. Moreover, it is a specific response to DNA damage not produced by general toxic effects to the cell. The use of DNA repair as a screening test on a large scale reveals it to be an effective approach (Williams, 1980c; IARC, 1980; Mitchell *et al.,* 1983).

The types of DNA repair (i.e. photoreactivation, excision and postreplication) and the variety of ways in which these can be measured have been the subject of numerous detailed reviews (Lehmann and Bridges, 1977; Cleaver, 1978; Roberts, 1978; Hanawalt *et al.,* 1979; Setlow, 1980). The major types of DNA damage all elicit excision repair and, at present, only this type of repair has significant application to carcinogen screening.

Excision DNA repair in mammalian cells was first demonstrated in cultured cells (Rasmussen and Painter, 1964; 1966). Subsequently, it has also been measured in whole animals (Brash and Hart, 1978, Mirsalis and Butterworth, 1980), organ fragments (Reiss and Williams, 1978; Ishikawa *et al.,* 1980) and in cell free assays (Mattern and Cerutti, 1975; Ciarrocchi and Linn, 1978). Cultured cells, however, have been the system most widely used for screening tests (IARC, 1980) and only their application to carcinogen screening will be considered here. This restriction, however, does not imply that other approaches might not also prove to be useful for testing.

B. METHODS OF MEASURING
DNA EXCISION REPAIR

Two main types of excision repair are now recognized: nucleotide excision and base excision. These two types of repair correspond to the long patch and short patch repair described by Regan and Setlow (1974). Another type of excision repair has been described for removal of alkylated purines, specifically 0^6 methylguanine. A mammalian liver enzyme can transfer the methyl group from the 0^6 position of guanine to cysteine, regenerating guanine directly in DNA (Pegg and Perry, 1981; Pegg *et al.,* 1982).

Screening tests for carcinogens have been developed that utilize the capacity of mammalian cells for nucleotide or base excision. The initial process in each of these differs, but both result in incision of the DNA strand in the vicinity of the DNA damage, excision of a stretch of DNA containing the region of damage, synthesis of a patch and rejoining of the strand. Each of these processes can be used as a measure of the DNA damage produced by a chemical (Table 3).

The first process in base excision is the spontaneous or N-glycosylase-mediated removal of the damaged base. This is followed by the action of an apurinic-apyrimidinic endonuclease. The first step in nucleotide excision repair

TABLE 1
Classification of Carcinogenic Chemicals[a]

Category and Class	Example
A. *DNA-reactive Carcinogens*	
1. Activation-independent	Alkylating agent
2. Activation-dependent	Polycyclic aromatic hydrocarbon
	Nitrosamine
3a. Inorganic[b]	Metal
B. *Epigenetic Carcinogens*	
3b. Inorganic[b]	Metal
4. Solid state	Plastics
	Asbestos
5. Immunosuppressor	Purine analog
	Antibody
6. Cytotoxin	Nitrilotriacetic acid
7. Hormone	Estrogen
	Androgen
8. Peroxisone-proliferation	Elsfibrate
9. Promoter	Phorbol ester
	Bile acid
C. Unclassified	Methapyrilene

[a]After Weisburger and Williams (1980)
[b]Some are tentatively categorized as genotoxic because of evidence for damage of DNA; others may operate through epigenetic mechanisms such as alterations in fidelity of DNA polymerases.

is an endonuclease incision in the vicinity of the DNA damage, producing discontinuities in the DNA chain which can be measured as reduction in the size of either single or double strand DNA. The size of single strand DNA can be determined by alkaline sucrose gradient centrifugation (McGrath and Williams, 1966; Lett *et al.,*1967) or by alkaline elution from polyvinyl chloride filters (Kohn, 1979); the size of double strand DNA can be measured by neutral sucrose gradient centrifugation (Lange, 1974). Alkaline elution is a relatively simple technique for measuring single strand breaks and has been applied to chemical screening (Swenberg *et al.,* 1976; Brambilla *et al.,* 1978; Bradley *et al.,* 1982). When used as a measure of this step in DNA repair, reduction in the size of DNA due to strand incision may not be distinguished from nucleolytic degradation or mechanical fragmentation of DNA. Accordingly, Kohn (1979) has urged caution in the interpretation of results with alkaline elution since this technique reveals DNA breaks with presumably innocuous agents such as ascorbic acid and visible light.

The next process in repair is excision of a portion of DNA by an exonuclease. The amount of removal varies in extent depending upon the type of damage and the type of excision repair that is provoked (Regan and Setlow, 1974). Specific determination of excision requires measurement of a loss of bases from DNA (Mattern *et al.,* 1973) or a reduction in the amount of carcinogen adducts in DNA (Crathorn and Roberts, 1966; Lieberman and Dipple, 1972; Walker and

TABLE 2
Observations Indicating that DNA is a Critical Target for Carcinogens

1. Biochemical studies:
   Many carcinogens or their metabolites are electrophiles that react with DNA.
2. *In vitro* and *in vivo* studies:
   Many carcinogens produce DNA damage and are gene or chromosomal mutagens.
3. Genetic diseases:
   a. Individuals with DNA repair defects such as xeroderma pigmentosum have an increased risk of cancer development.
   b. Individuals with some types of chromosomal abnormalities such as trisomy 21 have an increased risk of cancer development.
4. Studies of tumor cells:
   a. Cancer is heritable at the cellular level.
   b. Cancer cells may have chromosomal abnormalities.
   c. Cancer cells may display aberrant gene expression.

Ewart, 1973). The latter is more frequently done, but to accomplish this either carcinogen labelled with a radioisotope or some other means of measuring the amount of adduct such as radioimmunoassay (Poirier and Yuspa, 1977), fluorimetric techniques (Daudal *et al.,* 1975), high performance liquid chromatography (Goodman, 1976; Jeffrey *et al.,* 1976) or mass spectral analysis (Wiebers *et al.,* 1981) is required. Where such measurements are possible, they are usually employed to determine adduct formation rather than repair. For the screening of biological samples or complex mixtures, neither adduct formation nor removal can readily be used. An alternate approach more applicable to

TABLE 3
Methods for Studying DNA Excision Repair in Cultured Cells[a]

Process Involved in Excision Repair	Technique
Incision in region of DNA damage	Alkaline sucrose gradients
	Alkaline elution
Excision of damaged region	Loss of damaged bases
	Mass spectral analysis
	Radioimmunoassay
	Loss of enzyme-sensitive sites
Resynthesis of excised region	^{3}H-thymidine incorporation autoradiography, liquid scintillation counting
	Isopycnic gradients
	Bromouracil photolysis
	BND-cellulose chromatography
Rejoining of strand	Alkaline sucrose gradients
	Alkaline elution

[a]After Williams, 1979b.

monitoring adduct removal is the measurement of the loss of sites sensitive to enzymes that incise DNA in the region of damage (Peterson, 1978). In this approach, damaged DNA is incubated with purified endonucleases, and the number of damaged sites is measured by the action of these enzymes in reducing the size of DNA, usually revealed by alkaline sucrose gradient centrifugation. DNA damage by several types of carcinogens has been detected in this manner (Duker and Teebor, 1976; Heflich *et al.*, 1977; Hecht and Thielmann, 1978; and Paterson, 1978). Thus, reduction in enzyme-sensitive sites could be used to monitor DNA repair. The major limitations of this technique at present are the requirement for the appropriate nuclease and the minimal information available on the susceptibility of different types of chemical damage to incision by nucleases in vitro.

Following the excision of damaged segments of DNA, patches are synthesized using the opposite strand as template. This process can be measured by incorporation of nucleotides into the newly synthesized DNA by a variety of techniques. Originally, repair synthesis in mammalian cells was demonstrated by autoradiographic incorporation of ^{3}H-thymidine as unscheduled DNA synthesis (UDS), that is, DNA synthesis that is not confined to the DNA replicative phase of the cell cycle (Rasmussen and Painter, 1964; Painter and Cleaver, 1969). This procedure still remains the most frequently used technique for assessing repair synthesis provoked by carcinogens. Autoradiographic measurement of repair offers the advantage that only a light nuclear labelling due to ^{3}H-thymidine incorporation during repair is produced and this is easily distinguished from the heavy nuclear labelling of replicative DNA synthesis. Autoradiographic UDS has been shown to correspond to repair synthesis in the nonreplicating strands of parental DNA (Cleaver, 1969; Roberts *et al.*, 1971).

UDS can also be measured by liquid scintillation counting of radioactive thymidine incorporation into the DNA of cells in which replicative DNA synthesis has been suppressed by hydroxyurea (Evans and Norman, 1968), arginine deficiency (Stich and San, 1970), or a combination of both (Trosko and Yager, 1974). The hydroxyurea block has been extensively used (Cleaver, 1969; Lieberman *et al.*, 1971; Smith and Hanawalt, 1976; Martin *et al.*, 1978). Some difficulties, however, may arise with this technique. Replicative DNA systhesis may not be completely arrested by hydroxyurea (Roberts *et al.*, 1971) resulting in a lack of certainty regarding the significance of increases above the persisting background. The sensitivity of this approach may be limited, since DNA damage will inhibit persisting replicative synthesis, and, thus, repair will not become evident until the repair synthesis results in enough thymidine incorporation to equal the inhibited replicative synthesis and thereby exceed the control level. Another complication of this method is that hydroxyurea suppression of replicative DNA synthesis can be interfered with by other chemicals (Brandt *et al.*, 1972) resulting in a restoration of replicative synthesis which can be confused with repair. Finally, under some conditions, hydroxyurea has induced DNA repair (Clarkson, 1978; Andrae and Greim, 1979). Hydroxyurea has also been used to inhibit DNA synthesis for autoradiographic measurement of UDS (Lieberman *et al.*, 1971), but suffers from the same uncertainty regarding the determination.

Several definitive techniques which are not subject to confusion with replicative synthesis are available for assessing repair synthesis. Incorporation of the thymidine analog, 5-bromodeoxyuridine, into regions of repair does not significantly alter the density of parental DNA while newly replicated DNA will become denser due to more extensive incorporation. Because of the difference in density then, parental and replicated DNA can be separated on density gradients. Additional incorporation of either radioactive thymidine or 5-bromodeoxyuridine into the isolated parental DNA provides a measure of repair synthesis (Pettijohn and Hanawalt, 1964; Rasmussen and Painter, 1966; Roberts et al., 1968). Other elegant techniques for estimating the extent of repair involve the photolysis of 5-bromodeoxyuridine incorporated during repair (Regan et al., 1971) and the measurement of thymidine incorporation into DNA growing points which are retained on benzoylated naphthoylated DEAE-cellulose columns because of their single stranded regions (Scudiero et al., 1975). Despite their precision, these definitive techniques have not found wide usage in screening because of their more demanding technical requirements. Nevertheless, these techniques could be used on a select basis to confirm or extend results obtained in a general screening test. Furthermore, techniques that permit measurement of incorporation of precursors other than thymidine (Lieberman et al., 1971; Cleaver, 1973; McQueen and Williams, 1979; Andrae and Schwarz, 1981) may be important for detecting compounds that under some conditions produce specific types of repair (Hennings and Michael, 1976) or which might somehow block thymidine utilization during repair synthesis.

The final process in excision repair is rejoining of the strand by a ligase. This process can be followed by observing the restoration of fragmented DNA to full length using gradient centrifugation techniques (Lett et al., 1971; Omerod and Stevens, 1971; Michael and Williams, 1974) or alkaline elution (Bradley et al., 1978).

In addition to these biochemical techniques, repair can also be monitored by biological determinations. Techniques of this type include the reactivation of UV-irradiated DNA viruses (Day, 1974) and the enhancement of viral transformation of mammalian cells (Hirai et al., 1974, Casto et al., 1976). Although conceptually very intriguing, these approaches are rather involved for general screening. Nevertheless, their sensitivity is greater than that of direct measurements of DNA repair, and they could serve as a further step in the testing of a compound that was negative in standard assays.

Evaluation of all the approaches to the measurement of DNA repair has led to the conclusion that autoradiographic measurement of UDS is the most appropriate technique for screening (IARC, 1980). The EPA Gene-Tox review of the usefulness of DNA repair assays other than UDS also concluded that these techniques were less suitable for screening (Larsen, et al., 1982). Autoradiographic measurement of UDS is simple and reliable and also affords a quantification of the fraction of cells responding.

The quantification of repair synthesis has differed in an important regard from that used for other screening end points. For example, in mutagenesis or transformation studies, a cell or its colony-forming progeny is scored as either positive or negative and the data are expressed as the number of positive cells or their fraction in the popualtion. In contrast, DNA repair is usually quantified as the average response for the whole population, including both positive and negative cells. With this approach, repair in a fraction of cells comparable to that of induced mutation incidences (e.g. 100 per 10^6 cells) would probably not yield a significantly increased average. Fortunately, because DNA damage occurs at many sites throughout the genome and thus repair is a more general response than mutation or transformation, a greater fraction of cells engage in repair of chemical damage and positive results are recognized. Nevertheless, the sensitivity of autoradiographic UDS assays could be greatly increased by developing means of expressing the data that are similar to those used for other assays i.e., the fraction of responding cells.

C. CULTURED MAMMALIAN CELL TYPES FOR MEASURING DNA REPAIR

A variety of cell types from all species examined have been found to be capable of carrying out DNA repair (Table 4). Certain cell types are deficient in the ability to remove specific lesions from their DNA (Rajewsky et al., 1977) but, with the exception of human repair-deficient mutants, no species has been documented to be generally incapable of repairing DNA damage. Therefore, almost any cell type could in principle be used for screening. The usefulness of cell types for detection of carcinogens by DNA repair, however, is determined by two properties: 1) the activity of repair, and the status of replicative DNA synthesis, which obscures DNA repair in the cell type, and 2) the capability of the cell type to carry out biotransformation of chemicals requiring metabolism in order to exert their biologic effects.

The level of activity of excision repair processes in different cell types has been the subject of relatively few studies apart from those concerned with repair-deficient mutants. Certain post-replicative, differentiated cells have been reported to be incapable of DNA repair, leading to the concept that excision repair is most active in proliferating cells (Cleaver 1978). In some of the relevant studies, repair synthesis was monitored by thymidine (TdR) incorporation and the failure to observe it is attributable to poor utilization of TdR rather than inactive repair. Furthermore, it is clear that some nonreplicating cells, such as hepatocytes, have active repair systems both in vivo (Damjanov et al., 1973) and in vitro (Williams, 1976a). Species-dependent (Hart and Setlow, 1974; Maslansky and Williams, 1985) and age-dependent (Mattern and Cerutti, 1975) differences in the capability of cells to repair damage produced by radiation have been reported. However, in studies of repair of chemical damage, human HeLa cells and Chinese hamster V79 cells displayed the same amount of repair synthesis at equal levels of DNA damage by three alkylating carcinogens (Roberts et al., 1971) and rodent cells were as active as human cells in removing the DNA adducts of N-acetoxyacetyl-aminofluorene (Amacher et al., 1977). Although a recent extensive study (Kato et al., 1980) failed to confirm the correlation between repair potential and life span previously reported (Hart and Setlow, 1974), the experimental conditions between the two studies were not identical. Thus, current knowledge of species capabilities of repair of DNA damage by chemical carcinogens does not dictate the use of any specific species.

The cell types that have been used in most repair studies are proliferating lines, and, consequently, inhibition of replicative DNA synthesis has been necessary in the use of these cells. The techniques employed for this purpose have included hydroxyurea suppression of DNA synthesis (Evans and Norman, 1968; Lieberman et al., 1971), arginine deprivation (Stich and San, 1970; Casto et al., 1976) or a combination of both (Trosko and Yager, 1974). A severe limitation of these approaches is their inability to completely inhibit replicative DNA synthesis (Evans and Norman, 1968), leaving a variable background against which DNA repair must be evaluated. In addition, the possibility that the test compound may release the block, as Brandt et al. (1972) have shown, is always present. Thus, efforts have been made to obtain cell culture systems that do not engage in replicative DNA synthesis. Two such systems are lymphocytes (Evans and Norman, 1968; Lieberman et al., 1971; Gaudin et al., 1971; Mene-ghini, 1974) and hepatocytes (Williams, 1976a, 1977; Michalopoulos et al., 1978; Casciano et al, 1978; Yager and Miller, 1978). An advantage of using lymphocytes is that these cells can be obtained from both experimental animals and humans. The use of human cells is complicated, however, by the genetic heterogeneity of the donor population. Other factors such as age and sex have been shown to contribute to inter-individual variation in DNA repair in lymphocytes following exposure to DNA damaging agents (Pero et al., 1978; Pero and Ostlund, 1980). Nonreplicative hepatocytes can also be readily prepared from several species (Renton et al., 1978; Decad et al., 1979; Poiley et al., 1979; Klaunig et al., 1981a, b; Maslansky and Williams, 1981, 1982; McQueen et al., 1981a, 1982; Reese and Byard, 1981) and recently human cells have been prepared (Reese and Byard, 1981; Strom et al., 1982; Maekubo et al., 1982). Hepatocytes have found wider usage than lymphocytes mainly because of their intrinsic capacity for biotransformation.

Most DNA-reactive chemical carcinogens require metabolic activation by enzyme systems in order to exert their carcinogenic effects (Weisburger and Williams, 1982), and therefore, in addition to the relevence and reliability of the end point, another critical property determining the usefulness of a cell culture system for carcinogen detection is its capability for enzymatic activation of carcinogens. Unfortunately, virtually all culture systems are markedly deficient in biotransformation capability and thus respond to few activation-dependent carcinogens (San and Stich, 1975). To overcome this limitation such cell types require the addition of exogenous enzyme preparation to achieve significant metabolism (San and Stich, 1975; Martin et al., 1978). While this approach is valid, it is not particularly useful in the situation in which the DNA repair test is to be used as part of a screening battery (Williams, 1980a). The reason for this relates to the fact that bacterial mutagenesis assays are included in most test batteries because these tests are among the most sensitive and have shown a high correlation with carcinogenicity. Bacterial mutagenesis assays utilize enzyme preparations and therefore a DNA repair test that is dependent upon an enzyme preparation for metabolism provides no possible extension of biotransformation in such a battery.

Liver has the broadest capability for carcinogen metabolism (Weisburger and Williams, 1982) and for this reason liver culture systems were developed for carcinogen detection (Williams, 1976b). Evidence has been presented for activation of carcinogens by rat liver epithelial lines (Williams et al., 1973; Montesano et al., 1973; Tong and Williams, 1978), but, in particular, the hepatocyte primary culture system (Williams, 1976a; 1977; 1978) has been documented to preserve a broad intrinsic activation capability, as well as to retain the detoxification pathways that predominate in vivo. Thus, hepatocyte metabolism preserves similarities to that of the in vivo organ (Vadi et al., 1975; Billings et al., 1977; Yih and van Rossum, 1977; Schmeltz et al., 1978; McQueen et al., 1982; Williams, 1979a; Bates et al., 1981). By possessing a balanced enzymatic capability, hepatocyte primary cultures offer a system in which positive results greatly strengthen those obtained in bacterial mutagenesis assays supplemented with a subcellular enzyme preparation. Nevertheless, use of freshly isolated cells from other organs, such as colon (Freeman and San, 1980) may have specific applications to the study of organ selective carcinogens.

In summary, of the many cell types that have been studied, hepatocytes in primary culture have been recognized as being potentially the most useful for a DNA repair test to be included in a screening battery for chemical carcinogens (IARC, 1980; Mitchell et al., 1983; Andrae, 1984).

D. HEPATOCYTE PRIMARY CULTURE/DNA REPAIR TEST

Hepatocytes were developed as a screening system primarily in the expectation that they would retain the extensive ability of liver to metabolize chemical carcinogens. Hepatocytes in primary culture have indeed been found to possess a broad capability for xenobiotic biotransofrmation (Borek and Williams, 1980; Harris and Cornell, 1983). In addition, hepatocytes in primary cell culture have the advantage, unlike other cell types, that in the first 24 hours in culture less than 0.1% of the cells enter S-phase (Williams, 1976a; Laishes and Williams, 1976). With autoradiography, these few S-phase cells are easily indentified by their extensive incorporation of ^{3}H-thymidine during replicative DNA synthesis. These heavily labelled nuclei are excluded when the amount of DNA repair is quantified. Thus, inhibitors of replicative DNA synthesis such as hydroxyurea, do not have to be used in order to measure DNA repair in hepatocytes by autoradiographic techniques. However, despite the low level of cell replication in hepatocytes in primary culture, incorporation of ^{3}H-thymidine is still sufficient to require the use of hydroxyurea in techniques that do not distinguish DNA replication from DNA repair.

The original procedure described for the determination of DNA repair

TABLE 4
Cultured Cell Types Demonstrating DNA Repair[a]

Cell Type	Author
Human	
HeLa	Rasmussen and Painter (1964)
	Crathorn and Roberts (1966)
lymphocytes	Evans and Norman (1968)
	Lieberman et al. (1971)
fibroblasts	Stich and San (1970)
WI38	Lieberman and Poirier (1973)
	Mattern and Cerutti (1975)
AV$_3$ amnion	Trosko and Yager (1974)
RAJI lymphoblastoid	Scudiero et al. (1975)
primary hepatocytes	Strom et al. (1982)
	Reese and Byard (1981)
Nonhuman primate	
tree shrew lung	Kato et al. (1980)
macaque lung	Kato et al. (1980)
Mouse	
L fibroblasts	Reid and Walker (1969)
	Horikawa et al. (1972)
	Saito and Andoh (1973)
lymphoma L5178Y	Ormerod and Stevens (1971)
	Lange (1974)
Ehrlich ascites tumor 3T3	Lieberman and Poirier (1974)
skin fibroblasts	Hart and Setlow (1974)
embryo fibroblast C57BL/6J	Shinohara and Cerutti (1977)
primary hepatocytes	Maslansky and Williams (1981)
Rat	
Yoshida sarcoma cells	Ball and Roberts (1970)
liver epithelial cells	Michael and Williams (1974)
skin fibroblasts	Hart and Setlow (1974)
primary hepatocytes	Williams (1976a)
Hamster	
DFAF-33	Rasmussen and Painter (1964)
V79	Elkind and Kamper (1970)
	Roberts et al. (1971)
fibroblasts	Stich and San (1970)
skin fibroblasts	Hart and Setlow (1974)
embryo	Casto et al. (1976)
BHK 21	Stich and San (1970)
	Shinohora and Cerutti (1977)
primary hepatocytes	Maslansky and Williams (1981)
Rabbit	
Japanese hare lung	Kato et al. (1980)
primary hepatocytes	McQueen et al. (1982)

[a]After IARC Monograph, Supplement 2, 1980.

TABLE 5
Rat Hepatocyte Primary Culture/NDA Repair Test

Chemical Class	Carcinogen +	Carcinogen −	Non Carcinogen +	Non Carcinogen −	Unknown +	Unknown −
Alkylating Agents	5					
Polycyclic Aromatic Hydrocarbons	6		5			
Monocyclic Aromatic Amines	3	1				
Polycyclic Aromatic Amines and Amides	8	1	3	2		
Aminoazo Dyes	5					
Nitro-substituted Compounds	3	2		2	3	
Aza Aromatics	2		2	2	1	
Nitrosamines	7	1		3		
Mycotoxins	7	1		1		4
Pyrrolizidine Alkaloids	4				1	4
Intercalating Agents						5
TOTAL	50	6	0	16	7	13

produced in hepatocytes by carcinogens was that of autoradiographic measurement of UDS (Williams, 1976a), but DNA repair could in principle be monitored by any of the other techniques described above. Repair has, in fact, also been measured by ^{3}H-thymidine incorporation into acid precipitable macromolecules (Williams, 1978; Michalopoulos et al., 1978). As discussed, this approach is complicated by a fairly high background even in the presence of hydroxyurea suppression of replicative synthesis and, therefore, entails a lack of certainty regarding the significance of increased precipitable counts. The background can be reduced by isolating nuclei before acid precipitation of macromolecules (Althaus et al., 1982) or by isolating DNA on cesium chloride gradients (Machalopoulos et al., 1978; Oldham et al., 1980). This, however, does not eliminate the background due to replicative DNA synthesis, and thus, is still limited in specificity. Because of the background problem, positive results obtained by liquid scintillation counting techniques should always be confirmed by a more definitive procedure. With the autoradiographic determination of UDS, this is unnecessary and therefore it still appears to be the simplest technique for screening with hepatocytes.

The UDS produced in hepatocytes by UV or chemicals has been shown to be repair synthesis in density-labelled strands of parental DNA isolated by sodium iodide gradients (Yager and Miller, 1978) or cesium chloride density gradient centrifugation (McQueen and Williams, 1979, 1981b; Andrae and Schwarz, 1981). If the use of gradients for measurement of repair in hepatocytes is desired, the additional step of isolating parental DNA can be taken. This has the major advantage of completely eliminating replicative synthesis as the basis of incorporation and thereby provides high specificity. Furthermore, the sensitivity of the measurement can be increased by using radioactive deoxycytidine in place of thymidine for incorporation (McQueen and Williams, 1979; Andrae and Schwarz, 1981). This procedure is recommended as a second stage test for further study of chemicals negative in the primary screen.

Variations in the use of hepatocytes for repair have included the use of suspensions of freshly isolated hepatocytes (Nordenskjold et al., 1978; Michalopoulos et al., 1978; Brouns et al., 1979; Hsia and Kreamer, 1979) or cultures of longer duration on collagen membranes (Michalopoulos et al., 1978). Neither of these methods permits the simple autoradiographic measurement of repair synthesis. Furthermore, suspensions are mixtures of living and dead cells with very short survival periods. These limitations, therefore, make the primary culture system preferable for repair studies.

The protocol for the hepatocyte primary culture/DNA repair (HPC/DNA repair) test commences with the initiation of primary cultures of freshly dissociated hepatocytes on coverslips (Williams, 1976a, 1977). Since it is essential that hepatocytes of high initial viability be used, the percentage of cells excluding trypan blue is determined immediately following cell isolation. Only cell preparations having a viability greater than 80% are used. The techniques established for dissociation of rat liver (Williams et al., 1977; Williams et al., 1982) produce a selective recovery of hepatocytes and have been applied to mouse, hamster and rabbit with equally good results (Maslansky and Williams, 1981, 1982; McQueen et al., 1981, 1982). The dissociated hepatocytes are allowed 1.5 hours to attach in culture, which permits attachment of only viable cells (Williams et al., 1977). The cultures are washed to remove unattached cells and then exposed to the test compound plus ^{3}H-thymidine for incorporation during repair synthesis (Williams, 1977, 1978). After this, the cultures are washed and processed for autoradiography. The UDS is quantified as the net nuclear grains counted with an electronic counter with a microscopic attachment (Williams, 1978). The protocol has been described in detail (Williams et al., 1982).

In the HPC/DNA repair test the total nuclear grains are counted first by focusing the aperture of the counter on the nucleus and obtaining the digital count. Then the aperture is moved to three regions of the cytoplasm and the cytoplasmic background is recorded. Originally, the background counts were averaged and subtracted from the nuclear counts to obtain the net nuclear grains (Williams, 1976a). This procedure frequently resulted in a slight positive value for the nucleus. Since that seemed unrealistic and might bias the results with test compounds in favor of a positive result, the procedure was modified to that of subtracting the highest cytoplasmic background count from the nuclear count (Williams, 1978). This procedure resulted in a zero or net negative value for the nuclei of nonexposed hepatocytes and seemed more appropriate because it would not suggest a low level of repair (i.e. slight positive nuclear value) in nonexposed hepatocytes and, if anything, would slightly reduce the number of nuclear grains attributed to repair in exposed cultures.

The cytoplasmic background is the only significant problem that arises in the

TABLE 6
Evaluation of Drugs in the Rat Hepatocyte Primary Culture/DNA Repair Test

Drug	Carcinogenicity[a]	DNA Repair[a]
Pyrilamine maleate	U	+
Tripelennamine HCl	U	+
Hydralazine	+	+
Reserpine	+	−
Nicotinamide	U	−
Natulan	+	−
Cytoxan	+	−
Clofibrate	+	−
Nafenopen	+	−
Phenoazopyridine	U	−
Methapyrilene	+	−
Phenobarbital	+	−
Acetaminophen	−	−

[a] + = positive; − = negative; U = unknown.

conduct of this test. Several lines of evidence from both *in vivo* and *in vitro* studies with liver indicate that some radioactivity either in the form of thymidine or by tritium exchange is nonspecifically bound to various macromolecules (Yager and Miller, 1978). Another source could be incorporation into mitochondrial DNA (Lonati-Galligani *et al.*, 1983). Various measures such as isolation of DNA on gradients, isolation of nuclei or limiting ^{3}H-thymidine (Michalopoulous *et al.*, 1978; Williams and Laspia, 1979; Oldham *et al.*, 1980; Althaus, *et al.*, 1982) have been applied to reduce cytoplasmic background. However, even when it is high in autoradiographs, it does not impede the quantification of repair synthesis.

The recommended approach to screening is to test the compound over a range of concentrations separated by a factor of 10 from 10^{-1} molar (or the limit of solubility) down to 10^{-7} molar for 18 to 20 hours. An appropriate positive control, negative control, solvent control, and untreated cell control are included in each experiment. If a compound elicits repair, it should be rerun at the most active concentration and one concentration above and below that separated by a factor of 5. A negative compound should be rerun twice at doses up to the highest nontoxic doses to assure that adequate testing of cell preparations that are potentially different in metabolic capability has been conducted. Negative results are acceptable only when the positive controls are active.

Numerous carcinogens and noncarcinogens have been examined in the HPC/DNA repair test (Table 5). The correlation between UDS and carcinogenicity has been excellent. Reports from several other laboratories have confirmed these results (Michalopoulos *et al.*, 1978; Casciano *et al.*, 1978; Yager and Miller, 1978; Probst *et al.*, 1980, 1981). Over 250 chemicals of a variety of structural classes have now been tested (Williams, 1981a; Probst *et al.*, 1981; Williams *et al.*, 1982), establishing the usefulness of this test for screening.

A series of drugs including some that have been carcinogenic in animals has been evaluated in the HPC/DNA repair test (Table 6). Three drugs, pyrilamine maleate, tripelennamine HCl and hydralazine, induced DNA repair. An increased tumor incidence has been observed in mice receiving hydralazine (Toth, 1978). No data are available on the carcinogenicity of pyrilamine maleate and tripelennamine HCl. Several drugs such as phenobarbital and clofibrate which have produced neoplasms in rodent liver were negative (Williams, 1981b). Since these drugs are not mutagenic (Hollstein et al., 1979; Warren, 1980; Williams, 1980b) and did not induce DNA repair, they are thought to be epigenetic rather than genotoxic carcinogens (Williams, 1981b; 1983). Natulan, which did not induce DNA repair, has also been reported as negative in the standard Ames test using rat liver S-9 (Williams et al., 1982). In mouse and hamster hepatocytes, however, natulan was positive (McQueen et al., 1983).

E. CONCLUSIONS

DNA repair is a valuable end point for evaluation of chemical genotoxicity because it is a specific indicator of damage to DNA. It is not mimicked by any other toxic effect of chemicals. Therefore, the only concern in the interpretation of positive results is whether the method used is a reliable measurement of DNA repair. As discussed, autoradiographic measurement of UDS and techniques for demonstrating incorporation into parental DNA are reliable techniques.

A positive result in a reliable DNA repair assay is of considerable significance. The production of DNA repair indicates that the chemical is capable of producing covalent damage to DNA. Thus far, all chemicals that have been reported to elicit DNA repair are reliably carcinogenic. It is perhaps premature to suggest that production of DNA repair is a certain indication of carcinogenicity, although it seems highly probable that this could be true. The available data at present do support the suggestion (Williams, 1979b) that all chemicals that are mutagenic in bacterial tests and produce DNA repair in hepatocytes are carcinogenic. With these two systems, the balanced profile of metabolism performed by hepatocytes in particular, strengthens results in a test using a subcellular enzyme preparation, adding greater certainty to the significance of positive results in both. Considering the critical need to effectively allocate resources in carcinogen testing, it is, therefore, recommended that chemicals positive in both the Ames Salmonella/microsome test and HPC/DNA repair test either be considered carcinogens or, if further testing is desired, be submitted only to the limited in vivo bioassays recommended in the decision point approach to carcinogen testing (Weisburger and Williams, 1978; Williams and Weisburger, 1981).

Carcinogens may not elicit DNA repair for several reasons apart from simple technical failures of the test. The most obvious reason would be if the test system did not provide the required enzymatic activation of the chemical. This could occur with the HPC/DNA repair test in the case of activation-dependent carcinogens that require an activation step not performed by liver. One such chemical is dinitrotoluene which is primarily metabolized in rats by intestinal bacteria (Guest *et al.*, 1982). Dinitrotoluene did not induce DNA repair in hepatocytes in primary culture (Bermudez *et al.*, 1979), although DNA repair was observed in hepatocytes isolated after *in vivo* chemical exposure (Mirsalis and Butterworth, 1982). However, other nitroaromatics, including 4-nitrobiphenyl, were positive in the HPC/DNA repair test (Table 5) indicating that liver can activate some compounds of this type.

The capability of the HPC/DNA repair test to detect genotoxic chemicals can be extended to include the role of bacterial metabolism, by supplementation of the culture medium with specific enzymes (Williams *et al.*, 1981). Since the test can be performed with hepatocytes from a variety of species, and relatively few carcinogens do not affect to some extent the liver of either mice, rats, rabbits or hamsters, the number of compounds which are negative due to lack of activation is anticipated to be small.

Another cause for negative results is DNA interactions that do not provoke repair. An example of this is pure intercalating agents, but the number of these is small and the few that are tumorigenic produce neoplasms in low yield, generally locally upon subcutaneous injection. Thus, this type of chemical does not represent a significant limitation of DNA repair tests. To the contrary, the inability of certain bacterial mutagens such as intercalating agents and base analogs to elicit DNA repair may be considered an advantage of DNA repair tests in identifying bacterial mutagens that may not be reliably carcinogenic.

The most important reason for negative results is that some carcinogens apparently do not interact with DNA (Williams, 1980a, 1980b); that is, are not genotoxic. Such carcinogens are suggested to operate through epigenetic mechanisms and would be true negatives in short-term tests for genetic effects. Evidence has been presented that certain organochlorine hepatocarcinogens that have been negative in bacterial mutagenesis tests are also negative in the HPC/DNA repair test (Williams, 1979a; 1980b; Probst *et al.*, 1981). Certain carcinogenic drugs, as presented above, also appear to be non-genotoxic. For several of these organochlorine compounds and drugs, *in vivo* studies suggest that they produce liver tumors through a promoting action (Williams, 1981b; 1983; Williams and Numoto, 1984). The number of carcinogens accepted as epigenetic is expected to increase and it is important to recognize that they are not "false negatives" reflecting a limitation of short-term tests. Rather, the short-term tests provide information on the mechanism of action of such chemicals.

REFERENCES

Althaus, F.R., Lawrence, S.D., Sattler, G.L., Longfellow, D.G., Pitot, H.C.: Chemical quantification of unscheduled DNA synthesis in cultured hepatocytes as an assay for the rapid screening of potential chemical carcinogens. Cancer Res. **42**, 3010–3015 (1982).

Amacher, D.E., Eliott, J.A., Lieberman, M.W.: Differences in removal of acetylamino-fluorene and pyrimidine dimers from the DNA of cultured mammalian cells. Proc. Nat. Acad. Sci. USA) **74**, 1553–1557 (1977).

Andrae, U.: The DNA repair test with isolated hepatocytes. In: Critical Evaluation of Mutagenicity Testing, Bas, R., Gloclain, V., Grosdanoff, P., Henschler, D. Kolbey, B. Muller, D. and Neubert, N. (eds.) pp. 371–378, Munchen: MMV Medizen Verlag (1984).

Andrae, U., Greim, H.: Induction of DNA repair replication by hydroxyurea in human lymphoblastoid cells. Biochem. Biophys. Res. Comm. **87**, 50–58 (1979).

Andrae, U., Schwarz, L.R.: Induction of DNA repair synthesis in isolated rat hepatocytes by 5-diazouracil and other DNA damaging compounds. Cancer Lett. **13**, 187–193 (1981).

Ball, C.F., Roberts, J.J.: DNA repair after mustard gas alkylating by sensitive and resistant yoshida sarcoma cells *in vitro*. Chem. Biol. Interactions **2**, 321–329 (1970).

Bates, D.J., Foster, A.B., Jarman, M.: The metabolism of cyclophosphamide by isolated rat hepatocytes. Biochem. Pharmacol. **30**, 3055–3063 (1981).

Bermudez, E., Tillery, D., Butterworth, B. The effect of 2,4-diaminotoluene and isomers of dinitrotoluene on unscheduled DNA synthesis in primary rat hepatocytes. Environ. Mutagen. **1**, 391–398, 1979.

Billings, R.E., McMahon, R.E., Ashmore, J., Wagle, S.R.: The metabolism of drugs in isolated rat hepatocytes. Drug Metab. Dispo. **5**, 518–526 (1977).

Borek, C., Williams, G.M.: Differentiation and Carcinogenesis in Liver Cell Cultures. Annals of The New York Academy of Sciences, Vol. **349** (1980).

Bradley, M.O., Dysart, G., Fitzsimmons, K., Harbach, P., Lewin, J., Wolf, G.: Measurement by filter elution of DNA single- and double-strand breaks in rat hepatocytes: Effects of nitrosamines and γ-irradiation. Cancer Res. **42**, 2569–2597 (1982).

Bradley, M.O., Erickson, L.C., Kohn, K.W.: Non-enzymatic DNA strand breaks induced in mammalian cells by fluorescent light. Biochem. Biophys. Acta **590**, 11–20 (1978).

Brambilla, G., Caranna, M., Parodi, S.: Evaluation of DNA damage and repair in mammalian cells exposed to chemicals carcinogens. Pharmacol. Res. Commun. **10**, 693–717 (1978).

Brandt, W.N., Flamm, W.G., Bernheim, N.J.: The value of hydroxyurea in assessing repair synthesis of DNA in HeLa cells. Chem. Biol. Interact. **5**, 527–339 (1972).

Brash, D.E., Hart, R.W.: DNA damage and repair *in vivo*. J. Environ. Pathol. Toxicol. **2**, 79–114 (1978).

Brouns, R.E., Poot, M., de Vrind, R., v. Hoek-Kon, Th., Henderson, P.Th.: Measurement of DNA-excision repair in suspensions of freshly isolated rat hepatocytes after exposure to some carcinogenic compounds. Mutat. Res. **64**, 425–432 (1979).

Casciano, D.A., Farr, J.A., Oldham, J.W., Cave, M.D.: 2-acetylaminofluorene-induced unscheduled DNA synthesis in hepatocytes isolated from 3-methylcholanthrene treated rats. Cancer Lett. **5**, 173–178 (1978).

Casto, B.C., Pieczymski, W.J., Janosko, N., DiPaolo, J.A.: Significance of treatment interval and DNA repair in the enhancement of viral transformation by chemical carcinogens and mutagens. Chem. Biol. Interact. **13**, 105–125 (1976).

Ciarrocchi, G., Linn, S.: A cell-free assay measuring repair DNA synthesis in human fibroblasts. Proc. Natl. Acad. Sci. (USA) **75**, 1887–1891. (1978).

Cleaver, J.E.: Repair replication of mammalian cell DNA: effects of compounds that inhibit DNA synthesis or dark repair. Radiation Res. **37**, 334–348 (1969).

Cleaver, J.E.: DNA repair and its coupling to DNA replication in eukaryotic cells. Biochem. Biophys. Acta **516**, 487–516 (1978).

Cleaver, J.E.: DNA repair with purines and pyrimidines in radiation and carcinogen-damaged normal and xeroderma pigmentosum human cells. Cancer Res. **33**, 362–369 (1973).

Clarkson, J.M.: Enhancement of repair replication in mammalian cells by hydroxyurea. Mut. Res. **52**, 273–284 (1978).

Crathorn, A.R., Roberts, J.J.: Mechanism of the cytotoxic action of alkylating agents in mammalian cells and evidence for the removal of alkylated groups from deoxyribonucleic acid. Nature **211**, 150–153 (1966).

Damjanov, I., Cox, R., Sarma, D.S.R., Farber, E.: Patterns of damage and repair of liver DNA induced by carcinogenic methylating agents *in vivo*. Cancer Res. **35**, 1773–1778, (1973).

Daudel, P., Duquesne, M., Vigny, P., Grover, P.L., Sims, P.: Fluorescence spectral evidence that benzo(a)pyrene-DNA products in mouse skin arise from diol-epoxides. FEBS Lett. **57**, 250–253 (1975).

Day, R.S.: Studies on repair of adenovirus 2 by human fibroblasts using normal, xeroderma pigmentosum, and xeroderma pigmentosum heterozygous strains. Cancer Res. **34**, 1965–1970 (1974).

Decad, G.M., Dougherty, K.K., Hsieh, D.P.H., Byard, J.L.: Metabolism of aflatoxin B_1 in cultured mouse hepatocytes: comparison with rat and effects of cyclohexene oxide and diethylmaleate. Toxicol. Appl. Pharmacol. **50**, 429–436 (1979).

Duker, N.J., Teebor, G.W.: Detection of different types of damage in alkylated DNA by means of human corrective endonuclease (correndonuclease). Proc. Nat. Acad. Sci. (USA) **73**, 2629–2633 (1976).

Dunkel, V., Williams, G.M.: Biological significance of endpoints in *in vitro* test systems for carcinogenecity and mutagenicity. In: Proceedings of the Third Life Sciences Symposium on Health Risk Analysis, Richmond, C.R., Walsh, P.J., Copenhauer, E.D. (eds.), pp. 237–247, Philadelphia: The Franklin Press (1981).

Elkind, M.M., Kamper, C.: Two forms of repair of DNA in mammalian cells following irradiation. Biophysical J., **10**, 237–245 (1970).

Evans, R.G., Norman, A.: Radiation stimulated incorporation of thymidine into the DNA of human lymphocytes. Nature **217**, 455–456 (1968).

Flamm, W.G.: The role of repair in environmental mutagenesis. Environ. Health Persp. **6**, 215–220 (1973).

Freeman, H.J., San, R.H.: Use of unscheduled DNA synthesis in freshly isolated human intestinal mucosal cells for carcinogen detection. Cancer Res. **40**, 3155–3157 (1980).

Gaudin, D., Gregg, R.S., Yielding, K.L.: DNA repair inhibition: a possible mechanism of action of co-carcinogens. Biochem. Biophys. Res. Comun. **45**, 630–636 (1971).

Goodman, J.I.: Separation of the products of the reaction of deoxyguanosine with N-acetyoxy-2-acetylaminofluorene by high pressure liquid chromatography. Anal. Biochem. **70**, 203–207 (1976).

Guest, D., Schnell, S.R., Rickert, D.E., Dent, J.G.: Metabolism of 2,4-dinitrotoluene by intestinal microorganisms from rat, mouse and man. Toxicol. Appl. Pharmacol. **64**, 160–168 (1982).

Hanawalt, P., Cooper, P., Ganesan, A. Smith, C.: DNA repair in bacteria and mammalian cells. Ann. Rev. Biochem. **48**, 783–836 (1979).

Harris, R.A. and Cornell, N.W.: Isolation, Characterization and Use of Hepatocytes, Elsevier Science Publishing Co. (1983).

Hart, R.W., Setlow, R.B.: Correlation between deoxyribonucleic acid excision-repair and life-span in a number of mammalian species. Proc. Nat. Acad. Sci. (USA), **71,** 2169–2173 (1974).

Hecht, R., Theilmann, H.W.: Purification and characterization of an endonuclease from micrococcus luteus that acts on depurinated and carcinogen-modified DNA. Eur. J. Biochem. **89,** 607–618 (1978).

Heflich, R.H., Dorney, D.J., Maher, V.M., McCormick, J.J.: Reactive derivatives of benzo(a)pyrene and 7,12-dimethyl-benz(a)anthracene cause S_1 nuclease sensitive sites in DNA and "UV-like" repair. Biochem. Biophys. Res. Comm. **77,** 634–641 (1977).

Hennings, H., Michael, D.: Guanine-specific DNA repair after treatment of mouse skin cells with N-methyl-N'nitro-N-nitrosoguanidine. Cancer Res. **36,** 2321–2325 (1976).

Hirai, K., Defendi, V., Diamond, L.: Enhancement of Simian virus 40 transformation and integration by 4-nitroquinolin-1-oxide. Cancer Res. **34,** 3497–3500 (1974).

Hollstein, M., McCann, J., Angelosanto, F.A., Nichols, W.W.: Short-term tests for carcinogens and mutagens. Mutat. Res. **65,** 133–226 (1979).

Horikawa, M., Fukuhara, M., Suzuki, F., Nikaido, O., Sugahara, T.: Comparative studies on induction and rejoining of DNA single-strand breaks by radiation and chemical carcinogen in mammalian cells *in vitro*. Exptl. Cell Res. **70,** 349–359 (1972).

Hsia, M.T.S., Kreamer, B.L.: Induction of unscheduled DNA synthesis in suspensions of rat hepatocytes by an environmental toxicant, 3,3'4,4'-tetrachloroazobenzene. Cancer Lett. **6,** 207–212 (1979).

International Agency for Research on Cancer: Long-term and short-term screening assays for carcinogens: A critical appraisal. IARC Mongoraphs Suppl. 2, Int. Agency for Res. Cancer, Lyon, pp. 1–426 (1980).

Ishikawa, T., Takayama, S., Ide, F.: Autoradiographic demonstration of DNA repair synthesis in rat tracheal epithelium treated with chemical carcinogens *in vitro*. Cancer Res. **40,** 2898–2903 (1980).

Jeffrey, A.M., Blobstein, S.H., Weinstein, B. Harvey, R.G.: High-pressure liquid chromatography of carcinogen-nucleoside conjugates: separation of 7,12-dimethyl benzanthracene derivatives. Anal. Biochem. **71,** 378–385 (1976).

Kato, H., Harada, M., Tsuchiya, K., Moriwaki, K.: Absence of correlation between DNA repair in ultraviolet irradiated mammalian cells and life span of the donor species. Japan J. Genetics **55,** 99–108 (1980).

Klaunig, J.E., Goldblatt, P.J., Hinton, D.E., Lipsky, M.M., Chasko, J., Trump, B.F.: Mouse liver cell culture. I. Hepatocyte isolation. In Vitro, **17,** 913–925 (1981a).

Klaunig, J.E., Goldblatt, P.J., Hinton, D.E., Lipsky, M.M., Trump, B.F.: Mouse liver cell culture. II. Primary culture. In Vitro **17,** 926–934 (1981b).

Kohn, K.W.: DNA as a target in cancer chemotherapy: measurement of macromolecular DNA damage produced in mammalian cells by anticancer agents and carcinogens. Methods in Cancer Res. **XVI,** 291–345 (1979).

Laishes, B.A., Williams, G.M.: Conditions affecting primary cell cultures of functional adult rat hepatocytes: II. Dexamethasone-enhanced longevity and maintenance of morphology. In Vitro **12,** 821–832 (1976).

Lange, C.S.: The organization and repair of mammalian DNA. FEBS Letters **44,** 153–156 (1974).

Larsen, K.H., Brash, D., Cleaver, J.E., Hart, R.W., Maher, V.M., Painter, R.B., Saga, G.A.: DNA repair tests for environmental mutagens. A report of the U.S. EPA Gene-Tox Program. Mut. Res. **98,** 287–318 (1982).

Lehman, A.R., Bridges, B.A.: DNA repair assays. Biochem. **13,** 71–119 (1977).

Lett, J.T., Caldwell, I.R., Dean, C.J., Alexander, P.: Rejoining of x-ray induced breaks in the DNA of leukemia cells. Nature **214,** 790–792 (1967).

Lieberman, M.W., Sell, S., Farber, E.: Deoxyribonucleoside incorporation and the role of hydroxyurea in a model lymphocyte, system for studying DNA repair in carcinogenesis. Cancer Res. **31**, 1307–1312 (1971).

Lieberman, M.W., Dipple, A.: Removal of bound carcinogen during DNA repair in nondividing human lymphocytes. Cancer Res. **32**, 1855–1860 (1972).

Lieberman, M.W., Poirier, M.C.: Deoxyribonucleoside incorporation during DNA repair of carcinogen-induced damage in human diploid fibroblasts. Cancer Res. **33**, 2097–2103 (1973).

Lieberman, M.W., Porier, M.C.: Base repairing and template specificity during deoxyribonucleic acid repair synthesis in human and mouse cells. Biochem. **13**, 5384–5388 (1974).

Lonati-Galligani, M., Lohman, P.H.M. and Berends, F.: The validity of the autoradiographic method for detecting DNA repair synthesis in rat hepatocytes in primary culture. Mutat. Res. **113**, 145–160 (1983).

Maekubo, H., Ozaki, S., Mitmaker, B., Kalant, N.: Preparation of human hepatocytes for primary culture. In Vitro **18**, 483–491 (1982).

Martin, C.N., McDermid, A.C., Garner, R.C.: Testing of known carcinogens and noncarcinogens for their ability to induce unscheduled DNA synthesis in HeLa cells. Cancer Res. **38**, 2621–2627 (1978).

Maslansky, C.J., Williams, G.M.: Evidence for an epigenetic mode of action in organochlorine pesticide hepatocarcinogenicity: a lack of genotoxicity in rat, mouse and hamster hepatocytes. J. Toxicol. Environ. Health **8**, 121–130 (1981).

Maslansky, C.J., Williams, G.M.: Primary cultures and the levels of cytochrome P-450 in hepoatocytes from mouse, rat, hamster and rabbit liver. In Vitro **18**, 683–693 (1982).

Maslansky, C.J. and Williams, G.M.: Ultraviolet light-induced DNA repair synthesis in hepatocytes from species of differing longevities. Mech. Aging Develop. **29**, 191–203 (1985).

Mattern, M.R., Cerutti, P.A.: Age-dependent excision of damaged thymine from γ-irradiated DNA by isolated nuclei from human fibroblasts. Nature **254**, 450–452 (1975).

Mattern, M.R., Hariharen, P.V., Dunlap, P.E., Cerutti, P.A.: DNA degradation and excision repair in γ-irradiated Chinese hamster ovary cells. Nature **245**, 230–232 (1973).

McGrath, R.A., Williams, R.W.: Reconstruction *in vivo* of irradiated Escherichia coli deoxyribonucleic acid the rejoining of broken pieces. Nature **212**, 534–535 (1966).

McQueen, C.A., Williams, G.M.: Verification of unscheduled DNA synthesis as DNA repair in the hepatocyte primary culture/DNA repair test. Ann. N.Y. Acad. Sci. **349**, 404 (1979).

McQueen, C.A., Maslansky, C.J., Crescenzi, S.B., Williams, G.M.: the genotoxicity of 4,4′-methylene-bis-2-chloroaniline in rat, mouse and hamster hepatocytes. Toxicol. Appl. Pharmacol. **58**, 231–235 (1981a).

McQueen, C.A., Williams, G.M.: Characterization of DNA repair elicited by carcinogens and drugs in the hepatocyte primary culture/DNA repair test. J. Toxicol. Environ. Health **8**, 463–477 (1981b).

McQueen, C.A., Maslansky, C.J., Glowinski, I.B., Crescenzi, S.B., Weber, W.W., Williams, G.M.: Relationship between the genetically determined acetylator phenotype and DNA damage induced by hydralazine and 2-aminofluorene in cultured rabbit hepatocytes. Proc. Natl. Acad. Sci. (USA) **79**, 1269–1272 (1982).

McQueen, C.A., Kreiser, D.M., Hurley, P.M., Williams, G.M. The hepatocyte primary culture (HPC)/DNA repair test using mouse and hamster cells. Environ. Mutat. **5**, 483 (1983).

Meneghini, R.: Repair replication of opposum lymphocyte DNA: effect of compounds that bind to DNA. Chem. Biol. Interac. **8**, 113–126 (1974).

Michalopoulos, G., Sattler, G.L., O'Connor, L., Pitot, H.C.: Unscheduled DNA synthesis induced by procarcinogens in suspensions and primary cultures of hepatocytes on collagen membranes. Cancer Res. **38**, 1866–1871 (1978).

Michael, R.O., Williams, G.M.: Chloroquine inhibition of repair of DNA damage induced in mammalian cells by methyl methane-sulfonate. Mut. Res. **25**, 391–396 (1974).

Mirsalis, J.C., Butterworth, B.E.: Detection of unscheduled DNA synthesis in hepatocytes isolated from rats treated with genotoxic agents: an in vivo/in vitro assay for potential carcinogens and mutagens. Carcinogenesis **1**, 621–625 (1980).

Mitchell, A.D., Casciano, D.A., Meltz, M.L., Robinson, D.E., San, R.H.C., Williams, G.M., Von Halle, G.S.: Unscheduled DNA synthesis tests: A report of the Gene-Tox program. Mutat. Res. **123**, 363–410 (1983).

Montesano, R., Saint Vincent, L., Tomatis, L.: Malignant transformation in vitro of rat liver cells by dimethyl nitrosamine and N-methyl-N'nitrosoguanidine. Brit. J. Cancer **28**, 215–220 (1973).

Murray, A.W., Fitzgerald, D.J.: Tumor promoters inhibit metabolic cooperation in cocultures of epidermal and 3T3 cells. Biochem. Biophys. Res. Commun. **99**, 395–401 (1979).

Nordenskjold, M., Moldeus, P., Lambert, B.: Effects of ultraviolet light and cyclophosphamide on replication and repair synthesis of DNA in isolated rat liver cells and human leukocytes co-incubated with microsomes. Hereditas **89**, 1–6 (1978).

Oldham, J.W., Casciano, D.A., Cave, M.D.: Comparative induction of unscheduled DNA synthesis by physical and chemical agents in non-proliferating primary cultures of rat hepatocytes. Chem. Biol. Interac. **29**, 303–314 (1980).

Omerod, M.G., Stevens, U.: The rejoining of x-ray induced strand breaks in the DNA of a murine lymphoma cell. Biochem. Biophys. Acta. **232**, 72–82 (1971).

Painter, R.B.: DNA synthesis inhibition in HeLa cells as a simple test for agents that damage human DNA. J. Environ. Path. Toxicol. **2**, 65–78, (1978).

Painter, R.B., Cleaver, J.E.: Repair replication unscheduled DNA synthesis and the repair of mammalian DNA. Radiat. Res. **37**, 4151–4166 (1969).

Paterson, M.C.: Use of purified lesion-recognizing enzymes to monitor DNA repair in vivo. Adv. Radiation Biol. **7**, 1–53 (1978).

Pegg, A.E., Perry, W.: Stimulation of transfer of methyl groups from 0^6-methylguanine in DNA to protein by rat liver extracts in response to hepatotoxins. Carcinogenesis **2**, 1196–1200 (1981).

Pegg, A.E., Roberfroid, M., von Bahr, C., Foote, R.S., Mitra, S., Bresil, H., Likhachev, A., Montesano, R.: Removal of 0^6-methylguanine from DNA by human liver fractions. Proc. Natl. Acad. Sci. (USA) **79**, 5162–5164 (1982).

Pero, R.W., Bryngelsson, C., Mitelman, F., Kornfalt, R., Thulin, T., Norden, A.: Inter-individual variation in the responses of cultured human lymphocytes to exposure from DNA damaging chemical agents. Mut. Res. **53**, 327–341 (1978).

Pero, R.W., Ostlund, C.: Direct comparison, in human resting lymphocytes, of the inter-individual variation in unscheduled DNA synthesis induced by N-acetoxy-2-acetylaminofluorene and ultraviolet irradiation. Mut. Res. **73**, 349–361 (1980).

Pettijohn, D., Hanawalt, P.: Evidence for repair-replication ultraviolet damaged DNA in bacteria. J Mol. Biol. **9**, 395–410 (1964).

Probst, G.S., Hill, L.E., Bewsey, B.J.: Comparison of three *in vitro* assays for carcinogen-induced DNA damage. J. Toxicol. Environm. Hlth. **6**, 333–349 (1980).

Probst, G.S., McMahon, R.E., Hill, L.E., Thompson, C.Z., Epp, J.K., Neal, S.B.: Chemically induced unscheduled DNA synthesis in primary rat hepatocyte cultures. Environ. Mut. **3**, 11–32 (1981).

Rajewsky, M.F., Augenlicht, L.H., Biessmann, H., Goth, R., Hulser, D.F., Laerum, O.D., Ya, L.: Nervous system-specific carcinogenesis by ethylnitrosourea in the rat: molecular and cellular mechanisms. In: Hiatt, H.H., Watson, J.D., Winsten, J.A., eds, Origins of Human Cancer, Vol. 4, pp. 709–726. Cold Spring Harbor, New York: Cold Spring Harbor Laboratory (1977).

Rasmussen, R.E., Painter, R.B.: Evidence for repair of ultraviolet damaged deoxyribonucleic acid in cultured mammalian cells. Nature **203**, 1360–1362 (1964).

Rasmussen. R.E., Painter, R.B.: Radiation-stimulated DNA synthesis in cultured mammalian cells. J. Cell Biol. **29**, 1–19 (1966).

Reese, J.A., Byard, J.L.: Isolation and culture of adult hepatocytes from liver biopsies. In Vitro **17**, 935–940 (1981).

Regan, J.D., Setlow, R.B.: Two forms of repair in the DNA of human cells damaged by chemical carcinogens and mutagens. Cancer Res. **34**, 3318–3325 (1974).

Regan, J.D., Setlow, R.B., Ley, R.D.: Normal and defective repair of damaged DNA in human cells: a sensitive assay utilizing the photolysis of bromodeoxyuridine. Proc. Natl. Acad. Sci. (USA) **68**, 708–712 (1971).

Reid, B.D., Walker, I.G.: The response of mammalian cells to alkylating agents: II. On the mechanism of the removal of sulfur-mustard-induced cross-links. Biochem. Biophys Acta **179**, 179–188 (1969).

Reiss, B., Williams, G.M.: Induction of DNA repair and suppression of DNA synthesis by carcinogens in colon organ culture. Fed. Proc. **37**, 749 (1978).

Renton, K.W., DeLoria, L.B., Mannering, G.J.: Effects of polyriboinosinic acid, polyribocyticlylic acid and a mouse interferon preparation on cytochrome P-450-dependent mono-oxygenase systems in cultures of primary mouse hepatocytes. Mol. Pharmacol. **14**, 672–681 (1978).

Roberts, J.J., Crathorn, A.R., Brent, T.P.: Repair of alkylated DNA in mammalian cells. Nature **218**, 970–972 (1968).

Roberts, J.J., Pascoe, J.M., Smith, B.A., Crathorn, A.R.: Quantitative aspects of the repair of alkylated DNA in cultured mammalian cells: II. Non-semi-conservative DNA synthesis (repair synthesis) in HeLa and Chinese hamster cells following treatment with alkylating agents. Chem. Biol. Interactions **3**, 49–68 (1971).

Saito, M., Andoh, T.: Breakage of a DNA-protein complex induced by bleomycin and their repair in cultured mouse fibroblasts. Cancer Res. **33**, 1696–1700 (1973).

San, R.H.C., Stich, H.F.: DNA repair synthesis of cultured human cells as a rapid bioassay for chemical carcinogens. Int. J. Cancer, **16**, 284–291 (1975).

Schmeltz, I., Tosk, J., Williams, G.M.: Comparison of the metabolic profiles of benzo(a)pyrene obtained from primary cell cultures and subcellular fractions derived from normal and methyl-cholanthrene-induced rat liver. Cancer Lett., **5**, 81–89 (1978).

Scudiero, D., Henderson, E., Norin, A., Strauss, B.: The measurement of chemically-induced DNA repair synthesis in human cells by BND-cellulose chromatography. Mutation Res. **29**, 473–488 (1975).

Setlow, R.B.: DNA repair pathways. In: DNA Repair and Mutagenesis in Eukaryotes. Generoso, W.M., Shelby, M.D., de Serres, F.J. (eds.), pp. 45–54, New York: Plenum Publishing Corp. (1980).

Shinohara, K., Cerutti, P.A.: Excision repair of benzo(a)pyrene-deoxyguanosine adducts in baby hamster kidney 21/C13 cells and in secondary mouse embryo fibroblast C57BL/6J. Proc. Natl. Acad. Sci. (USA) **74**, 979–983 (1977).

Smith, C.A., Hanawalt, P.C.: Repair replication in human cells simplified determination utilizing hydroxyurea. Biochim. Biophys. Acta **432**, 336–347 (1976).

Stich, H.F., San, R.H.C.: DNA repair and chromatid anomalies in mammalian cells exposed to 4-nitroquinoline 1-oxide. Mutation Res. **10**, 389–401 (1970).

Stich, H.F., San, R.H.C., Kawazoe, Y.: DNA repair synthesis in mammalian cells exposed to a series of oncogenic and nononcogenic derivatives of 4-nitroquinoline 1-oxide. Nature **229**, 416–419 (1971).

Strom, S.C., Jirtle, R.J., Jones, R.S., Novicki, D.L., Rosenberg, M.R., Novotry, A., Irons, G., McLain, J.R., Michalopoulos, G.: Isolation, culture and transplantation of human hepatocytes. J.N.C.I. **68**, 771–778 (1982).

Swenberg, J.A. Petzold, G.L., Harback, P.R.: *In Vitro* DNA damage/alkaline elution assay for predicting carcinogenic potential. Biochem. Biophys. Comm. **72**, 732–738 (1976).

Tong, C., Williams, G.M.: Induction of purine analog resistant mutants in adult rat liver epithelial lines by metabolic activation-dependent and -independent carcinogens. Mutation Res. **58**, 339–352 (1978).

Toth, B.: Tumorigenic effect of 1-hydrazinophthalazine hydrochloride in mice. J. Natl. Cancer Inst. **61**, 1363–1365, (1978).

Trosko, J.D., Yager, J.D.: A sensitive method to measure physical and chemical carcinogen-induced "unscheduled DNA synthesis" in rapidly dividing eukaryotic cells. Exp. Cell Res. **88**, 47–55 (1974).

Vadi, H., Moldeus, P., Capdevila, J., Orrenius, S.: The metabolism of benzo(a)pyrene in isolated rat cells. Cancer Res. **35**, 2083–2091 (1975).

Walker, I.G., Ewart, D.F.: Repair synthesis of DNA in HeLa and L cells following treatment with methylnitrosourea or ultraviolet light. Can J. Biochem. **51**, 148–157 (1973).

Warren, J.R., Simmon, V.F., Reddy, J.K.: Properties of hyper lipidemic peroxisom proliferators in the lymphocyte [^{3}H] thymidine and Salmonella mutagenesis assays. Cancer Res. **40**, 36–41 (1980).

Weisburger, J.H., Williams, G.M.: Decision point approach to carcinogen testing. In: Structural Correlates of Carcinogenesis and Mutagenesis, Asher, I.M. and Zervos, C. (eds.) pp. 47–52, The Office of Science, FDA, Rockville, Md. (1978).

Weisburger, J.H., Williams, G.M.: Chemical Carcinogens. In: Toxicology: The Basic Science of Poisons, 2nd Ed., Doull, J., Klaassen, C.D., Amdur, M.O., (eds.), New York: Macmillan Publ. Co., Inc. (1980).

Weisburger, J.H., Williams, G.M.: Metabolism of chemical carcinogens. In: Cancer: A Comprehensive Treatise, 2nd Edition. Becker, E.F. (ed.), New York, Plenum Press, pp. 241–333, (1982).

Wiebers, J.L., Abbvott, P.J., Coombs, M.M., Livingston, D.C.: Mass spectral characterization of the major DNA-carcinogen adduct formed from the metabolically activated carcinogen 15,16-dihydro-11-methylcyclopento[a] phenanthren-17-one. Carcinogen. **2**, 637–643 (1981).

Williams, G.M.: Carcinogen-induced DNA repair in primary rat liver cell cultures; A possible screen for chemical carcinogens. Cancer Lett. **1**, 231–236 (1976a).

Williams, G.M.: The use of liver epithelial cultures for the study of chemical carcinogenesis. Amer. J. Pathol. **85**, 739–753 (1976b).

Williams, G.M.: The detection of chemical carcinogens by unscheduled DNA synthesis in rat liver primary cell cultures. Cancer Res. **37**, 1845–1851 (1977).

Williams, G.M.: Further improvements in the hepatocyte DNA repair test for carcinogens: Detection of carcinogen biphenyl derivatives. Cancer Lett. **4**, 69–75 (1978).

Williams, G.M.: Liver cell culture systems for the study of hepatocarcinogenesis. In: Advances in Medical Oncology, Research and Education. Proceedings of the XIIth International Cancer Congress. Vol. 1. Carcinogenesis. Margison, G.M. (ed.). pp. 273–280, N.Y., Pergamon Press (1979a).

Williams, G.M. The status of in vitro test systems utilizing DNA damage and repair for the screening of chemical carcinogens. J. Assoc. Off. Anal. Chem. **62**, 857–863 (1979b).

Williams, G.M.: The detection of chemical mutagens/carcinogens by DNA repair and mutagenesis in liver cultures, In: Chemical Mutagens, Vol. VI, DeSerres, F.J., Hollaender, A. (eds.), Plenum Press, New York (1980).

Williams, G.M.: Classification of genotoxic and epigenetic hepatocarcinogens using liver culture assays. Annals New York Acad. Sci. **349**, 273–282 (1980b).

Williams, G.M.: The predictive value of DNA damage and repair assays for carcinogenicity. In: The predictive value of in vitro short-term screening tests in carcinogenicity evaluation. Williams, G.M., Kroes, R., Wasijers, H.W., Van de Poll, K.W. (eds.) pp. 213–220. Elsevier/North-Holland Biomedical Press, Amsterdam (1980c).

Williams, G.M.: The detection of genotoxic chemicals in the hepatocyte primary culture/DNA repair test. In: Mutation, Promotion and Transformation, Inuii, N., Kuroki, T.,Yamada, M.A., Heidelberger, C., (eds.) Gann Monograph on Cancer Research **27**, 47–57 (1981a).

Williams, G.M.: The detection of genotoxic chemicals in the hepatocyte primary culture/DNA repair test. Gann **27**, 45–55 (1981c).

Williams, G.M.: Liver carcinogenesis: The role for some chemicals of an epigenetic mechanism of liver-tumor promotion involving modification of the cell membrane. Fd. Compet. Toxicol. **19**, 577–583 (1981b).

Williams, G.M.: Epigenetic effects of liver tumor promoters and implications for health effects. Environ. Health Perspec. **50**, 233–245 (1983).

Williams, G.M., Weisburger, J.H.: Systemic carcinogen testing through the decision point approach. Annual Review Pharmacol. Toxicol. **21**, 393–416 (1981).

Williams, G.M. and Numoto, S.: Promotion of mouse liver neoplasms by the organochlorine pesticides chlordane and heptachlor in comparison to dichlorodiphenyltrichloroethane. Carcinogen. **5**, 1689–1696 (1984).

Williams, G.M., Elliott, J.M., Weisburger, J.H.: Carcinoma after malignant conversion in vitro of epithelial-like cells from rat liver following exposure to chemical carcinogens. Cancer Res. **33**, 606–612 (1973).

Williams, G.M., Bermudez, E., Scaramuzzino, D.: Rat hepatocyte primary cell cultures. III: Improved dissociation and attachment techniques and the enhancement of survival by culture medium. In Vitro **13**, 809–817 (1977).

Williams, G.M., Laspia, M.F., Mori, H., Horono, I.: Genotoxicity of cycasin in the hepatocyte primary culture/DNA repair test supplemented with β-glucosidase. Cancer Lett, **12**, 329–333 (1981).

Williams, G.M., Laspia, M.F., Dunkel, V.C.: Reliability of the hepatocyte primary culture/DNA repair test in testing of coded carcinogens and noncarcinogens. Mut. Res. **97**, 359–370 (1982).

Yager, J.D., Miller, J.A.: DNA repair in primary cultures of rat hepatocytes. Cancer Res. **38**, 4385–4395 (1978).

Yih, T.D. and Van Rossum, J.M.: Isolated rat hepatocytes and 900g rat supernatant as metabolic systems for the study of the pharmacokinetics of barbiturates. Xenobiotica **7**, 573–582 (1977).

CHAPTER VII

MUTATION IN CULTURED MAMMALIAN CELLS

Kenneth A. Palmer*
Genetics Toxicology Branch
Division of Toxicology
Center for Food Safety and Applied Nutrition
Food and Drug Administration
Washington, D.C.

A. INTRODUCTION

The *in vitro* cultivation of somatic mammalian cells has provided a mechanism for developing model systems that have been used to evaluate the mutagenic potential of chemicals. Such information can then be used to infer carcinogenic potential because of the correlation between *in vitro* data and animal studies. Microbial systems are also used for this purpose; however, mammalian cell systems are believed to provide a more relevant model than the microbial systems since the genetic target is composed of a highly organized chromatin structure involving histones and residual proteins as is found in the whole animal, rather than simple circular DNA present in bacteria. The purpose of this chapter is to describe the most commonly used mammalian mutational assay systems, the genetic loci involved, the nature of the observed changes, and possible advantages and/or disadvantages of each system.

B. HISTORY OF MAMMALIAN CELL MUTAGENESIS SYSTEMS

The use of human cells, and later other mammalian cells, for *in vitro* genetic studies was developed by Puck et al. (1956) who employed the immortal HeLa cell line to develop a technique for cloning single cells *in vitro*. The technique is a quantitative method analogous to the plating techniques used in microbial

*Present Address: Office of Device Evaluation, Center for Devices and Radiological Health, Food and Drug Administration, Silver Spring, Maryland.

studies that permits the isolation of single cells capable of generating homogenous cell populations. Szybalski and Szybalska (Szybalski and Szybalska, 1962) and Szybalski et al. (Szybalski et al., 1964; Szybalski et al., 1962) first applied this technique using drug sensitivity as the genetic marker in human cells. Their studies were predicated on measuring an increase in the number of cells resistant to the purine analogues 8-azaguanine or 8-azahypoxanthine. Cells resistent to these analogues have low levels or completely lack the enzyme hypoxanthine-guanine phosphoribosyl tranferase (HGPRT). The studies of Szybalski tested a number of known bacterial mutagens including alkylating agents, purine and pyrimidine analogues, radiation, and several known carcinogens. These investigators concluded that no definite or consistent mutagenic effects were observed and that the background or spontaneous rate was so high that induction by chemical or physical mutagens was not possible. During this time Morrow (Morrow, 1964; Morrow, 1970) performed similar experiments using mouse cells and arrived at essentially the same conclusion. These investigators while recognizing several very important factors, such as expression time and different levels of resistance, failed to realize that the observed spontaneous mutation frequency was too high to allow the detection of an increase in the induced mutant frequency. Several years later Kao and Puck (Kao and Puck, 1968; Kao and Puck, 1969) demonstrated the induction of mutagenesis in nutritionally deficient Chinese hamster ovary (CHO) cells with the alkylating agents EMS and MNNG. At about the same time that Kao and Puck published their data, Chu and Malling (Chu and Malling, 1968) presented evidence that demonstrated the induction of mutagenesis in Chinese hamster V-79 cells using the alkylating agents MMS, EMS and MNNG. In this classic paper the authors recognize the importance of inoculum size, expression time and level of selective agents. These two studies, most notably the second, are the foundation on which future mutagenesis studies using mammalian cells are based. The nutritional markers developed by Kao and Puck (Kao and Puck, 1968) were not used to any great extent for mutagenesis testing; however the CHO cell line has been used by Hsie, one of Puck's former students, to develop a mutagenic assay system based on the induced loss of the enzyme hypoxanthine-guanine phosphoribosyl transferase (HGPRT). Hsie, along with his colleague O'Neill, has developed the CHO/HGPRT mutagen screening assay (O'Neill et al., 1977, O'Neill et al., 1977b; Hsie et al., 1979) which is widely used by industry to test chemicals. Chinese hamster V-79 cells are also used to detect mutations at the HGPRT locus but it has not been used to the same extent as the CHO/HGPRT. This may be because critical parameters have not been defined well enough for routine screening using V-79 cells. More recently, the cell line has been used by a number of laboratories for the mutagenesis studies (Bradley et al., 1981; Bartsch et al., 1980). While the same general protocol reported in earlier studies is still used, several critical changes have been made. These include extending the expression time from 3 days to 6-9 days, using a replating technique for dispersing the cells which allows a more efficient recovery of induced mutants and the inclusion of an exogenous metabolizing system. As stated above the HGPRT locus is used to the greatest extent; however, a multiple loci assay has

154

been developed by Carver and Adair (Carver et al., 1980; Adair et al., 1980) which used HGPRT, thymidine kinase (TK) and Na/K ATPase in CHO cells. It was believed that a multiple loci system would considerably increase the sensitivity of the assay for routine screening as any given chemical may exhibit a different response at the different loci, i.e., exhibiting a positive response at one locus and not at the other. By using multiple loci it should be possible to classify more accurately in a single test system a chemical with respect to its mutagenic potential. The use of multiple loci allows further characterization of this type of genetic lesion produced, i.e. frame shift or base pair substitution, since HGPRT and TK can detect both base pair substitution and frame shift mutations while Na/K ATPase can only detect base pair substitution. The use of multiple loci has not as yet gained wide acceptance for screening chemical mutagens, perhaps because of technical difficulties which arise when scoring several genetic loci at the same time. At the present time the HGPRT locus in both the CHO and V-79 cell lines is the preferred locus to use for screening potential mutagens.

Another cell line, the L5178Y mouse lymphoma, an ascites cell line, was originally isolated from a DBA/2 mouse treated with 3-methylcholanthrene by L.W. Law of the National Cancer Institute (Fischer, personal communication) and later grown in vitro by Glen Fischer who used the cells to study antitumor agents (Fischer and Sartorelli, 1964; Fischer, 1959). The cells have been used for several loci, including HGPRT, TK, Na/K ATPase, asparagine, and the fluctation test (Cole and Arlett, 1976; Cole, et al., 1976; Capizzi et al., 1973; Clive et al., 1972; Palmer et al., 1977). Although each of the listed loci have shown a significant response to known mutagens, the TK locus is the one commonly used for screening chemicals. Use of the TK locus was first described by Clive et al. (Clive et al., 1972) who utilized a presumed TK+/- L5178Y heterozygote originally isolated from L5178Y cells that were indirectly obtained from Fischer (Spaulding, personal communication). There has also been some exploration of a multiple loci assay by Cole and Arlett (Cole and Arlett, 1976) who compared the HGPRT, TK and Na/K ATPase loci in L5178Y cells. L5178Y cells were also used as indicator cells in the host mediated assay by Fischer (resistance to MTX, cystosine arabinoside, excess TdR) (Fischer, et al., 1974) and Cappizzi (L5178Y/Asn+) (Capazzi et al., 1973). The anticipated potential of this assay was never realized and it has been abandoned because of technical difficulties.

Human cells have also been used successfully to detect chemical mutagens. DeMars has used primary fibroblasts isolated from foreskin to detect mutation at the HGPRT locus and the adenine phosphoribosyl transferase locus (APRT) (DeMars, 1974; Jacobs and DeMars, 1978). These studies were mainly aimed at investigating the mechanisms of mutation rather than as an assay for screening chemicals. Another cell line, human lymphoblasts TK6 (Shopek, et al., 1978; Thilly, et al., 1980; Liber and Thilly, 1982) has recently been developed as a model in vitro human cell system similar to the L5178Y TK+/- assay described by Clive (Clive et al., 1972).

Human cells have also been used to compare the induced mutagenic response produced by chemicals at the HGPRT, Na/K ATPase and TK loci. Some attempts have also been made to use human cells like Xeroderma pigmentosum cells that are repair deficient to study chemical mutagenesis (Maher and McCormick, 1975; Maher and McCormick, 1976; Maher et al., 1976; McCormick and Maher, 1981). These have not been widely used because of the technical problems involved with culturing the cells. The cells have long generation times and poor cloning efficiencies making the experiments cumbersome and the data difficult to interpret. This is, in general, true of most human cell lines used for mutagenesis studies. At the present time the human cells do not appear to be as convenient for routine screening as the mouse or hamster cells. Generally, they are used for specific research purposes as opposed to routine testing.

The most important improvement in the development of *in vitro* models for mutation assays has been the inclusion of exogenous metabolic activation which can metabolize promutagens to active mutagens. These have developed along lines similar to the activation systems used for microbial assays. The most commonly used activation system is the 9000 x G supernant (S-9) from a rat liver homogenate, though mouse and hamster livers have also been used, along with the cofactors $NADP^+$ and isocitrate or glucose-6-phosphate. The S-9 can be prepared from animals previously treated with either arochlor or phenobarbital both of which induce an increased amount of microsomal drug metabolizing enzyme activity of the liver. Alternative approaches to activation include the cocultivation of the indicator cells with primary hepatocytes or irradiated feeder cells. Such systems have not been used widely to date because of technical complexities in preparing the activator cells.

C. GENETIC LOCI

This section focuses on those specific loci that are commonly used in mammalian cells mutagenesis assays, the biochemical system affected, location of the loci in the genome, level of sensitivity for detection, selective agents used and the possible target involved. Three routinely used loci are the HGPRT, TK and Na/K ATPase. Each will be discussed separately.

I. Hypoxanthine-Guanine Phosphoribosyl transferase locus (HGPRT)

The HGPRT locus was the locus chosen by the original mammalian mutagenesis workers (Szybalski and Szybalska, 1964; Szybalski et al., 1964; Szybalski et al., 1962; Morrow, 1964, Morrow, 1970; Chu and Malling, 1968). The enzyme HGPRT is referred to as a scavenger enzyme that catalyzes the reaction where the exogenous bases hypoxanthine and guanine react with phosphoribosyl pyrophosphate to form their respective nucleotides. Figure 1 illustrates the biochemical mechanism involved in the HGPRT pathway) or 6 thioguanine (6TG) from the natural substrate, hypoxanthine or guanine. When these analogues are phosphorylated they are lethal to the cells. Cells that lack HGPRT are able to grow in the presence of the analogues since they cannot phosphorylate the exogenous purines. The most effective purine analogues are 6TG and 8

Aza. 6TG is the prefered selective agent because of its higher affinity to the enzyme HGPRT (Caskey and Kruh, 1979) and therefore produces "cleaner selection." Mutation at the locus is measured by comparing the number of 8 Aza or 6TG resistant cells arising in a population after chemical exposure to an untreated control population.

The HGPRT locus is located on the X-chromosome and is present in a hemizygous state in the male which has only one X-chromosome or the hetero-zygous state in the female due to the inactivation of one of the X-chromosomes. The HGPRT locus has a human equivalent in the clinical disease called the Lesch-Nyhan syndrome. The Lesch-Nyhan syndrome is an inborn error in metabolism resulting in a deficiency in HGRPT and characterized by self-mutilation, choreoathetosis, developmental retardation, spasticity and an accelerated rate of *de novo* purine biosynthesis; it is inherited in an X-linked recessive manner. Gout is another human disease that is associated with a deficiency in HGPRT and is characterized by high blood levels of uric acid which result in painful swelling of joints.

The HGPRT locus has been shown to detect base pair substitutions as well as frame shifts in the genetic code. Also demonstrated is that the target (affected locus) is most likely the structural gene (Caskey and Kruh, 1979). While there is some evidence to suggest that control genes could be the target, the evidence is less than convincing and counter arguments point out that the authors failed to consider important factors such as the number of active X-chromosomes in the cell line used (DeMars, 1974) which could explain the observed results.

II. Thymidine Kinase (TK) Locus

The TK locus, like the HGPRT locus, is associated with a salvage pathway (Figure 2). While HGPRT catalyzes the formation of purine nucleotides from exogenous purines, TK catalyzes the formation of thymidine monophosphate (TMP) from exogenous thymidine. The TK locus is autosomal, located on chromosome number 11 in the mouse (Mc Breen et al., 1977) and number 17 autosome in the human (Willecke et al., 1977). Because the gene product, TK, is not essential for cell survival the locus can be used to detect frame shift mutations as well as base pair substitution. This has been demonstrated by an induced positive response for both types of mutagens in the TK+/- L5178Y assay (Clive et al., 1979; Amacher et al., 1980).

The TK locus is generally associated with the L5178Y cell line where the locus was originally utilized by Clive et al. (Clive et al., 1972) who isolated a cell line presumed to have heterozygous genotype (TK+/—). An attempt has been made by Carver and Adair (Carver et al., 1980; Adair et al., 1980) to isolate a TK+/-cell line from CHO cells but little work has been done with this system. Thilly's group at MIT have isolated a human TK+/- lymphoblast cell line but this work is still in the preliminary stage (Skopek et al., 1978; Thilly et al., 1980; Liver and Thilly, 1982).

Three selective agents have been used to detect changes at the TK locus. These include bromodeoxyuridine (BUdR), fluorodeoxyuridine (FUdR) and trifluorothymidine (F_3TdR). Original experiments employing this locus used BUdR for selection. Thymidine kinase competent cells are killed by BUdR by it first being phosphorylated and then incorporated into DNA. When both strands of DNA contain BUdR in place of thymidine the cell dies. BUdR can be used effectively to select for TK deficient cells; however, several cell divisions are required before the competent cells are killed and the selection is not clean in that some colonies are not true mutants. F_3TdR, however, is believed to be phosphorylated by TK and the F_3TdR monophosphate then inhibits thymidylate synthetase which quickly arrests cell growth. The mode of action F_3TdR is not completely understood but it is suggested that the effect may be cytostatic rather then cytotoxic (Thilly et al., 1980; Moore-Brown and Clive, 1979).

III. Na/K ATPase

Resistance to the cardiac glycoside, ouabain, is another selective system that has been used in mammalian cells to identify mutagens. The system involves the enzyme Na/K ATPase that is located on the plasma membrane of mammalian cells. This enzyme is inhibited when ouabain binds to the alpha subunit. Resistance to ouabain probably is the result of base pair substitutions occurring at only limited sites within the Na/K ATPase locus that affects binding of ouabain but does not destroy enzyme activity (Baker, et al., 1974). The susceptible mutagenic target would, therefore, be expected to be quite small resulting in a low spontaneous mutant frequency, lower than the HGPRT or TK loci. The gene that controls ouabain resistance has been mapped on chromosome 3 in the mouse (Kozak et al., 1979). The ouabain resistance phenotype is dominant and stable. Ouabain resistance cannot be induced by either ionizing radiation or the frame shift mutagen ICR 191 (Bradley et al., 1981) indicating that some NA/K ATPase activity is vital for cell survival and frame shift or other inactivating mutations which eliminate enzyme activity result in cell death.

D. ASSAY SYSTEMS

I. CHO/HGPRT Assay

The CHO/HGPRT assay is understood to detect single gene mutations occurring in the specific HGPRT locus of Chinese hamster ovary (CHO) cells; specifically, cell line $CHO-K_1-BH_3$ (O'Neill et al., 1977). The cell line is a proline auxotroph ideally suited for a rapid mutagenesis assay. The cells are grown as a monolayer, have a cloning efficiency of greater than 80%, a doubling time of 12-14 hrs and are well characterized genetically.

The assay measures a forward mutation indicated by an increased number of colonies that have lost almost all of the HGPRT activity following chemical treatment. This is detected by determining the number of cells resistant to the purine analogue 6TG, a compound that is lethal to cells containing normal levels of HGPRT activity. The spontaneous mutant frequency of the forward mutation is 0-20 mutants/10^6 cells. Hsie has reported that of 84 compounds identified as either carcinogens or non-carcinogens in animals, 77 were correlated with CHO/HGPRT mutagenicity results or 92% correlation with the animal carcinogenicity (Hsie et al., 1981).

A suggested protocol has been described in detail by O'Neill and Hsie et al. (O'Neill and Hsie, 1979; Hsie et al., 1981). They divide the assay into two segments, one for cytotoxicity and one for mutagenesis. In both segments the cells are exposed to varying chemical concentrations for 5 hours. The treatment can be performed either with or without exogenous metabolic activation; however, few compounds to date have been tested in this assay with activation. In the cytotoxicity segment the cells are immediately dispersed using trypsin and plated at 200-500 cells/60 mm petri dish following the 5 hour chemical treatment to determine the toxicity of the compound. In the mutagenicity segment treated cells are allowed a 7-9 day period to express their new phenotype, the time necessary for reduction of preexisting HGPRT enzyme and its m-RNA by the altered (mutated) form of HGPRT. During the phenotypic expression period the cultures are subcloned at 48 hr intervals. Selection for thioguanine resistant (TG^r) cells is carried out using hypoxanthine-free Hams F_{12} medium containing 5% heat-inactivated dialyzed fetal calf serum and 10 μM TG. There is some question whether the use of dialyzed serum is necessary if the concentration of TG is high enough. This medium will select colonies with greatly reduced HGPRT activity. The mutant selection plates are innoculated with 2 x 10^5 cells/100 mm plate and the plates for determining cloning efficency are seeded with 200 cells/60 mm plate. The plates are incubated at 37° for 7-8 days to allow visible colony formation and are then fixed, stained and counted. The mutant frequency is calculated by using the following equation: (total number or mutant colonies/number of cells innoculated) (cloning efficiency) equals mutant frequency. This is usually expressed as the number of mutants per 10^6 survivors. Several factors have been reported as important to optimal mutant recovery, including cell density, CO_2 concentration, and volume of medium.

The criteria for acceptance of data generated in this assay will vary somewhat, depending upon the laboratory where it was generated. These criteria can be expected to change as the experimental procedures become more defined. The following criteria would constitute an acceptance trial or test whether there was metabolic activation or not. The spontaneous mutant frequency should be within the historical range observed in the laboratory conducting the study. The cells should exhibit proper growth characteristics such as 80% or greater cloning efficiency for the CHO-K$_1$-BH$_4$ cell line and the culture should routinely be tested for and found free of mycoplasma contamination. The assay should contain appropriate positive control compounds as well as a solvent control with mutant frequencies for both types of controls within historical values. There should be a minimum of three dose levels with survivals of approximately 100, 50 or 10% of the solvent control.

In addition to the criteria for an acceptable trial, criteria must be established for classifying the observed response, i.e., positive, negative or questionable. These criteria should include: at least two acceptable trials that exhibit a

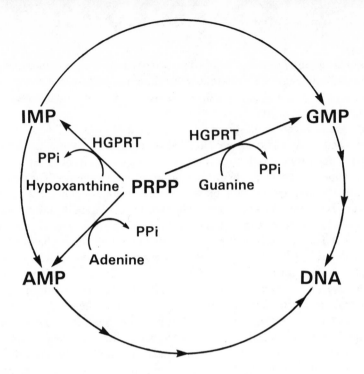

FIGURE 1: Purine Salvage Pathways

FIGURE 1: Diagrammatic illustration of the salvage pathway for free purines. Adenine, guanine and hypoxanthine are converted to nucleotides by the addition of ribosylphosphate through the action of either phosphoribosyltransferase or hypoxanthine guanine phosphoribosyltransferase.

Abbreviations: PRBB, phosyphoribosyl pyrophosphate; APRT, adenine phosphoribosyltransferase; HGPRT, hypoxanthine-guanine phosphoribosyltransferase; PPi, inorganic pyrophosphate; IMP, inosine monophosphate, GMP, guanosine monophosphate, AMP, adenosine monophosphate; DNA, deoxyribonucleic acid.

reproducible response, a positive response should be dose related over at least three different concentrations, and the data should be statistically significant (Snee and Irr, 1981).

The CHO/HGPRT assay appears to be fairly reproducible and sensitive to known mutagens. It has reasonably well defined parameters such as phenotypic expression time and selection conditions with sound genetic and biochemical basis. The protocol has been standardized for ready adaption in rapid mutagen screening. The assay suffers in that most of the compounds tested to date are direct acting mutagens and more work is required to test promutagens (requiring different types of metabolic activation) as well as establishment of a fully functional exogenous activation system. Another drawback is the long (7-9 days) phenotypic expression time which increases the level of effort needed to perform the assay because subculturing at 48 hour intervals during the expression period is required for maximal recovery of mutants.

II. V-79 Assay

This assay utilizes the established V-79 Chinese hamster cell line originally derived from embryonic lung tissue. Like the CHO cells, V-79 cells are quite easy to handle, have a short generation time, high cloning efficiency, stable karyotype and have been used to score both the HGPRT or Na/K ATPase loci. The cell line is the line originally employed by Chu and Malling (Chu and Malling, 1968) in their successful induction of chemical mutation in mammalian cells. The HGPRT locus has been more extensively used than the Na/K ATPase locus and is probably the best locus to use for mutagenesis screening because it can detect both frame shift mutations and base pair substitutions, whereas the Na/K ATPase locus is only sensitive to base pair substitutions and would not detect frame shift mutations.

The protocol used for the V-79 assay is fundamentally similar to that of the CHO/HGPRT assay (Bradley et al., 1981). Again, there are two segments, one to determine the toxicity of the compounds and another to determine the rate of induced mutations. The spontaneous mutant frequency of the stock culture used in the experiments should be low enough to detect induced mutants slightly above a historical background frequency of around 10 mutants/10^6 cells at the HGPRT locus and 2 mutants/10^6 cells at the Na/K ATPase locus (Bradley, et al., 1981). Should the mutant spontaneous frequency be too high in the stock culture it can be reduced for the HGPRT locus by growing the cells for 1-4 days in THMG (3.0 μg/ml thymidine, 5.0 μg/ml hypoxanthine, 0.1 μg/ml methotrexate, and 7.5 μg/ml) medium which selects against HGPRT deficient cells. The background mutant frequency at the Na/K ATPase locus can be reduced by recloning the stock culture and selecting a clone with a low spontaneous mutant frequency.

The criteria for acceptance of a test conducted either with or without metabolic activation in a V-79 assay are the same as that used for CHO/HGPRT: spontaneous mutant frequency controls which are within the historical range observed in the laboratory, proper growth characteristics, such as 80% or greater cloning efficiency, and routine checks for mycoplasma. Appropriate positive control compounds should be included in each trial as well as solvent control. There should be a minimum of 3 dose levels with survivals of 100, 50 or 10% relative to the concurrent control.

Classification of the observed response, i.e., positive, negative or questionable, are the same as those listed above for the CHO/HGPRT assay.

The toxicity segment of the protocol consists of testing a range of dose levels and choosing 3-5 doses that cover a range from relatively non-toxic (95% survival) to very toxic (10% survival). The dose levels selected in the toxicity segment are used in the mutagenesis segment of the assay which follows the same procedure used for CHO/HGPRT described above. Each segment should be performed either without or with an exogenous metabolic activation system.

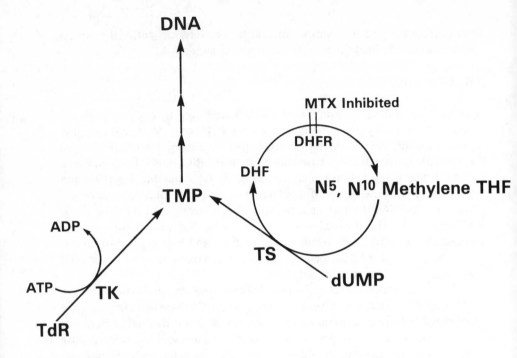

FIGURE 2: TMP Synthesis

FIGURE 2: Diagrammatic illustration of the biochemical basis for the TK +/-assay. Cells that synthesize TK are selected against by growing them in medium containing thymidine analogues (BuDR or F_3TdR) that when phosphorylated are toxic to the cells. This allows only thymidine kinase deficient cells to survive. Likewise thymidine kinase deficient cells are selected against by growing them in medium containing methotrexate which blocks the reduction of dihydrofolate to N^5, N^{10} methylene tetrahydrofolate.

Abbreviations: TdR, thymidine; ATP, adenosine triphosphate; TK, thymidine kinase; TMP, thymidine monophosphate; ADP, adenosine diphosphate; MTX, methotrexate; DHFR, dihydrofolate reductase; DHF, dihydrofolate; THF, tetrahydrofolate; TS, thymidylate synthetase; dUMP, deoxyuridine monophosphate.

There are two type of activation systems that have been used for the V-79 assay. They include the cell mediated activation system (Huberman and Sachs, 1974; Huberman and Sachs, 1976) or tissue homogenate mediated activation system (Krahn and Heidelberger, 1977). Sufficient data are not available to date that would show that one activation system is superior to the other. However, the tissue homogenate activation system appears to be better adapted to routine mutagenesis screening because it is technically easier to perform.

The first demonstration of induced chemical mutagenesis in mammalian cells was carried out in the V-79 assay by Chu and Malling (Chu and Malling, 1968). Over the years, the assay has been well characterized and now has a large and impressive data base indicating its suitability as a mutagenesis screening assay. In addition to the HGPRT locus, the Na/K ATPase locus has also been used to measure chemical mutagenesis in V-79 cells. The V-79 cells are easy to handle, have a short generation time, high cloning efficiency and a stable karyotype. Although the Na/ATPase locus has a short 2 day expression time, this locus most likely detects only base pair substitution type mutational events limiting its sensitivity. The HGPRT locus has the advantage of being able to detect both frame shift type mutational events and base pair substitution type mutational events. The long expression time detracts from this advantage by increasing the level of effort. The assay also lacks data about critical parameters involved in exogenous metabolic activation systems.

III. L5178YTK+/- Assay

L5178Y mouse lymphoma cells were originally isolated from DBA/2 mice treated with 3 methylcholanthrene (Fischer, Personal communication) and later established as an *in vitro* suspension culture (Fischer, 1959). The utilization of the thymidine kinase locus was reported by Clive et al. (Clive et al., 1972; Clive et al., 1973), who isolated an L5178Y cell line that was in a presumed heterozygous state at the TK locus. The L5178YTK+/- assay which has evolved from these early experiments is now recognized by industry and government as a mutagenesis assay that can be used to screen chemicals for their mutagenic potential. The cells are routinely grown in either Fischer's medium or RPMI 1640 medium supplemented with 5% or 10% horse serum (Amacher et al., 1979; Amacher et al., 1980; Clive and Spector, 1979). Cloning is performed in soft agar containing growth medium (i.e., Fischers or RPMI 1640), 5%-20% horse serum and 0.37% Nobel agar. The cells are handled in a similar manner as bacterial suspension cultures. They have a short, 10-12 hour, generation time and high (> 70%) cloning efficiency in soft agar. The assay has been extended to include exogenous metabolic activation which allows the detection of promutagens, agents found non-mutagenic when tested without activation (Clive et al., 1979; Amacher et al., 1979; Amacher et al., 1980).

The L5178YTK+/- assay is typically performed using 50ml centrifuge tubes with the cells maintained in suspension culture by placing the tubes in a roller drum. A detailed procedure has been described by Moore-Brown and Clive, 1979. The assay normally consists of two segments, one to access the toxicity of the test chemical and to establish dose levels to be tested in the mutagenesis segment, the second segment. A typical mutagenesis assay should include a solvent control, a positive control and at least three dose levels of the chemical which cover a dose range from non-toxic (80% survival) to very toxic (10% survival). The assay should be conducted in the presence and absence of exogenous metabolic activation. In addition test results should be confirmed by repeat experiments.

An experimental trial must fulfill certain minimum criteria in order to be accepted. If the criteria are not met then the trial is considered an invalid test.

Minimum criteria included the following: a) the spontaneous mutant frequency within the historical control of the laboratory (this, however, should never exceed 100×10^{-6} mutants/cell); b) a range of toxicity observed for the dosage levels used, unless the compound was non-toxic at very high concentrations i.e., 5,000 to 10,000 μg/ml.; c) an appropriate positive control used which demonstrates a positive response within a historical mutual frequency range and; d) the absolute cloning efficiency of the solvent control must be at least 70%. If the trial meets the criteria for acceptance then the data can be evaluated. Certain additional criteria must be met to establish whether the observed response is positive, negative or questionable. The exact criteria that are considered usually vary depending upon the investigator. A general rule-of-thumb used by many investigators defines a positive response as one which is twice the spontaneous mutant frequency. This, however, should be supported by statistical analysis for which several models have been proposed (Clive et al., 1979; Amacher et al., 1980; Irr and Snee, 1982). The compound must be tested in the presence and absence of metabolic activation. The response must be reproducible in at least duplicate experiments. There may be instances where a compound will produce a weak reproducible response at a single dose level; this type of response should be considered questionable and confirmed in another system.

It has been suggested that the L5178YTK+/- assay has the capacity to identify both point mutation and chromosomal aberrations produced by exposure to chemical mutagens (Clive et al., 1980; Hozier et al., 1981). This is exhibited by the presence of large and/or small colonies arising in the soft agar in the presence of selective agent F_3TdR. Small colonies, it is suggested, represent chromosomal aberrations which produce a slow growing cell and hence a small colony. Large colonies on the other hand are believed to be the result of single point mutations occurring in the structural gene. These are interesting interpretations of L5178YTK+/- assay data; however, there are certain elements to these observations that are troubling. These include: a) lack of stability of colony size and generation time of small F_3TdR^r colonies, b) lack of data concerning generation time of large F_3TdR^r colonies to THMG, d) lack of cytogenetic analysis of large as well as small F_3TdR^r colonies derived as spontaneous variants, e) classification of slow growth as having a generation time of 12 hours or longer when a 12 hour generation time is within the reported normal range for this cell line (Clive et al., 1972; Clive et al., 1973), f) the cytostatic mode of action of F_3TdR^r (Thilly et al., 1980; Moore-Brown and Clive, 1979), and g) many of the induced small F_3TdR^r colonies fail to exhibit stable cytogenetic damage (Hozier et al., 1981). The existence of large and small colonies was noted in the early mammalian mutagenesis assay (Kao and Puck, 1968; Kao and Puck, 1969; Chu and Malling, 1968). They are of interest in mutagenesis mechanism studies but at this point seem to add very little to a mutagenesis screening assay. The important requirement of a mutagenesis screening assay is to identify an induced heritable alteration in the genome of the indicator cell. On its face, it does not seem to matter whether the change results in the formation of a large colony or small colony as long as the change is permanent and heritable.

The L5178YTK+/- assay is well suited for mutagenesis screening of unknown chemicals. The techniques used in conducting of the assay are easy as the cells grow in suspension allowing them to be manipulated like bacteria. The phenotypic expression time is short (48-72 hours), permitting a short turn-around time and also increasing the efficiency of the effort expended. The activation system coupled with the L5178YTK+/- assays has been used to examine a much larger number of chemicals than in the other assays discussed in this work and is therefore regarded as the best characterized. The assay can detect chemicals which induce base pair substitution as well as frame shift type compounds and has the capacity to identify certain classes of chemical carcinogens, i.e. chlorinated compound, metals, or the nitrosamine, dimethylnitrosamine (Clive et al., 1979; Amacher et al., 1980) that presently go undetected in the Salmonella assay.

The L5178YTK+/-assay utilizes the TK locus, which is not well characterized. While some efforts have been made to better understand the mechanisms involved in mutagenesis at the TK locus, the results are a bit confusing (Clive and Voytek, 1977). In the original isolation and characterization of the TK+/- heterozygote it was concluded that the TK gene was expressed as a single gene because the TK+/- clones isolated exhibited approximately half of the TK activity exhibited in the TK+/+ wild type parent (Clive et al., 1973). Later data were presented as support that the genetic target was a structural gene, where TK activity in a TK+/- cell line, TK+/-3.1.1, was twice that of the TK+/+ wild type parent. This is in conflict with the original hypothesis where the expected TK activity would have been half that of the TK+/+ wild type parent. These experiments lead the authors to conclude that the target of the L5178YTK+/- assay is the TK structural gene; however, in view of the conflict of these data with those of earlier studies it seems premature to make this conclusion without further investigations. Experiments conducted in our laboratory indicate that the genetic target of the L5178YTK+/-assay may not be a structural gene. These studies are being expanded to better understand the nature of mutation at the TK enzyme.

The observation that small colonies are characteristic in this assay requires that a stringent protocol be followed which will prevent loss of the small colonies and enhance their detection. The critical elements of such a protocol have not been clearly established.

The mode of action of F_3TdR is not clearly understood and has been reported to be cytostatic rather than cytotoxic (Thilly et al., 1980; Moore-Brown and Clive, 1979). F_3TdR has also been reported to be labile under the conditions used for mutant selection (Liber and Thilly, 1982). These characteristics of F_3TdR could allow formation of non-mutant colonies if an adequate concentration of F_3TdR is not present in the selective medium.

The L5178YTK+/-assay is a mammalian mutagenesis assay that appears to detect direct acting mutagens and promutagens. The results presented to date indicate that it can detect certain classes of compounds not detected in the Salmonella assay (Clive et al., 1979; Amacher et al., 1980). It is recognized by industry and government as an *in vitro* mutagenesis system that can be used in a testing battery to identify potentially hazardous environmental chemicals but more needs to be learned with regard to its genetic and biochemical basis.

IV. Other Mutagenesis Assays

There are two additional assay systems that deserve mention. These are the human fibroblast/HGPRT, APRT (DeMars, 1974) system and the human lymphoblast TK6TK+/-assay (Skopek et al., 1978; Thilly et al., 1980; Liber and Thilly, 1982). Human fibroblasts have been mainly used to investigate mutagenic mechanisms and have not been used to any extent for mutagenesis screening. The TK6 TK+/- assay is still in developmental stages and will require more extensive validation before it will reach the point of the better established mutagenesis screening systems.

E. DISCUSSION

The *in vitro* mammalian mutagenesis screening systems discussed above have been developed to a point where any of them could be used to evaluate the mutagenic potential of unknown chemicals. The assays CHO/HGPRT, V-79, L5178YTK+/-all have been used to identify mutagens. The loci employed are scored for the presence or absence of specific enzyme activity, i.e. 6-TG^r for HGPRT$^{(-)}$, Oua^r for Na/K ATPase and F$_3$TdR^r for TK$^{-/-}$. The use of one or all of the loci and/or systems might be indicated for testing certain chemicals and should be an important element in the development of any screening battery for unknown chemicals. The L5178YTK+/-assay appears to be the most widely used *in vitro* mammalian mutagenesis screen and has the largest data base for testing chemicals both with and without activation. The Na/K ATPase locus is not recommended for general screening because the locus does not appear to detect frameshift mutations. The HGPRT locus is probably the best characterized but requires a long phenotypic expression time increasing the amount of effort required to perform a study. There are two human mutagenesis systems available; however, they lack either the ease of handling or their development is incomplete and are used mainly for mechanism studies.

The *in vitro* mammalian mutagenesis systems offer some advantages over both bacterial systems and *in vitro* systems. These include their ability to detect certain classes of mutagenic compounds missed by the *Salmonella* assay. They are higher on the phylogenetic ladder containing an organized nucleus, not naked DNA, as is found in bacteria; therefore the data are more relevant to man. They are cheaper to perform and have a shorter turn-around time than *in vivo* assays, and the data are more reliable because the *in vitro* loci are better characterized than the *in vivo* systems.

Disadvantages to the *in vitro* mammalian systems include the fact that the end-point in the *in vitro* systems is genetic and not carcinogenic, the *in vitro* data are less relevant to man than the *in vivo* data, metabolic activation cannot mimic that found in the whole animal, *in vitro* assays require stringent control of the protocol to obtain valid data, and *in vitro* mammalian assay systems are very difficult if not impossible to use in underdeveloped countries.

Mammalian *in vitro* mutagenesis assays are recognized for their ability to predict potential mutagenesis and carcinogenesis. Resistance to the selective agents does not, however, distinguish between genotoxicity or non-genotoxicity. The results from these studies are still useful since a genotoxic response could indicate mutagenic effects on somatic and germinal cells *in vivo* and a non-genotoxic effect could indicate a stable phenotypic change that could cause cancer. With this in mind it should be recognized that *in vitro* mammalian mutagenesis assays are an important and an intergral part of any tier/battery test approach used to screen chemicals.

REFERENCES

Adair, G.M., Carver, J.H. and Wandres, D.L. Mutagenicity testing in mammalian cells. I. Derivation of a Chinese hamster ovary cell line heterozygous for the adenine phosphoribosyl transferase and thymidine kinase loci. *Mutat. Res.* **72**:177–205 (1980).

Amacher, D.E., Paillet, S. and Ray, V.A. Point mutations at the thymidine kinase locus in L5178Y mouse lymphoma cells. I. Applications to genetic toxicological testing. *Mutat. Res.* **64**:391–406 (1979).

Amacher, D.E., Paillet, S.C., Turner, G.N., Ray, V.A., and Salsburg, D.S. Point mutations at the thymidine kinase locus in L5178Y mouse lymphoma cells. II. Test validation and interpretation. *Mutat. Res.* **72**:447–474 (1980).

Baker, R.M., Burnette, D.M., Mankovitz, R., Thompson, L.H., Whitmore, G.F, Siminovitch, L., and Till, J.E. Ouabain-resistant mutants of mouse and hamster cells in culture. *Cell* **1(1)**:9–21 (1974).

Bartsch, H., Malavielle, C., Camus, A.N., Mortel-Planche, G., Brun, G., Hautefeville, A., Sabadie, N., and Barbin, A. Validation and comparative studies on 180 chemicals with *S. Typhimurium* strains and V-79 Chinese hamster cells in the presence of various metabolizing systems. *Mutat. Res.* **76**:1–50 (1980).

Bradley, M.O., Bhuyan, B., Frances, M.C., Langenbach, R., Peterson, A., and Huberman, E. Mutagenesis by chemical agents in V-79 Chinese hamster cells: A review and analysis of the literature. A report of the Gene-Tox program. *Mutat. Res.* **87**:81–142 (1981).

Capazzi, R.L., Smith, W.J., Field, R. and Papirmeister, B.A. Host-mediated assay for chemical mutagens using the L5178YAsn murine leukemia. *Mutat. Res.* **21**:6 (1973).

Carver, J.H., Adari, G.M., and Wandres, D.L. Mutagenicity testing in mammalian cells. II. Validation of multiple drug-resistance markers having practical application for screening potential mutagens. *Mutat. Res.* **72**:207–230 (1980).

Caskey, T.C. and Kruh, G.D. The HGPRT Locus. *Cell* **16**:1–9 (1979).

Chu, E.H.Y. and Malling, H.V. Mammalian cell genetics, II. Chemical induction of specific locus mutation in Chinese hamster cells in vitro. *Proc. Nat. Acad. Sc.* **61**:1306–1312 (1968).

Clive, D., Flamm, W.G., Machesko, M.R., and Bernheim, N.J. A mutational assay system using the thymidine kinase locus in mouse lymphoma cells. *Mutat. Res.* **16**:77–87 (1972).

Clive, D., Flamm, W.G., and Patterson, J.B. Specific-locus mutational assay systems for mouse lymphoma cells. In: Chemical Mutagens: Principles and Methods for Their Detection. (ed. A. Hollaender) Vol. 3, pp. 79-103 (1973).

Clive, D. and Spector, J.F.S. Laboratory procedure for assessing specific locus mutations at the TK locus in cultured L5178Y mouse lymphoma cells. *Mutat. Res.* **31**:17-29 (1975).

Clive, D. and Voytek, P. Evidence for chemically induced structural gene mutations at the thymidine kinase locus in cultured L5178Y mouse lymphoma cells. *Mutat. Res.* **44**:269-278 (1977).

Clive, D., Johnson, D. K., Spector, J.F.S., Batson, A.G. and Brown, M.M.M. Validation and characterization of the L5178Y/TK+/- mouse lymphoma mutagen assay system. *Mutat. Res.* **59**:61-108 (1979).

Clive, D., Batson, G.A., and Turner, N.T. The ability of L5178Y/TK/+/-mouse cells to detect single gene and viable chromosome mutation: Evaluation and relevance to mutagen and carcinogen screening. In: the Predictive Value of Short-Term Screening Tests in Carcinogen Evaluation. (ed. G.M. Williams et al.) pp. 103-123, Elsevier/North-Holland Biomedical Press (1980).

Cole, J. and Arlett, C.F. Ethyl methanesulphonate mutagenesis with L5178Y mouse lymphoma cells: A comparison of ouabain, thioguanine, and excess thymidine resistance. *Mutat. Res.* **34**:507-526 (1976).

Cole, J., Arlette, C.F., and Green, M.H.L. The fluctuation test as a more sensitive system for determining induced mutation in L5178Y mouse lymphoma cells. *Mutat. Res.* **41**:377-386 (1976).

DeMars, R. Resistance of cultured human fibroblasts and other cells to purine and pyrimidine analogues in relation to mutagenesis detection. *Mutat. Res.* **24**:335-364 (1974).

Fischer, G.A. Nutritional and amethopterin-resistance characteristics of leukemic clones. *Cancer Res.* **19**:372-376 (1959).

Fischer, G.A. and Sartorelli, A.C. Development, maintenance and assay of drug resistance. *Meth. Med. Res.* **10**:247-262 (1959).

Fischer, G.A., Lee, S.Y. and Calbresi, P. Detection of chemical mutagens using host-mediated assay (L5178Y) mutagenesis system. *Mutat. Res.* **26**:501-511 (1974).

Hozier, J., Swayer, J., Moore, M., Howard, B. and Clive, D. Cytogenetic analysis of the L5178Y/TK+/- TK-/- mouse lymphoma mutagenesis assay system. *Mutat. Res.* **84**:169-181 (1981).

Hsie, A.W., Couch, D.B., O'Neill, J.P., San Sebastian, J.R., Brimer, P.A., Machanoff, R., Riddle, J.C., Li, A.P., Fuscoe, J.C., Forbes, N., and Hsie, M.H. Utilization of a quantitative mammalian cell mutation system, CHO/HGPRT, in experimental mutagenesis and genetic toxicology. In: Strategies for Short-Term Testing for Mutagens/Carcinogens (ed. B.E. Butterworth) pp. 39-54 CRC Press, West Palm Beach, FL. (1979).

Hsie, A.W., Casciano, D.A., Couch, D.B., Krahn, D.F., O'Neill, J.P., and Whitfield, B.L. The use of Chinese hamster ovary cells to quantify specific locus mutation and to determine mutagenicity of chemicals. A report of the Gene-Tox. program. *Mutat. Res.* **86**:193-214 (1981).

Huberman, E. and Sachs, L. Mutability of different genetic loci in mammalian cells by metabolically activated carcinogens/polycyclic hydrocarbons (ouabain, temperature, and 8-azaguanine resistance) membrane mutants/ aminophylline/chinese hamster cells. *Int. J. Cancer* **13**:326-333 (1974).

Huberman, E. and Sachs, L. Cell mediated mutagenesis of mammalian cells with chemical carcinogens. *Proc. Natl. Acad. Sci. (USA)* **73**:188-192 (1976).

Irr, J.D. and Snee, R.D. A statistical method for analysis of mouse lymphoma L5178Y cell TK locus forward mutation assay. *Mutat. Res.* **97**:371–392 (1982).

Jacobs, L. and DeMars, R. Quantification of chemical mutagenesis in diploid human fibroblasts: induction of azaguanine-resistant mutants by N-methyl-N'-nitrosoquanidine. *Mutat. Res.* **53**:29–53 (1978).

Kao, F.T. and Puck, T.T. Genetics of somatic mammalian cells, VII. Induction and isolation of nutritional mutants in Chinese hamster cells. *Proc. Nat. Acad. Sc.* **60**:1275–1282 (1968).

Kao, F.T. and Puck, T.T. Genetics of somatic mammalian cells, IX. Quantitation mutagenesis by physical and chemical agents. *J. Cell. Physiol.* **74**:245–258 (1969).

Kozak, C.A., Fowinier, R.E.K., Lwinwand, L.A., and Ruddle, F.H. Assignment of the gene governing cellular ouabain resistance to *Mus Musculus* chromosome 3 using human/mouse mirocell hybrids. *Biochem. Genet.* **17**:23–34 (1979).

Krahn, D.F. and Heidelberger, C. Liver homogenate mediated mutagenesis in Chinese hamster V-79 cells by polycyclic aromatic hydrocarbons and aflatoxins. *Mutat. Res.* **46**:27–44 (1977).

Liber, H.L. and Thilly, W.G. Mutation assay at the thymidine kinase locus in diploid human lymphoblasts. *Mutat. Res.* **94**:467–485 (1982).

Maher, V.M. and McCormick, J.J. Cytotoxic and mutagenic effects of carcinogenic aromatic amides and polycyclic hydrocarbons and ultraviolet irradiation in normally repairing and repair-deficient (Xeroderma pigmentosum) diploid human skin fibroblasts. *Basic Life Sci.* **58**:785–787 (1975).

Maher, V.N. and Mccormick, J.J. Effect of DNA repair on the cytoxicity and mutagenicity of UV irradiation and of chemical carcinogens in normal and Xeroderma pigmentosum cells. In: Biology and Radiation Carcinogenesis (eds. J.M. Yuhas, R.W. Tennant and J.D. Regan) pp. 129–145, Raven Press, N.Y. (1976).

Maher, V.M., Curren, R.D., Quellette, L.M. and McCormick, J.J. Effect of DNA repair on the frequency of mutations induced in human cells by ultraviolet irradiation and by chemical carcinogens. In: Fundamentals in Cancer Prevention (ed. P.N. Magee et al.) pp. 363–382, Univ. of Tokyo Press, Tokyo/Univ. Park Press, Baltimore (1976).

McBreen, P., Orkwiszewski, K.G., Chern, C.J., Mellman, W.J. and Croce, C.M. Synteny of the genes for thymidine kinase and galactokinase in the mouse and their assignment to mouse chromosome II. *Cytogenet. Cell. Genet.* **19**:7–13 (1977).

McCormick, J.J. and Maher, V.M. Mutagenesis studies in diploid human cells with different DNA-repair capacities. Short-Term Tests, Chem. Carcinogens. pp. 264–276 (1981).

Moore-Brown, M.M. and Clive, D. The L5178Y/TK+/- mutation assay system: *In situ* results. In: Banbury Report 2 Mammalian Cell Mutagenesis: The Maturation of Test Systems. (Eds. A.W. Hsie, J.P. O'Neill, V.K. McElheny) pp. 71–88 (1979).

Morrow, K.J., Jr. An investigation into the basis of variation of purine analogue resistance in an established murine cell line. Ph.D. Thesis, University of Washington (1964).

Morrow, J. Genetic analysis of azaguanine resistance in an established mouse cell line. *Genetics* **65**:279–287 (1970).

O'Niell, J.P., Brimer, P.A., Machanoff, R., Hirsch, G.P., and Hsie, A.W. A quantitative assay of mutation induction at the hypoxanthine-guanine phosphoribosyl transferase locus in Chinese hamster ovary cells (CHO/HGPRT system): Development and definition of the system. *Mutat. Res.* **45**:91–102 (1977a).

O'Neill, J.P., Couch, D.B., Machanoff, R., San Sebastian, J.R., Brimer, P.A., and Hsie, A.W. A quantitative assay of mutation induction at the hypoxanthine-guanine phosphoribosyl transferase locus in Chinese hamster ovary cells (CHO/HGPRT system): utilization with a variety of mutagenic agents. *Mutat. Reg.* **45**:103–115 (1977b).

O'Neill, J.P. and Hsie, A.W. The CHO/HGPRT mutation assay: Experimental procedure. In: Banbury Report 2 Mammalian Cell Mutagenesis: The maturation of Test Systems. (eds. A.W. Hsie, J.P. O'Neill, V.K. McElheny) pp. 55–69 (1979).

Palmer, K.A., Denunzio, A., and Green, S. The mutagenic assay of some hair dye components using the thymidine kinase locus of L5178Y mouse lymphoma cells. *J. Environ. Path.* **1**:87–91 (1977).

Puck, T.T. and Marcus, P.I. A rapid method for viable cell titration and clone production with HeLa cells on tissue culture; the use of X-irradiated cells to supply conditioning factors. *Proc. Nat. Acad. Sc.* **41**:432–437 (1955).

Puck, T.T., and Marcus, P.I., and Cieciura, S.J. Clonal growth of mammalian cells in vitro. Growth characteristics of colonies from single HeLa cells with and without a "feeder" layer. *J. Exptl. Med.* **103**:273–289 (1956).

Skopek, T.R., Leber, H.L., Penman, B.W. and Thilly, W.G. Isolation of a human lymphoblastoid line heterozygous at the thymidine kinase locus: Possibility for a rapid human cell mutation assay. *Biochem. Biophys. Res. Commun.* **84**:411–423 (1978).

Snee, R.D., and Irr, J.D. Design of a statistical method for the analysis of mutagenesis at the hypoxanthinguanine phoshoribosyl transferase locus of cultured chinese hamster ovary cells. *Mutat. Res.* **85**:77–93 (1981).

Szybalski, W. and Szybalska, E.H. Drug sensitivity as a genetic marker for human cell lines. *U. Mich. Med. Bull.* **28**:277–293 (1962).

Szybalski, W., Szybalska, E.H. and Ragni, G. Genetic studies with human cell lines. *Natl. Cancer Inst. Monograph* **No. 7**:75–88 (1962).

Szybalski, W., Ragni, G. and Cohn, N.K. Mutagenic response of human somatic cell lines. *Symp. Internat. Soc. Cell Biol.* **3**:209–221 (1964).

Thilly, W.G., DeLuca, J.G., Furth, E.E., Hoppe IV, H., Kaden, D.A., Krolewski, J.J., Liber, H.L., Skopek, T.R., Slapikoff, S.A., Tizard, R.J. and Perman, B.W. Gene-locus mutation assays in diploid human lymphoblast lines. In: Chemical Mutagens: Principles and Methods for Their Detection (eds. F.J. deSerres and A. Hollaender) Vol. 6, Plenum, New York, pp. 331–364 (1980).

Willecke, K., Reber, T., Kucherlapatic, R.S. and Ruddle, F.H. Human Mitochondrial thymidine kinase is coded for by a gene on chromosome 16 of the nucleus. *Somatic Cell Genet.* **3(3)**:237–245 (1977).

CHAPTER VIII

COMPARISON OF CARCINOGENESIS AND MUTAGENESIS OF MAMMALIAN CELLS IN CULTURE

J. Carl Barrett and Eugene Elmore[1]
Environmental Carcinogenesis Group
Laboratory of Pulmonary Function & Toxicology
National Institute of Environmental Health Sciences
National Institutes of Health
Research Triangle Park, N.C. 27709

A. INTRODUCTION

An examination of the relationship between mutagenesis and carcinogenesis requires that each process be quantitated and that the mechanism of each process be defined. The process of somatic mutation can be studied reliably by examining various heritable phenotypic alterations of mammalian cells, particularly resistance to certain drugs. Additionally, the basis of somatic mutation can be defined at the molecular level in biochemical terms. Neoplastic transformation, in contrast, is less well understood, a fact partially attributable to the lack of a definitive phenotypic alteration characteristic of malignancy. Although tumor formation *in vivo* serves to define neoplastic transformation of cells *in vitro*, tumorigenicity is a multi-faceted phenomenon which is difficult to analyze at the molecular or cellular level. Accordingly, several other *in vitro* phenotypic characteristics which are associated with transformed cells have been studied extensively. Thus, somatic mutation and neoplastic transformation can be investigated by the same experimental approach, i.e., by studying heritable phenotypic alterations of cells in culture.

There have been several excellent reviews of the experimental systems to study neoplastic transformation of cells in culture. One review (Hollstein, et al, 1979) is an extensive side by side comparison of short-term tests and collates results with numerous chemicals tested in more than one system. A second review prepared by an *ad hoc* working group of the IARC presents a more

1. Current Address: Northrop Services, P.O. Box 12313, Research Triangle Park, NC 27709.

detailed description of different *in vitro* transformation systems (IARC, 1980). The third review, which was prepared by a committee for the Gene-Tox Program of the U.S. Environmental Protection Agency (Heidelberger, et al, 1983), is the most complete survey of the literature on chemical carcinogenesis in cell culture. Barrett and Thomassen (1984) also provide a detailed description of quantitative assays. These reviews describe the types of systems available, give the advantages and disadvantages of each, and indicate the current validation of each as a screen for carcinogens. That information will not be repeated here. In an earlier review by Barrett and Ts'o (1978a) which has been updated (Barrett, et al, 1984), a discussion of mechanistic studies of neoplastic transformation of cells was presented. Therefore, in this chapter we will focus on the comparison between neoplastic transformation and somatic mutation of cells in culture. A description of the experimental systems to measure oncogenesis in culture will be given with the aim of understanding the biological significance of these systems and the possible role of mutation in the cell transformation process.

The origin of the somatic mutation theory of carcinogenesis is generally credited to Theodor Boveri, who in 1914 published a book entitled, *Zur Frage der Entstehung Maligner Tumoren* ("On the Problem of the Origin of Malignant Tumors") (Boveri, 1914). Today, this is still a major theory of carcinogenesis, although it is not proven and many cancer biologists favor an epigenetic basis for the neoplastic alteration of tumor cells (Barrett, et al, 1981a). There are several lines of evidence which support the somatic mutation theory of carcinogenesis and these are discussed in detail in Chapter 2 of this volume and elsewhere (Barrett, et al, 1981a; Barrett, et al, 1983).

One of the difficulties in elucidating the role of mutagenesis in carcinogenesis is the limited number of studies in which somatic mutation and neoplastic transformation are examined concomitantly. The correlation between mutagenicity and carcinogenicity of a number of chemicals, which provides major experimental support for the somatic mutation theory, has been demonstrated primarily using bacterial mutagenicity assays (Ames, et al, 1973). While this correlation can be nearly 90% in some studies (McCann and Ames, 1976; McCann, et al, 1975), chemicals have been reported that are carcinogenic but not mutagenic, or mutagenic but not carcinogenic (Barrett, et al, 1983; Barrett, et al, 1981a; Metzler, et al, 1980; Trainin, et al, 1964). These exceptions to this correlation may provide insight into the mechanisms of neoplastic transformation and the relationship of this process to somatic mutation. On the other hand, these exceptions may not be real, but simply result from the use of different assay systems to measure each process (e.g., mutagenicity in bacteria versus carcinogenicity in man). A correlation between mutagenicity and carcinogenicity might be observed with all chemicals, if both processes were measured in the same target cell. The use of mammalian cells in culture allows the concomitant study of somatic mutation and neoplastic transformation measured in the same target cell (Barrett, et al, 1981a). During the past years several laboratories have completed such studies and these will be discussed in detail in a later section.

172

Systems which measure neoplastic transformation of cells in culture also provide short-term assays for potential carcinogens. In contrast to several other short-term tests, cell transformation assays for carcinogens are not predicated on a theoretical correlation between carcinogenesis and mutagenesis or other genotoxic endpoints. Of course, cell transformation assays are based on the assumption that neoplastic transformation induced in cells in culture occurs by the same mechanism as neoplastic alteration of cells *in vivo*. This is an important point to which we will return in the discussion of different cell transformation systems.

Before discussing experimental systems using cells in culture for the study of neoplastic transformation, an essential feature of cancer development *in vivo* needs to be addressed. There is now considerable evidence that neoplastic development occurs as a progressive process through qualitatively different stages (Barrett, et al, 1981a; Foulds, 1969). Experimental support for a multi-stage model of carcinogenesis is provided from many diverse studies (Table 1 and Barrett, et al, 1981a). Studies with cells in culture have clearly demonstrated the progressive nature of neoplastic development (Barrett and Ts'o, 1978a; Barrett, et al, 1981a). For example, if one starts with a culture of normal, diploid embryo fibroblasts, these cells will progress to a preneoplastic stage prior to conversion of the cells to a neoplastic or tumorigenic stage (Barrett, et al, 1981a; Barrett and Ts'o, 1978b; Barrett, 1980). This process will occur either spontaneously or following carcinogen treatment, which increases the rate and frequency of the process. A preneoplastic cell is defined as one which is altered from the normal cell in that it has an increased propensity to become neoplastic as measured by tumorigenicity *in vivo*. In culture, preneoplastic cells often acquire some, but not all of the properties needed for a tumor cell. In addition, these cells acquire a number of other phenotypic changes which may or may not be necessary for the malignant phenotype (Barrett and Ts'o, 1978a; Barrett, 1980).

There are two essential points that need to be emphasized here. First, it is important in studies of transformation of cells in culture to consider whether one is studying the transformation of normal cells to a preneoplastic state or the transformation of preneoplastic cells to the neoplastic or some other state. Second, the mechanisms of transformation of cells from one stage to another may vary depending on the starting point of the cells. Thus, the mechanism of transformation of normal cells to preneoplastic cells may be different than that for the change of preneoplastic cells to neoplastic cells. These two points should be considered in any discussion of the biological significance of cell transformation systems.

B. EXPERIMENTAL MODELS TO STUDY NEOPLASTIC TRANSFORMATION OF CELLS IN CULTURE

A number of experimental systems utilizing cells from a variety of species have been employed for studies of cell transformation by chemical carcinogens (Hollstein, et al, 1979; IARC, 1980; Heidelberger, et al, 1983; Barrett and Thomassen, 1984). Neoplastic transformation *in vitro* of both epithelial-like

TABLE 1
Evidence for Multistage Models of Neoplastic Development

1. Pathological Observations of Tumors (Tumor Progression, Foulds)
2. Two-Stage Model of Chemical Carcinogenesis in Mouse Skin
3. Individuals with Genetic Traits Manifested by an Early Occurrence of Cancer
   (eg. familial retinoblastoma, adenomatosis of the colon and rectum).
4. Mathematical Models Based on Age Specific Tumor Incidence Curves
5. Cell Culture Studies

and fibroblast-like cells has been reported. Fibroblast-like cells are easier to grow in culture and hence most studies have employed this cell type. Studies with epithelial-like cells are also now possible (Barrett and Thomassen, 1984).

Table 2 lists some of the experimental systems which have been used for quantitative studies of cell transformation by chemical carcinogens. In addition to these systems, virally infected cultures of rat, mouse, and hamster cells have been employed (Hollstein, et al, 1979; IARC, 1980; Heidelberger, et al, 1983). Viral and chemical carcinogenesis appears to be a sensitive assay for carcinogens (Hollstein, et al, 1979; IARC, 1980; Heidelberger, et al, 1983). However, this represents the enhancement of viral carcinogenesis, at least in some systems (Hollstein, et al, 1979; IARC, 1980; Heidelberger, et al, 1983), and the significance of these observations to the mechanism of chemical carcinogenesis is unclear.

Of the systems listed in Table 2, Syrian hamster embryo cells, BHK cells, mouse Balb/c 3T3 and mouse C3H 10T½ cells have been studied most extensively (Hollstein, et al, 1979; IARC, 1980; Heidelberger, et al, 1983). Hence, a further discussion of these systems will be given. Due to the obvious importance of human cells, a discussion of the studies with human cell transformation also will be presented.

TABLE 2
Fibroblast-Like Cell Culture Systems to Study Neoplastic Transformation of Cells in Culture

I. Hamster Cells
    A. Syrian Hamster
        1. Syrian Hamster Embryo (SHE) Cells
        2. Baby Hamster Kidney (BHK) Cells
    B. Chinese Hamster
II. Ray Embryo Cells
III. Guinea Pig Fetal Cells
IV. Murine Cells
    A. Ventral Prostate Cell Line
    B. Balb/c 3T3 Cell Line
    C. C3H 10T½ Cell Line
    D. C3H M2 Cell Line
V. Human Cells

I. Studies With Cells From Syrian Hamsters

The first unequivocal demonstration of chemical carcinogen induced neoplastic transformation of cells in culture was by Berwald and Sachs (1963; 1965). They demonstrated that Syrian hamster embryo cells exposed in culture to benzo(a)pyrene or other carcinogens give rise to morphologically altered cells which, if isolated or passaged a number of times, are tumorigenic when injected into Syrian hamsters. The cell cultures consist predominantly of fibroblasts and the tumors from carcinogen exposed cells are generally fibrosarcomas (Berwald and Sachs, 1963; 1965). Untreated cells fail to produce tumors *in vivo* even when 10^9 cells were injected while as few as 1–10 transformed cells can produce tumors in newborn hamsters (Huberman and Sachs, 1966; Barrett, et al, 1979; Benedict, et al, 1975).

Berwald and Sachs (1965) were able to quantitate the number of morphologically transformed colonies that resulted in 1–8 days following exposure of cells to a carcinogen. Studies by DiPaolo and colleagues (1969; 1971a; 1971b; 1971c; 1972a) and Pienta and co-workers (1977; 1980) demonstrated that morphological transformation of Syrian hamster embryo cells occurs following treatment with a variety of chemical carcinogens, but not after treatment with structurally related non-carcinogens. In fact, this is now one of the most sensitive and selective short-term tests for carcinogens (Pienta, et al, 1977; 1980).

The number of morphologically transformed colonies observed is dependent on the dose of the carcinogen employed and the number of cells at risk (DiPaolo, et al, 1971a; Barrett and Ts'o; 1978a). Statistical analysis of the dose response curve of the chemically induced morphological transformation indicates that it fits very well with a "one hit" model for this transformation (Gart, et al, 1979). Results with this system also demonstrate that this process results from the induction of transformed cells as opposed to selection of pre-existing neoplastic cells (DiPaolo, et al, 1971b; Barrett and Ts'o, 1978a). There is also no evidence to support a role for endogenous viruses in the chemically induced neoplastic transformation in this or any of the other cell transformation systems (Barrett and Ts'o, 1978a). DNA is at least one of the critical targets for neoplastic transformation of Syrian hamster embryo cells since a perturbation specific for DNA is sufficient to induce neoplastic transformation of these cells (Barrett, et al, 1978a; Tsutsui, et al, 1979).

Morphological transformation is the earliest observed change in the transformation process of these cells, but morphologically transformed cells are not tumorigenic (Barrett and Ts'o, 1978a; 1978b; Barrett, et al, 1981a). Rather these cells undergo a series of progressive changes ultimately resulting in neoplastic conversion of the cells (Barrett and Ts'o, 1978b). Barrett and Ts'o (1978b) and Barrett (1980) have presented evidence that both spontaneous and carcinogen induced neoplastic transformation of these cells *in vitro* is a progressive process, in analogy to the process of neoplastic development *in vivo* (IARC, 1980; Barrett, et al, 1981a; Foulds, 1969; Barrett and Ts'o, 1978b). Preneoplastic cells have been isolated and exhibit some but not all of the phenotypes associated with neoplastic cells (Table 3). Morphological alterations are observed in some but not all preneoplastic and neoplastic cells (Barrett, 1980). Anchorage independent growth, as measured by the ability to grow in semisolid media such as agar, is an *in vitro* phenotype which is closely associated with tumorigenicity in Syrian hamster cells. Preneoplastic cells do not grow in semisolid agar, but can give rise to cells which are able to grow in agar and are not tumorigenic *in vivo* (Barrett, 1980). The transition from anchorage dependent to anchorage independent growth can occur in a single step with preneoplastic cells, but is not measurable with normal, diploid cells (Barrett and Ts'o, 1978b; Barrett, 1980). Normal cells following carcinogen exposure give rise to preneoplastic cells with one or more of the characteristics of such cells listed in Table 3 and these preneoplastic cells progress to neoplastic cells with further growth in culture (Barrett and Ts'o, 1978b).

In addition to early passage Syrian hamster embryo cells, extensive studies have been done with a Syrian hamster fibroblast cell line, BHK, which was derived from the kidney of a young hamster (Stoker and MacPherson, 1964). This cell line has the properties of preneoplastic cells listed in Table 3 and undergoes neoplastic conversion in apparently a single step (Bouck and diMayorca, 1976). In fact, frequently the cells transform spontaneously and more than 10^4 cells are often tumorigenic in animals. By subcloning, cells can be isolated with a relative low frequency (10^{-5}) of spontaneous growth in soft agar. This *in vitro* phenotype can be induced following treatment with chemical carcinogens and this technique is employed as a short-term assay for potential carcinogens (Bouck and diMayorca, 1976; Styles, 1980).

II. Mouse Cell Lines

Cultures of Syrian hamster embryo cells generally have a limited life span in culture and senesce after less than 20 passages (Barrett and Ts'o, 1978b).

TABLE 3
Characteristics of Cell Populations During Neoplastic Progression of Syrian Hamster Embryo Cells

Normal Cells	Preneoplastic Cells	Neoplastic Cells
Diploid	Aneuploid	Aneuploid
Low fibrinolytic activity	Enhanced fibrinolytic activity	Enhanced fibrinolytic activity
Definite lifespan	Indefinite lifespan	Indefinite lifespan
Anchorage dependent growth	Anchorage dependent growth	Anchorage independent growth
Nontumorigenic in suspension	Nontumorigenic in suspension	Tumorigenic in suspension
Nontumorigenic when attached to plastic substrate	Tumorigenic when attached to plastic substrate	Tumorigenic when attached to plastic substrate

Establishment of a permanent cell line with an indefinite lifetime in culture occurs only rarely with hamster cells in the absence of carcinogen treatment (Barrett and Ts'o, 1978b; Barrett, 1980). In contrast, cultures of mouse embryo cells escape cellular senescence spontaneously with a high frequency and continue to grow *in vitro* (Todaro and Green, 1963; Aaronson and Todaro, 1968a). These cell lines often progress to malignancy if grown continuously in culture (Aaronson and Todaro, 1968b). The rate at which the cells become tumorigenic is dependent on the density at which they are grown *in vitro*. If maintained at low cell densities and passaged at confluence, nontumorigenic cell lines can be isolated (Aaronson and Todaro, 1968b). For example, Aaronson and Todaro (1968a) established the 3T3 cell line from a Balb/c mouse embryo by transferring the culture every 3 days at 3×10^5 cells per 60mm dish. (The nomenclature of the cell line designates this growth regimen.) Balb/c3T3 cells are nontumorigenic whereas Balb/c 3T12 cells (subcultured every 3 days at 12×10^5 cells) are tumorigenic (Aaronson and Todaro, 1968b). By the same basic principle Reznikoff, et al (1973a) were able to obtain a nontumorigenic C3H mouse embryo cell line designated C3H 10T½, i.e. passaged every 10 days at 0.5×10^5 cells per 60mm dish.

The Balb/c 3T3 and the C3H 10T½ cell lines are similar in that both are morphologically normal, contact inhibited and nontumorigenic when injected *in vivo* as a cell suspension (Reznikoff, et al, 1973a). However, the cells are aneuploid with a subtetraploid model chromosome number and readily become neoplastic *in vitro* if treated with carcinogens (Reznikoff, et al, 1973a; 1973b). If maintained *in vivo* attached to a plastic or glass substrate for approximately 6 months, the cells also neoplastically transform (Boone, 1975; Boone and Jacobs, 1976). Therefore, the cell lines possess properties of preneoplastic cells and should be considered as such.

Both the Balb/c 3T3 and the C3H 10T½ cells are very useful for assays of cell transformation. Clones of either cell type can be isolated which have a low rate of spontaneous transformation but transform with a high frequency when exposed to chemical carcinogens (Hollstein, et al, 1979; IARC, 1980; Heidelberger, et al, 1983; Reznikoff, et al, 1973b; DiPaolo, et al, 1972b; Kakunaga, 1973). The transformation process can be easily monitored by the emergence of morphologically transformed foci of piled up, criss-crossed cells which are quite distinct from the surrounding contact inhibited monolayer of nontransformed cells. Isolated cells from transformed foci are tumorigenic when injected into syngeneic mice (Reznikoff, et al, 1973b; DiPaolo, et al, 1972b; Kakunaga, 1973).

Recently, certain aspects of the transformation process in C3H 10T½ cells have become evident which complicate the quantitation of the cell transformation. Haber and Thilly (1978), Haber, et al (1977), Kennedy and Little (1980; Kennedy, et al, 1980) and Fernandez, et al (1980) have followed up the original observation by Reznikoff, et al (1973b) that the transformation frequency (i.e., number of transformed foci per cell treated after correcting for cells killed) is dependent upon the initial cell number. Extensive studies by Kennedy and Little (1980) with x-ray induced transformation have demonstrated that the absolute yield of transformed cells is constant over a wide range of initial cell numbers. For example, if an initial expression time of 12–14 population doublings after carcinogen treatment is completed and the cells are then resuspended and plated at different densities from 1 to 10,000 cells per plate, the number of transformed foci per dish is approximately 1 for all groups; hence, the apparent transformation frequency varies from 0.01–100% depending on the conditions employed. Also, for a given dose of carcinogen, the number of transformed foci per dish is independent of the number of cells treated. This is in contrast to the results with the Syrian hamster embryo cells (DiPaolo, et al, 1971a).

According to Kennedy, et al (1980), these observations suggest that the transformed clones do not occur as the direct consequence of carcinogen treatment. Rather, these authors propose a two step model to explain the results. The initial change induced by the carcinogen apparently occurs in a large number, perhaps all of the cells. This change does not directly result in the transformation of the cells, but rather, increases the probability that the transformation of these cells will occur as a rare, secondary event. Since the initial cell number and the number of population doublings do not appear to influence the number of transformed foci, Kennedy, et al (1980) initially suggested that this process occurs at confluence, because the number of cells at confluence is constant in the density inhibited C3H 10T½ cell line regardless of the initial cell density. The authors further proposed that these observations are inconsistent with a mutational mechanism and suggested that an epigenetic process is involved in the carcinogen induced transformation of C3H 10T½ cells (Kennedy, et al, 1980).

Heidelberger and co-workers (Fernandez, et al, 1980) have made similar observations with the C3H 10T½ cells and have proposed a "probabilistic theory" to explain the formation of transformed foci by these cells following 3-methylcholanthrene treatment. Their theory is similar to that proposed by Kennedy, et al (1980) in that two steps must occur for cell transformation. The first step is the "activation" of a large percentage of the cells by the carcinogen, which occurs with a probability p_1 and the second step is the transformation of the activated cells, which occurs with a probability of p_2 per cell generation. The authors have derived a mathematical equation which predicts the frequency of foci formation based on the probability of these two steps (p_1 and p_2) plus the probability of deactivation per cell generation of the carcinogen activated cells, which is termed p_3. This approach has the advantage of allowing the determination of these probabilities based on experimental results. The equation derived to describe focus formation is $\log(F/N) = \log[2p_1p_2(1-p_3)/2(1-p_3)-1] + n\log(1-p_3)$, where F = mean number of foci per dish, and N = number of cells in a dish at confluence, and p_1, p_2, and p_3 are the probabilities described above. This equation has been verified experimentally with 3-methylcholanthrene induced C3H 10T½ transformation and the values of $p_3 = 0.24$ and $p_1p_2 = 3.8 \times 10^{-6}$ were calculated.

Unfortunately, the values of p_1 and p_2 could not be determined uniquely (Fernandez, et al, 1980). However, based on the results of these authors (Fernandez, et al, 1980), as well as Kennedy, et al (1980), the probability of activation, p_1, must be nearly equal to 1, since transformation is commonly observed with 1–5 cells at risk. This means that following carcinogen treatment, most, if not all, of the cells are activated, but only a few of the activated cells subsequently transform ($p_2 \geq 3.8 \times 10^{-6}$) per cell generation.

Unfortunately, the probabilistic theory of Fernandez, Mondal, and Heidelberger (1980) for 3-methylcholanthrene induced transformation is insufficient to describe the results of Kennedy, et al (1980) with X-ray induced cell transformation of C3H 10T½ cells (Fernandez, et al, 1980). The reasons for this are not clear. Furthermore, the activation process following X-ray irradiation appears to be stable for 26 generations according to the experiments of Kennedy, et al (1980). This appears to conflict with the p_3 value of 0.24 calculated by Fernandez, Mondal, and Heidelberger for 3-methylcholanthrene treated cells (Fernandez, et al, 1980). We will return to this point in the section of this review on mutational mechanisms and will further analyze these results.

III. Human Cells

There have been several reports of chemical or radiation induced *in vitro* neoplastic transformation of human fibroblasts (Table 4); however, quantitation of the process with these cells is limited. The long latency period and number of cell doublings required for neoplastic expression (Kakunaga, 1978; Milo and DiPaolo, 1978; Namba, et al, 1978; Borek, 1980) and its enhancement by multiple treatments (Namba, et al, 1978) indicate that neoplastic transformation of human cells occurs as a multistage, progressive process. Therefore, isolation and characterization of preneoplastic cells during neoplastic development is required for quantitative studies of this process. Morphological transformation is an important marker for carcinogen altered rodent cells and occurs following carcinogen treatment of human cells (Benedict, et al, 1975; Kakunaga, 1978; Namba, et al, 1978; Borek, 1980; McCormick, et al, 1980; Sutherland, et al, 1980; DeMars and Jackson, 1977; Freedman and Shin, 1977; Tejwani, et al, 1981; Milo, et al, 1981; Silinskas, 1981; Greiner, 1981; Zimmerman and Little, 1981). However, this phenotypic transformation occurs with a low frequency and it not reproducible. The degree of morphological change is less than with rodent cells and the scoring of these changes is more subjective. Anchorage independent growth in semisolid media, a late event in the progressive transformation of rodent cells (Barrett and Ts'o, 1978b) and a reliable indicator of tumorigenicity (Barrett and Ts'o, 1978a; Barrett, et al, 1979), is a relatively early event during neoplastic development in human cells (McCormick, et al, 1980; Sutherland, et al, 1980; DeMars and Jackson, 1977; Freedman and Shin, 1977). However, there are several reports of chemically induced morphological transformation of human cells which grow in soft agar but do not form tumors in nude mice (Table 4). This introduces another problem: that of finding a good experimental model for determining tumorigenicity of human cells, since the use of syngeneic animals is not possible. The occurrence of false negatives and variation in the latency for the growth of human tumor cells in nude mice (Sharkey, et al, 1978) leads one to doubt the suitability of using nude

TABLE 4 Reports of *In Vitro* Transformation of Human Fibroblasts

	Number of Transformants Reported	Transformed Phenotypes			
		Morphological Foci	Growth in Soft Agar or Methyl Cellulose	Infinite Lifespan	Tumorigenicity**
CELLS FROM NORMAL INDIVIDUALS					
Benedict et al. 1975	1	+	+	+	+
Kakunaga 1978	7	+	+	+	+
Milo and DiPaolo 1978	10	NR*	+	NR	+
Milo and DiPaolo 1980	numerous	NR	+	NR	+
Namba et al. 1978	1	+	+	+	+
Borek 1980	5	+	+	NR	+
McCormick et al. 1980	2	+	+	NR	+
Sutherland et al. 1980	numerous	+	+	NR	–
DeMars and Jackson 1977	1	+	+	–	–
Tejwani et al. 1981	numerous	NR	+	NR	+
Freedman and Shin 1977	10	+	+	–	–
Milo et al. 1981	numerous	NR	+	NR	+
Silinkas et al. 1981	numerous	NR	+	NR	NR
Greiner et al. 1981	numerous	NR	+	NR	+
Zimmerman and Little	numerous	NR	+	NR	NR
CELLS FROM INDIVIDUALS WITH XP					
Shimada et al. 1976	1	+	NR	NR	–
CELLS FROM INDIVIDUALS WITH ACR					
Kopelovich et al. 1979		+	+	NR	+
Rhim et al. 1980		+	+	NR	–
Miyaki et al. 1980		+	+	NR	NR
Miyaki et al. 1980		+	+	NR	–

*Were not reported.

**As defined by tumor formation in nude mice, or invasiveness on chick membranes.

mice for quantitative tumorigenicity assays for human cells. A review of other alternatives can be found in Freedman and Shin (1978), but these alternative methods also give many possibly false negatives.

One key problem in studying neoplastic progression in any cellular system is the characterization and isolation of altered cells, which represent intermediate stages of development between normal cells and malignant cells. These "preneoplastic" cells appear to have a selective growth advantage in cultures of rodent fibroblast-like cells and can be isolated readily from carcinogen treated cultures. These cells also persist in untreated cultures following senescence of the normal cells and hence, preneoplastic cell lines can be obtained spontaneously as well. These preneoplastic rodent cells progress to malignancy if maintained in culture for a sufficient time period. Hence, neoplastic transformation of rodent cells in culture is readily observable. However, it is possible that preneoplastic populations of human cells differ from preneoplastic rodent cells and this may relate to the difficulty in studying human cell transformation in culture. If preneoplastic human cells cannot be identified in carcinogen treated cultures and they have no growth advantage in culture, then these cells will be only a minor population of the treated culture. The rate of neoplastic conversion of the preneoplastic cells is relatively low and hence, the probability of neoplastic transformation of a human cell culture is extremely small, since it is the result of two rare events. Rodent cells transform frequently because the preneoplastic cells have a selective growth advantage and become the major population in a culture. Therefore, the limiting factor for neoplastic transformation of carcinogen treated rodent cells is mainly the rate of the second transformation event, i.e., preneoplastic to neoplastic. As stated earlier the results with human cell transformation indicate that it is a multistage, progressive process as observed with rodent cells; however, the lack of studies that have isolated and characterized intermediate cells in this process indicates that preneoplastic cells either occur at a very low frequency, that they do not have a selective growth advantage, or that they do not display an obvious phenotypic alteration, such as morphological transformation.

One approach to this problem would be to use cells from genetically altered individuals who inherit preneoplastic cellular alterations and hence show an increased frequency and shorter latency for the appearance of certain neoplasms. These cells would be useful for the study of progressive neoplastic development *in vitro* and to define the conditions necessary for isolation and characterization of preneoplastic human cells.

Kopelovich and co-workers have proposed (1979a; 1979b) that cells from patients with adenomatosis of the colon or rectum (ACR) are preneoplastic. Experiments by Kopelovich and co-workers (1979a; Rhim, et al, 1980) suggest that the latency period for neoplastic transformation in culture may be reduced for these cells as compared to normal cells. Further studies with this and other such cell types should improve the quantitation of *in vitro* neoplastic transformation of human cells.

It should be noted that not all types of genetic defects which increase the incidence of cancer in the individual will necessarily result in an increased probability of transformation *in vitro*. If selection of preneoplastic cells is the limiting factor in transformation in culture, cells which are not preneoplastic will not have a shorter latency period for transformation *in vitro*. For example, repair deficient cells from patients with Xeroderma pigmentosum (XP), should transform with a lower dose of certain carcinogens than normal cells. In the individual this is important, but in cell culture equally effective doses of carcinogen can be given to both normal and XP cells. Both cell types may yield the same frequency of preneoplastic cells, but at different doses. The time required for these cells to progress to tumorigenicity should be similar. Without selection for preneoplastic cells the occurrence of neoplastic transformation of XP cells will be very rare as observed with normal cells. The results to date indicate that this is the case (Shimada, et al, 1976). This is in contrast to the results with ACR cells (Kopelovich, et al, 1979a; 1979b) which are possibly preneoplastic and transform more readily in culture.

IV. Epithelial Cells

Several experimental systems are currently available for the *in vitro* study of chemical induction of neoplastic transformation of epithelial cells. Since 80% of all human cancers are of epithelial cell origin (Barrett and Ts'o, 1978a; Barrett and Thomassen, 1984), systems employing epithelial cells are very important in understanding human malignancies. At present, neoplastic transformation by chemical carcinogens of epithelial cells derived from liver, skin, salivary gland, bladder, kidney, mammary gland, pancreas, and trachea have been reported (Barrett and Thomassen, 1984). One major advantage in using fibroblast-like cell culture systems is that chemical carcinogens induce changes in the morphology of the cells.

These changes occur shortly after exposure to the carcinogen and can be quantitated. Such quantitative indices of transformation of epithelial cells are lacking (Barrett and Thomassen, 1984), thus making the study of these cells more difficult. Furthermore, neoplastic transformation of epithelial cells is not readily detectable until several months after treatment with carcinogen, reflecting the progressive nature of neoplastic development of these cells in culture.

As with human fibroblast cells, progress in the study of epithelial cell transformation is impeded by the lack of suitable markers which can be used to identify, quantitate, and select preneoplastic cells. One early change induced by carcinogens in a number of different epithelial cells is a growth alteration which can be measured by increased growth capacity of the cells *in vitro* (Nettesheim, et al, 1981; Slaga, et al, 1978; Colburn, et al, 1978; Nettesheim and Barrett, 1984). This alteration is induced in tracheal epithelial cells exposed to a carcinogen *in vivo* as well as *in vitro* (Nettesheim, et al, 1981). Normal epithelial cells have a limited survival with conventional cell culture conditions, i.e., tissue culture media supplemented with fetal bovine serum and certain hormones. Neoplastic and preneoplastic cells have growth alterations which allow for extended *in vitro* growth of the cells including establishment as cell lines (Nettesheim and Barrett, 1984). Normal epithelial cells can be maintained in culture for longer time periods if grown in low concentrations of calcium (Hennings, et al, 1980) or with co-cultures of lethally irradiated fibroblasts, which serve as metabolic "feeder" cells (Rheinwald and Green, 1977). With either of these conditions, reduced differentiation of the epithelial cells is observed, which suggests that the limited maintenance of normal epithelial cells under conventional conditions is due to the terminal differentiation of these cells in these conditions. Therefore increased growth of preneoplastic and neoplastic epithelial cells relative to normal cells in conventional tissue culture growth media may be due to either increased proliferation, decreased differentiation, or both. It is possible to grow normal epithelial cells with reduced calcium ion concentrations or on fibroblast feeder layers, to expose the cells to carcinogens, to allow further growth for expression of the carcinogen induced alterations, and then to expose the cells to culture conditions which do not allow for growth of normal cells but will select for cells with carcinogen induced growth alterations (Hennings, et al, 1980; Kulesz-Martin, et al, 1980; Thomassen, et al, 1983). This approach has led to the development of a quantitative transformation system for epithelial cells (Barrett and Thomassen, 1984). Another potential assay for selecting altered epithelial cells is based on the induction of terminal differentiation of normal epithelial cells when the cells are suspended in a semisolid medium (Green, 1977; Rheinwald and Becket, 1980). Survival of neoplastic or possibly preneoplastic cells under these conditions may allow for the selection of cells with a defect in differentiation which may be an important step in neoplastic progression of epithelial cells (Barrett, 1982).

C. ANALYSIS OF SOMATIC MUTATION AND NEOPLASTIC TRANSFORMATION OF CELLS IN CULTURE

As stated in the introduction of this chapter, the study of cells in culture uniquely permits one to compare directly the processes of mutagenesis and carcinogenesis concomitantly in the same target cell. In analyzing such comparisons, one should remember that transformation of cells in culture is a multistep process. Therefore, the transformation events studied represent different types of changes with different cell systems; for example, morphological transformation of diploid Syrian hamster embryo cells is the expression of the transition of a normal cell to a preneoplastic cell, whereas morphological transformation of C3H 10T½ cells is the expression of the transition of a preneoplastic cell to a neoplastic cell or another preneoplastic cell which progresses to malignancy. (It has not been conclusively proven that morphologically transformed cells of C3H 10T½ are tumorigenic when detected or whether they progress more rapidly than untreated cells to this stage and therefore are tumorigenic after isolation.) Since different transformation processes are measured with different cellular systems, the mechanisms of these processes may differ. Hence, different results may be observed in comparing cell transformation and mutation with different transformation systems, even though the same mutational markers or transformed phenotype (i.e., morphology) are studied.

Another important point to consider in the analysis of transformation and mutation is the choice of mutational markers. Two mutational changes are commonly studied with mammalian cells: resistance to ouabain (oua^R), which involves a dominant mutation at the $Na^+/K^+ATPase$ locus, and resistance to 6-thioguanine (TG^r), which involves an X-linked, recessive mutation at the hypoxanthine phosphoribosyl transferase (HPRT) locus (Siminovitch, 1976; Robbins and Baker, 1977; Baker, 1979; O'Neill and Hsie, 1979; Jacobs and DeMars, 1977; Arlett, et al, 1975). $Na^+/K^+ATPase$ function is required for cell viability, therefore ouabain resistance cannot arise from loss of this enzyme function. Rather, ouabain resistant mutants result from a lowered affinity of the mutant enzyme for ouabain (Robbins and Baker, 1977; Baker, 1979). The types of gene mutations responsible for this alteration are limited (Baker, 1979). Deletion mutations, for example, may inactivate the enzyme and, hence, ouabain resistant mutants are not induced by certain mutagens like gamma irradiation (Arlett, et al, 1975). The HPRT function of cells is a purine salvage pathway and loss of this enzyme does not impair cell viability, because purines can be synthesized *de novo* by a separate enzyme pathway. 6-Thioguanine resistance can and often does arise from total loss of HPRT enzyme function (Siminovitch, 1976; O'Neill, Hsie, 1979; Jacobs and DeMars, 1977; Arlett, et al, 1975). In contrast to ouabain resistance, 6-thioguanine resistance can arise from both point mutations and deletion mutations (Arlett, et al, 1975).

However, these two mutational markers do not measure all types of genetic damage. Genetic damage can be categorized into three general types (de Serres, 1979): (1) Gene mutations (point mutations, frameshift mutations, and deletion mutations); (2) Chromosome aberrations (translocations, dicentrics, inversions and terminal deletions); (3) Aneuploidy (abnormal numbers of chromosomes). The Oua^R & TG^r markers detect gene mutations and chromosome aberrations in the case of TG^r (Cox and Masson, 1978), but fail to detect aneuploidy changes. Therefore, comparing transformation to mutation with these two mutational markers limits the comparison to gene mutations and chromosome aberrations and does not allow a comparison of transformation and aneuploidy (Barrett, 1982; Barrett, et al, 1981b; Barrett, et al, 1984).

In 1977 Parodi and Brambilla (1977) presented an analysis of the published literature on quantitative studies of the frequencies of mutation and transformation induced by carcinogens and mutagens. No direct measurements of both processes in the same cellular system were analyzed, but the authors were able to compare the activities of a number of chemicals at equitoxic doses in different systems. The authors observed that the frequency of induced transformation was about 10^2–10^3 times greater than the frequency of mutation induction. The observation that cell transformation occurs at a much higher frequency than gene mutations indicates, according to these authors, that an absolute difference exists between these two processes. They conclude that "epigenetic" phenomena are involved in the process of cell transformation (Parodi and Brambilla, 1977). Since Parodi and Brambilla's review was published, several studies on the concomitant measurement of transformation and mutation have been published (Table 5) and these will be considered in the following two sections.

TABLE 5

Studies with Direct Comparisons of Cell Transformation and Somatic Mutation in Some Target Cell

Authors	Cells	Carcinogens	Mutational[9] Markers	Transformation Phenotype	Transformation Frequency/ Mutation Frequency
Huberman, Mager & Sachs 1982	SHE	B(a)P[3]	Oua^R	Morphology	15–24
Barrett & Ts'o 1983	SHE	B(a)P-diol B(a)P	Oua^R	Morphology	25–540
		MNNG[4]	TG^r Oua^R		
Barrett, Wang & McLachlan 1980	SHE	DES[5]	TG^r	Morphology	> 10^4
Barrett 1984		Modified	Oua^R		
	SHE	Purines B(a)P	TG^r Oua^R	Morphology	3–12.5
Spandidos & Siminovitch 1986	Chinese Hamster	urethane	TG^r	Morphology	170–4050
McCormick et al. 1953	Human	Propane sultone	TG^r	Soft agar growth	20
Crawford et al. 1985–86	FOL-2[2]	MNNG	Oua^R	Soft agar growth	< 0.01
Chan & Little 1978	C3H 10T½	UV[6]	Oua^R	Morphology	9–17
Landolph and Heidelberger 1976	C3H 10T½	B(a)P N-AcoAAF[7]	Oua^R	Morphology	12–21
Lang 1979		B(a)P			
Kakunaga 1973	Balb/c 3T3	MNNG	Oua^R	Morphology	100
	Balb/c 3T3	UV	Oua^R	Morphology	100
Marquardt 1980	C3H M2	MNNG	Oua^R	Morphology	24–1118

[1]SHE—Syrian hamster embryo
[2]FOL-2—A preneoplastic cell line derived from Syrian hamster embryo cells (Barrett, 1980)
[3]B(a)P—benzo(a)pyrene
[4]MNNG—N-methyl-N'-nitro-N-nitrosoguanidine
[5]DES—diethylstilbestrol
[6]UV—ultraviolet light
[7]N-Aco-AAF—N-acetoxy-N-a-acetylaminofluorene
[8]7-MBA—7 methylbenz(a)anthracene
[9]Oua^R—ouabain resistance
TG^r—6-thioguanine resistance

185

I. Comparison of Cell Transformation and Mutation in Diploid, Fibroblast Cells

Extensive studies have been made on the comparison of gene mutations to morphological transformation of diploid Syrian hamster embryo cells (Table 5). Huberman, et al (1976) were the first to report a direct comparison of transformation and mutation measured in the same cellular system. The authors reported that the ratio of the frequency of morphological transformation to mutation (Oua^R) was ~ 20. This is lower than the ratio predicted by Parodi and Brambilla (1977) based on their comparison of measurements made in a number of different studies. Parodi and Brambilla (addendum to Parodi and Brambilla, 1977) note that the transformation and mutation data of Huberman, et al (1976) fall at the extreme low and high ends of their respective distributions for combined experiments of several laboratories. Hence, the ratio of 20:1 may be the lower estimate for this comparison (Parodi and Brambilla, 1977).

Barrett and Ts'o (1978c) published a more detailed study which included two classes of carcinogens, different embryo cell preparations, two mutational markers, and an analysis of the characteristics of the mutants and the factors which influence quantitation of the mutation frequency (Barrett, et al, 1978b). In these studies the ratio of transformation to gene mutation varied from 25–540 (Barrett and Ts'o, 1978c). This range of results is in general agreement with both Huberman, et al (1976) and the predictions of Parodi and Brambilla (1977). Barrett and Ts'o (1978c) show that, although some variation does occur with different conditions, the process of morphological transformation occurs with a much higher frequency than gene mutations at a given dose of certain carcinogens. The magnitude of the increase of cell transformation relative to gene mutations is at least 20-fold and most often 100-fold. Similar results have been reported with diploid Chinese hamster cells (Spandidos and Siminovitch, 1978).

At least four explanations can be offered for these results. The high frequency of morphological transformation may be due to (1) a large target size for this phenotype, (2) mutational "hot spots" in the gene (or genes) controlling this phenotype, (3) a different mutational basis for this phenotypic alteration than the mutations measured at the other loci, or (4) a nonmutational alteration in gene expression (Barrett, et al, 1981a; Barrett, 1982; Barrett and Ts'o, 1978c). The above experiments cannot distinguish between these possibilities.

One of the advantages of being able to measure mutation and transformation in the same cellular system is that one can study compounds that have been reported to be carcinogenic but not mutagenic or mutagenic but not carcinogenic (Barrett, 1982; Barrett, et al, 1984). Exceptions to the correlation between mutagenicity and carcinogenicity of some chemicals have been reported (Barrett, 1982). These exceptions may provide insight into the role of mutagenesis in carcinogenesis. However, these exceptions may not be real, but simply result from the use of different assay systems (bacterial vs. mammalian) to measure each endpoint. Measuring both processes in the same cellular system allows a critical analysis of the relationship between mutagenesis and carcinogenesis without the complications that exist in comparing the two processes with vastly different assay systems (Barrett, 1982).

Using this approach, we have studied representative examples of possible mutagens which are not carcinogens, and carcinogens which are not mutagens (Barrett, 1982; Barrett, et al, 1981b; Barrett, 1981; Barrett, et al, 1984). The compounds studied are 2-aminopurine, a nucleic acid base analog, which is a classical mutagen in prokaryotic systems, but not a carcinogen in animal studies, and diethylstilbestrol, a synthetic estrogen, and asbestos. The latter are known human carcinogens, but are inactive as mutagens in many systems. We have studied the ability of these compounds to induce neoplastic transformation and/or somatic mutation in the Syrian hamster embryo cell assays.

2-Aminopurine (2AP) is a well-defined mutagen in bacteriophages and bacteria and can induce base pair changes in DNA. However, 2-AP is inactive as a carcinogen in rats following weekly subcutaneous injections (Sugiura, et al, 1970) and in mice following skin painting with croton oil as a promoter (Trainin, et al, 1964). Although 2-AP is a very active mutagen in prokaryotic systems (Ronen, 1979), it was only a weak mutagen in Syrian hamster embryo cells (Barrett, 1981). 2-AP is a mutagen in other eukaryotic organisms, although not potent, and is not effective in some organisms (Ronen, 1979). Another modified purine, 6-N-hydroxylaminopurine (6-HAP), is like 2-AP in that it induces base pair changes in prokaryotic and eukaryotic cells. Although 6-HAP is less potent than 2-AP in inducing rII mutants of page T_4 (Freese, 1968), Brockman, et al (1979) have reported that 6-HAP is much more potent than 2-AP in inducing ad-3 mutants in *Neurospora crassa*. Also, 6-HAP is a weak carcinogen under conditions where 2-AP is not a carcinogen (Sugiura, et al, 1970). These findings prompted us to examine the effects of 6-HAP in Syrian hamster embryo cells. 6-HAP was a potent mutagen in these cells, and the relative mutagenicity of 6-HAP and 2-AP in Syrian hamster embryo cells is consistent with their mutagenicity in *Neurospora*.

Since 2-AP is mutagenic in bacteria, but not carcinogenic in animals, it is of interest to compare the ability of 2-AP, as well as 6-HAP, to induce somatic mutation and transformation in hamster embryo cells. 2-AP failed to induce neoplastic transformation of Syrian hamster embryo cells in our studies and only one morphologically transformed colony was observed following 2-AP exposure. Although no morphologically transformed colonies were observed in controls, one cannot declare the significance of the transformed colony in the 2-AP treated cultures. Further experiments are needed, but the results of this study indicate that 2-AP is, at best, a weak transforming agent. The inability to induce tumors with 2-AP in two animal species is consistent with these observations. In contrast to the results with 2-AP, 6-HAP induced morphological and neoplastic transformation of hamster cells in a dose dependent manner (Barrett, 1981). This correlates with the greater mutagenic activity in these cells of 6-HAP than 2-AP. These experiments indicate that the mutagenicity of modified purines correlates with their ability to induce transformation when these end-points are measured in the same cellular system. Thus, this class of compounds is not an exception to the correlation of mutagenesis and carcinogenesis.

There are, however, quantitative differences in the relative ability of 6-HAP to induce transformation and mutation when compared to B(a)P or MNNG (Barrett, 1981). In contrast to the ratio of approximately 100 in the transformation to mutation frequencies observed with the latter carcinogens, the ratio following 6-HAP treatment was only 3–12. Although 6-HAP can induce both transformation and mutation, it is much less potent than other carcinogens in inducing transformation when compared at equal levels of mutagenicity. This suggests a difference in the two processes.

Diethylstilbestrol (DES) is known to be a carcinogen in humans and rodents (IARC, 1979). However, DES and its metabolites are inactive as mutagens in the Ames test, even with a variety of metabolic activating systems (Metzler, et al, 1980). In collaboration with John McLachlan and Annette Wong of our Institute, we have examined the ability of DES to induce neoplastic transformation and somatic mutation of Syrian hamster embryo cells (Barrett, et al, 1981b). We observed that DES was capable of inducing morphological and neoplastic transformation of these cells. Under the same conditions, however, DES failed to induce measurable somatic mutation at either of two loci (HPRT or $Na^+/K^+ATPase$). This is the first example of a definitive dissociation of gene mutation and cell transformation measured in the same cellular system (Barrett, et al, 1981b).

Our results with DES may indicate a nonmutational basis for morphological transformation; however, we have proposed an alternative mechanism based on the ability of DES to induce aneuploidy in a number of systems including dysplastic lesions in women exposed to DES prenatally. We have proposed that a mutation at the chromosomal level, attributable to nondisjunction, may be one cause of morphological transformation and possibly cancer (Tsutsui et al, 1983).

Our hypothesis that a chromosomal type mutation is involved in the transformation of Syrian hamster embryo cells provides an explanation for several observations. First, it explains the ability of DES to induce neoplastic transformation without measurable somatic mutations at two loci. The Oua^R and TG^r systems do not detect changes in chromosome number. Therefore, the lack of mutagenicity of DES with these markers indicates that DES fails to induce gene mutations under the conditions that it induces neoplastic transformation; but such results are still consistent with morphological transformation resulting from a chromosomal mutation. Second, the frequency of chromosomal lesions is high in carcinogen treated cells (Benedict, 1972), which might explain the high frequency of morphological transformation. Third, this hypothesis provides an explanation for the variation in the ratio of transformation to mutation induced by different classes of carcinogens and mutagens. Chemicals which induce aneuploidy readily, but not gene mutations, would have a high ratio of transformation to mutation (e.g., DES). Chemicals which are effective inducers of point mutations would have a low ratio of transformation to mutation (e.g., 6-HAP and possibly 2-AP). Nucleic acid base analogs can induce chromosome aberrations and aneuploidy in mammalian cells (Biesele, et al, 1952, Tsutsui, et al,

1984). Therefore, it is possible that induction of transformation by these compounds also occurs by a chromosomal type mutation (Tsutsui, et al, 1984).

Asbestos and other mineral dusts also are able to transform SHE cells (Hesterberg and Barrett, 1984). Fiber dimensions, length and diameter, are important determinants in potency for cell transformation, which is similar to the findings for induction of mesotheliomas *in vivo*. Chrysotile and crocidolite asbestos are potent inducers of numerical chromosome changes and weak inducers of structural chromosome aberrations (Oshimura, et al, 1984). The dose-response relationship and fiber size dependence for chromosome mutations and cell transformation are very similar, which supports the hypothesis that these changes are mechanistically related (Barrett, et al, 1983; Hesterberg and Barrett, 1984; Oshimura, et al, 1984). Other chemical carcinogens also induce aneuploidy (Barrett, 1981; Barrett, et al, 1983) indicating that this is possibly a general mechanism of cell transformation. However, there are also data to support the role of other types of genetic damage in carcinogenesis. The most reasonable view is that there are many mechanisms which may lead to the same final phenotypic changes and a series of pathways rather than a single mechanism should be considered.

Sachs and co-workers have proposed that the tumorigenic response in Syrian hamster embryo cells is controlled by a balance of suppressor and expressor chromosomes (Yamamoto, et al, 1973). Our hypothesis is consistent with this model as well as any other model based on a chromosomal-type lesion (Barrett, 1982). There is also reason to believe that genetic damage at the chromosome level is important in neoplastic development *in vivo* (Barrett, 1982).

Only limited studies of the comparison of mutation and transformation of human cells have been published. This is due to the lack of quantitative studies of human cell transformation. McCormick, et al (1980) observed a ratio of propane sultone induced transformation (measured by growth in soft agar) to mutation (HPRT locus) of 20. This is similar to the results with rodent cells (Table 5).

II. Comparison of Cell Transformation and Mutation in Aneuploid Cell Lines

From the preceding section it can be seen that in the absence of induced gene mutation, DES induces the neoplastic transformation of diploid Syrian hamster cells. The induction of transformation of these cells by DES and other carcinogens is most consistent with a chromosome mutation rather than a gene mutation. Whether gene mutations play a role in later steps of neoplastic progression is a separate question. Examination of the results of all cell transformation studies with preneoplastic cells and the relationship of this process to gene mutation is one approach to this problem.

Bouck and DiMayorca (1976) have presented evidence for somatic mutation as the basis for "malignant" transformation of BHK cells (actually growth in a soft agar is measured but this phenotype does correlate well with tumorigenicity in these cells (Barrett, et al, 1979)). Their conclusion that this transformation is a mutagenic process is based on the following observations: BHK cells have a low frequency of spontaneous transformation to the ability to grow in soft agar; the frequency of this phenotype is increased by treatment with mutagens, this phenotype is stable and has a low frequency for reversion; and the phenotype is often temperature sensitive, which suggests that it arises from a temperature sensitive gene product, typically a protein derived from a missense mutation (Bouck and Dimayorca, 1976).

There are certain limitations in the data of Bouck and DiMayorca (1976) which weaken their conclusions. Very little can be concluded from the measurement of the spontaneous transformation frequencies. As the authors state, this frequency can vary from 10^{-7} to 5×10^{-4} (many laboratories have observed even higher frequencies) depending on the culture conditions and age of the cultures. One would need to measure the spontaneous transformation rate, that is, the number of transformants per cell per generation, to obtain a number to compare with spontaneous mutation rates. The authors also indicate that the induced transformation frequencies are similar to induced mutation frequencies, but no direct measurements of the mutation frequencies in these cells are made.

It is reasonable to assume that revertants of transformed BHK cells in culture have a selective disadvantage relative to transformed cells; therefore, the instability of the transformants and the frequency of reversion may be greater than suggested by Bouck and DiMayorca (1976). In fact, the mutagen induced reversion frequency calculated from Bouck and DiMayorca's data of the cells surviving three cycles of the selection procedure employed by them for isolation of revertants is 4.6×10^{-4} rather than the reported value 4×10^{-6} which was determined by the number of isolated, stable revertants. The temperature sensitivity of a large percentage of the transformants is an interesting observation, but the proposed mechanism of this observation is only speculation.

The induction of transformation in BHK cells by mutagens and carcinogens was demonstrated with a limited number of chemicals by Bouck and DiMayorca (1976), but further work by Styles (1980) and Ishii, et al (1977) has demonstrated that these cells are sensitive to a number of carcinogens, most of which are known mutagens. Interestingly, BHK cells are not induced to grow in agar by DES, which does not induce gene mutations, but which does induce transformation of diploid Syrian hamster embryo cells (Barrett, et al, 1981b). This observation further illustrates the difference in the induction of the transformation process in normal, diploid cells vis-á-vis preneoplastic, aneuploid cells.

Even though the evidence with BHK cells is not unequivocal, it is consistent with the transformation of these cells resulting from a gene mutation and this is the best explanation for the observations. Whether this conclusion can be extrapolated to other systems remains to be demonstrated. Recently, Crawford, et al (1983) studied the mechanism of transformation of another preneoplastic cell line, FOL-2 (Barrett, 1980). This cell line, like BHK cells, was spontaneously derived from a culture of Syrian hamster cells and transformation of these cells from anchorage dependent to anchorage independent growth in agar correlates with neoplastic conversion of the cells (Barrett, 1980), again in analogy to BHK cells. However, in contrast to the near diploid BHK cells, FOL-2 cells are subtetraploid (Barrett, 1980). Crawford, et al (1983; Barrett, et al, 1981a) have measured the spontaneous transformation rate (to the ability to grow in agar) of these cells by a Luria-Delbruck fluctuation analysis (1943) and observed that transformants arise at a rate ($0.57 - 5.5 \times 10^{-7}$ transformants/cell/generation) which is consistent with a single locus gene mutation in these cells (7.8×10^{-8} Oua^R mutants/cell/generation).

Several experiments have demonstrated that the frequency of transformants of FOL-2 cells is not increased by treatment with mutagens (Barrett, et al, 1981a; Crawford, et al, 1983). Thus, despite the apparent similarity of the spontaneous rates of transformation and gene mutation in these cells, these two processes are clearly distinct in terms of their sensitivity to mutagen treatment. Crawford, et al (1983) have proposed that the transformation and neoplastic conversion of FOL-2 cells is the result of chromosome segregation. This hypothesis is supported by their studies on the rate of nondisjunction in aneuploid Syrian hamster cells and the behavior of cell-cell hybrids which suppress or express agar growth and tumorigenicity depending on chromosome segregation.

Comparisons of mutation and transformation frequencies of the preneoplastic mouse cell lines, Balb/c 3T3, C3H 10T½ and C3H M2 have also been made (Table 5). The ratio of transformation to mutation in these cells varies from 10–4000. Only ouabain resistance has been measured as a mutational marker in these cells because the cells are near tetraploid; HPRT mutants are recessive and will not be detected in cells with more than one X-chromosome unless all the genes are mutated. The other problem with these studies is the ambiguity in determining the transformation frequency of the cells. This problem exists clearly with the C3H 10T½ cells and very likely with the other cell lines. As stated earlier in the description of the C3H 10T½ cells, the frequency of transformation can vary by several orders of magnitude depending on the initial cell number (Haber, et al, 1977; Haber and Thilly, 1978; Kennedy, et al, 1980). Thus, a comparison of transformation to mutation frequency with these cells is difficult to interpret.

In fact, the observations that the transformation process is independent of the number of cells treated has been cited as evidence for an epigenetic mechanism as the basis for this transformation. To repeat the hypothesis of Kennedy, et al (1980) and Fernandez, et al (1980) exposure of C3H 10T½ cells to a carcinogen results in the "activation" of a large number, perhaps 100%, of the cells. The activated cells then have an increased probability to transform under the conditions of confluence. It is clear from the data of these authors that this activation step is occurring in a large number of the cells. This can be deduced from the observations that even weeks after carcinogen exposure (X-irradiation), 1–5 cells can be plated in a dish and will give rise to transformed cells after growth to confluence. Untreated cells fail to transform under these conditions. What is not clear from observations is the timing and the mechanism of the second step. Kennedy, et al (1980) propose that it occurs at confluence because it is not influenced by the number of generations which precede the attainment of confluence by the cells. An alternative hypothesis is that the second step is the result of a spontaneous transformation process, which is enhanced by the activation step. This spontaneous transformation may be similar to spontaneous mutations. If this is the case, then it should occur during the growth phase of the culture; it should occur randomly during this time; and the rate of this change should be similar to the rate of spontaneous mutations.

We have analyzed the data of Kennedy and Little (1980) (kindly provided to us in preprint form), to determine if this type of mechanism is consistent with their results. Mutation rate analysis is commonly performed by a Luria-Delbruck fluctuation analysis (1943). In this procedure, a large number of cultures are seeded with a low number of cells. The number of initial cells per culture is chosen so that no preexisting mutants are contained in the dishes. The cells are allowed to grow for a period of time and then each culture is assayed to determine whether or not any mutants were generated during the time of the experiment. The probability that a culture will or will not contain a mutant can be calculated from the Poisson distribution. The probability that a culture will have no mutants (P_o) is equal to e^{-m} where m is the average number of mutational events per culture. If the fraction of cultures having no mutants is known, one can then calculate a value for m. From m the mutation rate, a, (mutations/cell/generation) can be calculated from the formula.

$$a = \frac{\ln 2m}{N_t - N_i}$$

where N_t is the final cell number and N_i is the initial cell number in the cultures.

In addition to calculating a mutation rate by the Luria-Delbruck analysis, one can determine whether the mutational phenotype arose spontaneously during the growth period or was induced by the selection agent or procedure. For example, it is possible with drug resistant mutants that the drug used as a selective agent turns on the drug resistant phenotype by an epigenetic mechanism and these nonmutated cells would appear to be mutants. One can distinguish between these two mechanisms, random mutation-like event versus induction by the selective agent, by the Luria-Delbruck fluctuation analysis (1943). If the variant phenotype is the result of induction by the selective agent then the event should occur with a Poisson distribution, which predicts that the variance between cultures should equal to the mean number of mutants per culture (variance/mean = 1). If a mutation like event occurs randomly during the growth of the culture, then most mutants will occur when the cell number is the greatest, i.e. at the last division, however, some mutants will arise early when the cell number is small. In the latter case the mutants will expand with the nonmutant population and when assayed this culture will have a large percentage of mutant cells. If the culture conditions are chosen properly, many cultures, ideally one half, will have no mutants and the P_o can be used to calculate the mutation rate. Other cultures will have a large number of mutants and the variance between cultures will be great, i.e. variance/mean > 1. The measurement of the variance/mean in these cultures can be used to distinguish a random occurring event (variance/mean > 1) versus one induced by the selection method (variance/mean $= 1$).

The experiments of Kennedy and Little (Kennedy, et al, 1980) are amenable to analysis by the Luria-Delbruck method. After treating the cells and allowing an expression period, the cells are replated at various densities, all of which are below the level of preexisting transformations. (This is known because only a fraction of the dishes have transformants and only one foci per dish is usually observed rather than the entire dish consisting of transformed cells.) The authors also report the fraction of cultures of dishes without transformants or P_o. Knowing P_o, the number of initial cells (N_i) per culture, and assuming that the final cell number per dish (N_t) is the number of cells at confluency (2×10^6 cells), which is constant in this density inhibited cell line, we can use the Luria-Delbruck equations to calculate the apparent transformation rates of the C3H 10T½ cells under different experimental conditions.

The first experiment of Kennedy, et al (1980) that we analyzed by this method was the effect of varying the initial cell number from 5 to 400 cells on the transformation induced by 600 rads of X-ray (Table 6). Little effect on the number of transformed foci per dish was observed with an 80-fold change in initial cell number. Therefore, the transformation frequency for such an experiment varied 80-fold. It is of interest to determine if a calculated transformation *rate* would be constant or vary greatly. The transformation rate for this experiment, calculated from the P_o, varied from only $1.3 - 1.8 \times 10^{-7}$ transformants per cell per generation (Table 6). No significant difference in the transformation rates is apparent with different initial cell numbers.

If the estimated transformation rate of $\sim 10^{-7}$ transformants per cell per generation is correct, then the results with different initial cell numbers are not surprising. At this rate, the probability of a transformation occurring during the division of 5 or 400 cells is very low. Hence, most of the transformation events in the transformation process must occur at or near the last cell division when 10^6 cells are at risk. This also explains the results with the replating experiments of Kennedy, et al (1980). In these experiments, the same number of foci were observed whether the cells were allowed to form foci without replating or were replated at dilutions of $1/10$ to $1/10,000$. The dilution of $1/10$ is apparently sufficient to exclude any transformants that occurred during the initial growth phase. The diluted cell populations then spontaneously transform in this model with the same rate as the original treated cells. The number of cells plated, i.e., the dilution factor, is of little consequence because the transformation event is improbable until a sufficient cell number is achieved. Indeed, the calculated transformation rate with 400 rads of x-ray is 2.3×10^{-7} for non-replated cells and $0.77 - 3.2 \times 10^{-7}$ for replated cells (Table 7). The larger variability in this rate compared to that observed in Table 6 may be due to the smaller number of cultures employed in some of the experimental groups.

The same calculation can be performed for the data with transformation with

TABLE 6
Calculation of Apparent Induced Transformation Rates of C3H 10T½ Cells

Treatment	Initial number of cells per culture (N_i)	Fraction of Dishes Without Transformants (P_o)	Estimated Transformation Frequency (transformants) per cell plated	Calculated Transformation[2] Rate (Transformants/cell/ Generation)
600 Rads	100–400	65/99 = 0.66	2.4×10^{-3}	1.4×10^{-7}
600 Rads	50–100	44/64 = 0.69	4.1×10^{-3}	1.3×10^{-7}
600 Rads	1–30	21/35 = 0.60	2.3×10^{-2}	1.8×10^{-7}
600 Rads	5	48/75 = 0.64	1.4×10^{-1}	1.6×10^{-7}

[1]Data taken from Table 2. Kennedy $et\ al.$ (1980)
[2]Calculated from the Luria-Delbruck (1943) fluctuation analysis equations (where: $P_o = e^{-m}$ and

$$a = \frac{\ln 2m}{N_t - N_i}$$

P_o = fraction of the dishes without transformants
M = mean number of transformation events per culture
N_i = initial number of cells per dish
N_t = final number of cells per dish ($= 2 \times 10^6$ as estimated by Kennedy $et\ al$ 1980)
a = transformation rate per cell per generation

100 rads of X-ray plus the tumor promoter, TPA (Table 8). The transformation rate with this treatment is $0.77 - 5.6 \times 10^{-7}$.

There does not appear from this data to be a dose dependent increase in the transformation rate with 400–600 rads. However, this is consistent with the results of Terzaghi and Little (1976) in that the dose response curve for the transformation frequency, measured with a constant viable cell number, increase exponentially from 100 to 400 rads but is constant from 400 to 1500 rads. The transformation rate for 100 rads calculated by us from the data of Kennedy and Little (1980) is $0.35 - 2.1 \times 10^{-8}$ (Table 8) or approximately 10 fold less than with 400–600 rads. Addition of the tumor promoter, TPA, to cultures irradiated with 100 rads increases the apparent transformation rate to that observed with 400–600 rads alone (Table 8). Kennedy and Little (1980) report data on spontaneous transformation of C3H 10T½ in these experiments. Unfortunately, very little other data exist in the literature on spontaneous transformation of these cells. The calculated spontaneous transformation rate for C3H 10T½ cells from the data of Kennedy and Little (1980) is $3.4 - 7 \times 10^{-9}$ transformants per cell per generation for untreated cultures and $0.7 - 4.0 \times 10^{-8}$ for TPA treated cultures (Table 8). From these data it appears that carcinogen treatment increases the spontaneous transformation rate of C3H 10T½ cells from $\sim 5 \times 10^{-9}$ to 5×10^{-7} transformants per cell per generation.

While these calculations are very interesting and can lead to much speculation on the mechanism of C3H 10T½ cell transformation, they do not distinguish between spontaneous transformation during growth of carcinogen activated cells and transformation of the cells after reaching confluence (Kennedy, et al, 1980). Both models are consistent with the data. As stated earlier, the Luria-Delbruck fluctuation experiment can be used to distinguish between random change during growth and induction by the selective agent (confluence in the case of C3H 10T½ cells) by comparing the variance of the cultures to the mean number of transformants. Analysis of the variance in the

TABLE 7
Calculation of Apparent Induced Transformation Rates C3H 10T½ Cells[1].

Treatment	Replating Dilution	N_i	Fraction of Dishes Without Transformants	Calculated Transformation Rate[2] Transformants/cell/generation
400 rads	No replating	270(96–440)	53/104 = 0.51	2.3×10^{-7}
400 rads	1/10	31000	8/20 = 0.40	3.2×10^{-7}
400 rads	1/30	9000	7/10 = 0.70	1.2×10^{-7}
400 rads	1/100	3100	11/20 = 0.55	2.0×10^{-7}
400 rads	1/10000	25	8/10 = 0.80	0.77×10^{-7}

[1]Data taken from Table 1 of Kennedy et al. (1980)
[2]Calculated as described in Table 6
[3]Data in original table showed an unusually high ratio of foci to dishes with foci which is not indicative of Poisson distribution

experiments of Kennedy, et al (1980; Kennedy and Little, 1980) is not possible. This is due to the fact that a focus that appears on a dish may arise from one transformant or from a colony of many transformants. Therefore the actual number of transformed cells in a culture at confluence is not measured. Some experiments (Kennedy, et al 1980; Kennedy and Little, 1980) do note a non Poisson distribution of foci in dishes. For example in one experiment (Kennedy and Little, 1980) which consisted of 8 out of 10 dishes with foci, more than half of the 83 observed foci were in 2 dishes (distribution among 10 dishes was 0,0,1,1,4,8,8,11,19,31). Experiments with cells redispersed at confluence to measure the variance accurately need to be done to distinguish between these two models. If the variance to mean ratio is greater than one in these experiments, this would support our model that the transformation event occurs randomly during growth to confluence.*

The probabilistic model of C3H 10T½ transformation of Fernandez, Mondal and Heidelberger (1980) is consistent with our model for the results of Kennedy, et al (1980), although the equation derived for 3-methylcholanthrene induced transformation is not applicable for X-ray induced transformation (Fernandez, et al, 1980). We were able to calculate a "transformation rate" from the results of Fernandez, Mondal and Heidelberger (1980) with 3-methylcholanthrene induced transformation of C3H 10T½. The transformation rate was established from the mean number of transformants per culture by the method of Capizzi and Jameson (1973). The calculated transformation rate (Table 9) was $1 - 6 \times 10^{-7}$ transformants per cell per generation for methylcholanthrene induced transformation which is in close agreement with the results with high doses of X-ray irradiation (Tables 6 and 7). Calculation of the transformation rate from the mean number of transformants per culture is more subject to error than a determination based on the P_o method. This is due to secondary factors such as selective growth advantage and satellite colony formation, which will influence the number of variants per culture. Considering that the experiments were done in different laboratories with different transforming agents and calculated on a different basis, the similarity in the calculated transformation rates from the studies of Kennedy, et al (1980) and Fernandez, Mondal and Heidelberger (1980) is quite interesting. In fact, the original experiments of Mondal and Heidelberger (1970) on transformation of single cells of mouse prostate fibroblasts with 3-methylcholanthrene can also be analyzed by this method. The calculated transformation rate based on the P_o calculation for these experiments is $2 - 6 \times 10^{-7}$/cell/generation.

*Footnote: Since the submission of this manuscript, Kennedy et al (1984) have successfully completed experiments to distinguish between two models. Their studies, using redistribution analysis with C3H 10T½ cells, indicate that the transformation step occurs during the growth phase following X-ray induced activation (initiation). The redistribution analysis suggest that the transformation event was dependent upon the number of cellular divisions and therefore could be expressed as a rate/cell/generation. Evaluation of the Kennedy et al, data (Table 1) using fluctuation analysis by the P_o method gave similar transformation rates (2 to 3.8×10^{-7}/cell/generation) to those reported in our manuscript.

TABLE 8
Calculation of Apparent Induced and Spontaneous Transformation Rates of C3H 10T½ Cells[1].

Treatment		N_i/Dish (range)	Fraction of Dishes Without Transformants (P_o)	Calculated Transformation Rate[2] (Transformants/Cell/Generation)
Irradiation 100 Rads	TPA			
+	+	370(330–396)	65/115 = 0.59	2.0×10^{-7}
+	+	63(53–72)	10/48 = 0.21	5.0×10^{-7}
+	+	1(0–3)	8/66 = 0.12	7.3×10^{-7}
+	0	308(145–428)	67/68 = 0.99	3.5×10^{-9}
+	0	8(3–11)	29/31 = 0.94	2.1×10^{-8}
0	0	296(201–391)	121/122 = 0.99	3.4×10^{-9}
0	0	3(1–6)	105/107 = 0.98	7.0×10^{-9}
0	+	262(154–525)	49/50 = 0.98	7.0×10^{-9}
0	+	4(1–9)	94/106 = 0.89	4.0×10^{-8}

[1]Data taken from Kennedy and Little (1980)
[2]Calculated as described in Table 6

TABLE 9
Transformation Rates of Methylcholanthrene Treated C3H 10T½ Mouse Embryo Fibroblasts[1,2].

Survivors per Dish	Number of Dishes	Number of Transformants	Transformants per Dish	Transformation Rate Transformants/Cell/Generation[3,4]
1	22	1	0.045	1.0×10^{-7}
1	26	2	0.077	1.1×10^{-7}
2.9	18	1	−.056	1.2×10^{-7}
7.2	28	2	0.071	1.0×10^{-7}
15	20	2	0.01	1.5×10^{-7}
29	20	3	0.15	1.8×10^{-7}
58	25	13	0.52	3.4×10^{-7}
116	29	4	0.14	1.4×10^{-7}
231	25	8	0.32	2.5×10^{-7}
434	26	12	0.46	3.1×10^{-7}
868	31	25	0.81	4.3×10^{-7}
1736	31	32	1.03	5.1×10^{-7}
3472	33	42	1.21	5.8×10^{-7}
6943	38	36	0.95	4.5×10^{-7}
13886	36	53	1.45	6.3×19^{-7}

[1]Treatment—1 μg/ml methylcholanthrene for 24 hours
[2]Taken from Tables 1 and 3, Fernandez et al. (1980)
[3]Calculated using the Capizzi and Jameson Method and Formulas: a = CaN_t/CN_t, where a = the transformation rate/cell/generation; C = the number of dishes, N_t = the number of cells per dish at confluence; r = the mean number of transformants per dish, and CaN_t was determined from Cr using Table 1, Capizzi and Jameson (1973)
[4]The spontaneous transformation rate is estimated to be $< 0.58 \times 10^{-7}$

The transformation rate that we have calculated is a function of the three probabilities that Fernandez, Mondal and Heidelberger describe in their paper. Their method of analysis has the advantage of calculating a value for p_3, the probability of deactivation, and the product of $p_1 \times p_2$. Our method of analysis yields a single number, the transformation rate, but hopefully this number will provide a basis for comparing the affects of different doses and types of transforming agents.

Keeping in mind that our model is only a hypothesis, it is still interesting to speculate on its significance. First, it should be reiterated that we concur with Kennedy, et al (1980) and Fernandez, et al (1980) that the initial carcinogen induced activation occurs in a large percentage, perhaps all, of the cells. This is apparently a nonmutational event and the understanding of its mechanism will be of fundamental importance to cancer research. Our model is that the result of this activation is to increase the spontaneous transformation rate of the cells by -100 fold. The second event in this process, the spontaneous transformation to the ability to form a morphologically altered focus, is similar to a spontaneous mutation. The rate of this change (after activation) is within the measured ratio of spontaneous mutations at single gene loci. It will be very interesting to learn if this step is enhanced by a secondary treatment with mutagens. MNNG, which mutates but does not transform asynchronous C3H 10T½ cells will be an interesting compound to study with X-ray activated C3H 10T½ cells. If mutagens fail to increase the frequency of transformation of activated C3H 10T½ cells, then an interesting analogy exists with the results of Crawford, et al (1983; Barrett, et al, 1981a) with the preneoplastic, subtetraploid Syrian hamster cell line, FOL-2. These cells have a spontaneous transformation rate similar to that of activated C3H 10T½ cells. Transformation of FOL-2 cells is not increased by mutation treatment and Crawford, et al (1983; Barrett, et al, 1981a) have suggested that chromosome segregation of this subtetraploid cell is the mechanism of this event. If this model is correct for C3H 10T½, then it is possible that untreated C3H 10T½ have a very low rate of spontaneous transformation due to a stable chromosome constitution. Treatment of the cells with carcinogens activates the cells by increasing the rate of nondisjunction. With near tetraploid cells more than one nondisjunction type of event may be needed. In this regard it is interesting that Saxholm and Digernes (1980) reported a progressive loss of DNA and lowering of the chromosomal model in chemically transformed C3H 10T½ cells during development of their oncogenic potential. The normal C3H 10T½ cells maintain a stable hypotetraploid DNA content and treated cells display a decrease in DNA content and chromosome number during neoplastic progression. The above discussion is certainly speculative and open to criticism but it is hoped that it will stimulate further thought and research on the C3H 10T½ transformation system.

D. CONCLUSION AND FUTURE DIRECTIONS

The following conclusions can be summarized from this discussion:
1. Neoplastic transformation in cell culture is a multistage process and the

role of mutagenesis may vary with different steps in this process.

2. Aneuploid cell lines, which are nontumorigenic, have acquired some properties of neoplastic cells and progress to neoplastic cells more readily than normal, diploid cells. These aneuploid cell lines should be considered as preneoplastic cells.

3. Cell transformation of normal, diploid cells to aneuploid, preneoplastic cells may occur by a mechanism different from the transformation of preneoplastic cells to neoplastic cells.

4. Cell culture studies offer the advantage of directly comparing the processes of mutagenesis and carcinogenesis in the same target cells.

5. Genetic damage can occur by gene mutations, chromosomal aberrations, or by aneuploidy. Conventional somatic mutation assays do not detect all three types of genetic damage.

6. Induction of transformation in normal, diploid cells can occur in the absence of measurable gene mutations. Aneuploid conversion has been proposed as a mechanism for transformation of these cells to the preneoplastic state.

7. The difficulty in transforming human cells may be due to the lack of good assays to select preneoplastic cells and to the chromosome stability of cells of this species in culture.

8. The only cells in culture which transform by a gene mutation like process are BHK cells. The evidence for a gene mutation in the malignant transformation of these cells is not conclusive, but highly suggestive. The transformation of a subtetraploid cell line (FOL), which like BHK was derived from the Syrian hamster, is distinctly different from the BHK cells in its response to mutagens.

9. The transformation of the aneuploid mouse cell line, C3H 10T½ and possibly other similar cell lines occurs in a two-step process. The first step, termed activation, involves a large percentage of carcinogen treated cells and appears to be a nonmutational event. The second step occurs with a low probability and may involve a mutational event, but there is no evidence at present to support this conclusion.

Several areas for future research are evident from these conclusions. First, increased knowledge about the control of chromosome aberrations and segregation is needed. Assays to study mitotic aneuploidy in mammalian cells should be developed. These assays may offer the potential for short term tests for carcinogens like DES and possibly many other carcinogens. The nature of factors which control chromosome aberrations needs to be defined. The role of transposable genetic elements in mammalian cells and their response to chemical carcinogens may be important in this process. Further studies on the fibroblast cell culture system are needed. The role of gene mutations and chromosomal mutations needs to be studied in these systems. The activation step in C3H 10T½ cells, which appears to be nonmutational, is an intriguing problem that needs exploration. Development of transformation systems to study human cells and epithelial cells are needed. Recognition of the need to develop new markers for preneoplastic cells, which can be used to select these altered cells, should facilitate work in this area. The use of preneoplastic cells derived from genetically altered individuals should advance our understanding of such cell populations.

ACKNOWLEDGEMENTS

We would like to thank Dr. John Drake for his confirmation of our calculations of the transformation rates of C3H 10T½ cells and his valuable discussions on this problem. We would also like to thank Drs. Ann Kennedy and John Little for sharing with us their unpublished data.

REFERENCES

Aaronson, S.A., and Todaro, G.J. Development of 3T3-like lines from Balb/c mouse embryo cultures: Transformation susceptibility to SV40. J. Cell Physiol. **72**, 141–148 (1968a).

Aaronson, S.A., and Todaro, G.J. Basis for the acquisition of malignant potential by mouse cells cultivated *in vitro*. Science **162**, 1024–1026 (1968b).

Ames, B.N., Durston, W.E., Yamasaki, E. and Lee, F.D. Carcinogens are mutagens: A simple test system combining liver homogenates for activation and bacteria for detection. Proc. Nat. Acad. Sci., U.S.A. **70**, 2281–2285 (1973).

Arlett, C.F., Turnbill, D., Harcourt, S.A., Lehmann, and Colella, C.M. A comparison of the 8-azaguanine and ouabain-resistance systems for the selection of induced mutant chinese hamster cells. Mutation Res. **33**, 261–278 (1975).

Baker, R.M. Nature and use of ouabain-resistant mutants. In: *Banbury Report 2: Mammalian Cell Mutagenesis*, ed. A.W. Hsie, J.P. O'Neill, V.K. McElheny, pp. 237–248 (1979). Cold Spring Harbor Laboratory, New York.

Barrett, J.C. A preneoplastic stage in the spontaneous neoplastic transformation of Syrian hamster embryo cells in culture. Cancer Res. **40**, 91–94 (1980).

Barrett, J.C. Gene mutation and cell transformation of mammalian cells induced by two modified purines, 2-aminopurine and 6-N-hydroxylaminopurine, Proc. Nat. Acad. Sci., U.S.A. **78**, 5685–5689 (1981).

Barrett, J.C. Cell Transformation, Mutation, and Cancer. In: *The Use of Mammalian Cells for the Detection of Environmental Carcinogens: Mechanisms and Applications*, eds. C. Heidelberger, N. Inui, T. Kuroki and M. Yamada. Gann Monograph on Cancer Research, **27**, 195–200 (1982).

Barrett, J.C., Hesterberg, T.W. and Thomassen, D.G. Use of cell transformation systems for carcinogenicity testing and mechanistic studies of carcinogenesis. Pharmacol. Rev. **36**, 53S–70S (1984).

Barrett, J.C. and Thomassen, D.G. Use of quantitative cell transformation assays in risk estimation. In: Vouk, V.B., Butler, G.C., Hoel, D.G., and Peakall, D.B. (eds.), Methods of Estimating Risk in Human and Chemical Damage in Non-Human Biota and Ecosystems, SCOPE, SGOMSEC 2, IPCS Joint Symposia 3, John Wiley and Sons, Chichester, New York, Brisbane, Toronto, Singapore, in press, (1984).

Barrett, J.C., Thomassen, D.G. and Hesterberg, T.W. Role of gene and chromosomal mutations in cell transformation. New York Acad. of Sci. **407**, 291–300 (1983).

Barrett, J.C. and Ts'o, P.O.P. Evidence for the progressive nature of neoplastic transformation *in vitro*. Proc. Nat. Acad. Sci., U.S.A. **75**, 3761–3765 (1978a).

Barrett, J.C. and Ts'o, P.O.P. Mechanistic studies of neoplastic transformation of cells in culture. In: *Polycyclic Hydrocarbons and Cancer*, eds. H. Gelboin and P.O.P. Ts'o, pp. 235–267 (1978b). Academic Press, N.Y., Vol. 2.

Barrett, J.C. and Ts'o, P.O.P. The relationship between somatic mutation and neoplastic transformation. Proc. Nat. Acad. Sci., U.S.A. **75**, 3297–3301 (1978c).

Barrett, J.C. and Ts'o, P.O.P. Neoplastic transformation, DNA damage, and chromosomal aberrations induced by a direct perturbation of DNA. Nature **274**, 229–232 (1978a).

Barrett, J.C., Bias, N.E., and Ts'o, P.O.P. A mammalian cellular system for the concomitant study of neoplastic transformation and somatic mutation. Mutation Res. **50**, 121–136 (1978b).

Barrett, J.C., Crawford, B.D., Mixter, L.O., Schechtman, L.M., Ts'o, P.O.P., and Pollack, R. Correlation of *in vitro* growth properties and tumorigenicity of Syrian hamster cell lines. Cancer Res. **39**, 1504–1510 (1979).

Barrett, J.C., Crawford, B.D. and Ts'o, P.O.P. The role of somatic mutation in a multistage model of carcinogenesis. In: *Mammalian Cell Transformation by Chemical Carcinogens*, eds. V.C. Dunkel and R.A. Mishra (1981a). Senate Press, Princeton.

Barrett, J.C., Wong, A., and McLachlan, J.A. Diethylstilbestrol induces neoplastic transformation of cells in culture without measurable somatic mutation at two loci. Science, **212** (1981b).

Benedict, W.F. Early changes in chromosomal number and structure after treatment of fetal hamster cultures with transforming doses of polycyclic hydrocarbons. J. Natl. Cancer Inst. **49**, 585–590 (1972).

Benedict, W.F., Jones, P.A., Laug, W.W., Igel, H.J., and Freeman, A.E. Characterization of human cells transformed *in vitro* by urethane. Nature **256**, 322–324 (1975a).

Benedict, W.F., Rucker, N., Mark, C. and Kouri, R.E. Correlation between balance of specific chromosomes and expression of malignancy. J. Natl. Cancer Inst. **54**, 157–162 (1975b).

Berwald, Y. and Sachs, L. *In vitro* cell transformation with chemical carcinogens. Nature **200**, 1182–1184 (1963).

Berwald, Y. and Sachs, L. *In vitro* transformation of normal cells to tumor cells by carcinogenic hydrocarbons. J. Natl. Cancer Inst. **35**, 641–661 (1965).

Biesele, J.J., Berger, R.E., Clarke, M., and Weiss, L. Effects of purines and other chemotherapeutic agents on nuclear structure and function. Exp. Cell Res., Suppl. **2**, 279–300 (1952).

Boone, C.W. Malignant hemangioendotheliomas produced by subcutaneous inoculation of Balb/3T3 cells attached to glass beads. Science **188**, 68–70 (1975).

Boone, C.S. and Jacobs, J.B. Sarcomas routinely produced from putatively non-tumorigenic Balb/3T3 and C3H 10T½ cells by subcutaneous inoculation attached to plastic platelets. J. Supramolecular Structure **5**, 131–137 (1976).

Borek, C. X-ray-induced *in vitro* neoplastic transformation of human diploid cells. Nature **283**, 776–778 (1980).

Bouck, N., and DiMayorca, G. Somatic mutation as the basis for malignant transformation of BHK cells by chemical carcinogens. Nature **264**, 722–727 (1976).

Boveri, T.H. *Zur frage der entstehun maligner tumoren*. Fischer, Jena (1914).

Brockman, H.E., Hung, C.Y., deSerres, F.J., and Ong, T.M. Potent mutagenicity of 6-N-hydroxyl-amino purine and 2-amino-N^6-hydroxyadenine at the ad-3 region of *Neurospora crassa*. Environ. Mut. **1**, 133 (1979).

Cairns, J. On the origin of human cancers. Nature **289**, 353–357 (1981).

Capizzi, R.L. and Jameson, J.W. A table for the estimation of the spontaneous mutation rate of cells in culture. Mutation Res. **17**, 147–148 (1973).

Chan, G.L. and Little, J.B. Induction of ouabain-resistant mutations in C3H 10T½ mouse cells by ultraviolet light. Proc. Natl. Acad. Sci. U.S.A. **75**, 3363–3366 (1978).

Colburn, N.H., Bruegge, W.F.V., Bates, J.R., Gray, R.H., Rossen, J.D., Kelsey, W.H. and Shimada, T. Correlation of anchorage-independent growth with tumorigenicity of chemically transformed mouse epidermal cells. Cancer Res. **38**, 624–634 (1978).

Cox, R. and Masson, W.K. Do radiation-induced thioguanine-resistant mutants of cultured mammalian cells arise by HGPRT gene mutation of X-chromosome rearrangement? Nature **276**, 629–639 (1978).

Crawford, B.D., Barrett, J.C., and Ts'o, P.O.P. Neoplastic conversion of preneoplastic Syrian hamster cells: Rate estimation by fluctuation analysis. Mol. and Cell Biol. **3**, 931–945 (1983).

DeMars, R., and Jackson, J.L. Mutagenicity detection with human cells. J. Environ. Pathol. Toxicol. **1**, 55–77 (1977).

deSerres, F.J. Problems associated with the application of short-term tests for mutagenicity in mass screening programs. Environmental Mutagenesis **1**, 203–208 (1979).

DiPaolo, J.A., Donovan, P., and Nelson, R. Quantitative studies of *in vitro* transformation by chemical carcinogens. J. Natl. Cancer Inst. **42**, 867–874 (1969).

DiPaolo, J.A., Donovan, P.J., and Nelson, R.L. *In vitro* transformation of hamster cells by polycyclic hydrocarbons: factors influencing the number of cells transformed. Nature New Biology **230**, 240–242 (1971a).

DiPaolo, J.A., Donovan, P.J., and Nelson, R.L. Transformation of hamster cells *in vitro* by polycyclic hydrocarbons without cytotoxicity. Proc. Natl. Acad. Sci. **68**, 2958–2961 (1971b).

DiPaolo, J.A., Nelson, R.L. and Donovan, P.J. Morphological, oncogenic, and karyological characteristics of Syrian hamster embryo cells transformed *in vitro* by carcinogenic polycyclic hydrocarbons. Cancer Res. **31** 1118–1127 (1971c).

DiPaolo, J.A., Nelson, R.L. and Donovan, P.J. *In vitro* transformation of Syrian hamster embryo cells by diverse chemical carcinogens. Nature **235**, 278–280 (1972).

DiPaolo, J.A., Takano, K., and Popescu, N.C. Quantitation of chemically induced neoplastic transformation of Balb/3T3 cloned cell lines. Cancer Res. **32** 2686–2695 (1972).

Fernandez, A., Mondal, S. and Heidelberger, C. Probabilistic view of the transformation of cultured C3H 10T½ mouse embryo fibroblasts by 3-methylcholanthrene. Proc. Natl. Acad. Sci., U.S.A. **77**, 7272–7276 (1980).

Foulds, L. *Neoplastic Development*, Vol. 1 (1969), Academic Press, London.

Freedman, V.H., and Shin, S. Isolation of human diploid cell variants with enhanced colony-form efficiency in semi-solid medium after a single step chemical mutagenesis: Brief communication. J. Natl. Cancer Inst. **58**, 1873–1875 (1977).

Freedman, V.H., and Shin, S. Use of nude mice for studies on the tumorigenicity of animal cells. In: *The Nude Mouse in Experimental and Clinical Research*, eds. J. Fogh and B.C. Giovanella pp. 353–384 (1978). Academic Press, N.Y.

Freese, E.B. The mutagenic effect of hydroxyaminopurine derivatives on phage T$_4$. Mutation Res. **5**, 299–301 (1968).

Gart, J.J., DiPaolo, J.A., Donovan, P.J. Mathematical models and the statistical analyses of cell transformation experiments. Cancer Res. **39**, 5069–5075 (1979).

Green, H. Terminal differentiation of cultured human epidermal cells. Cell **11**, 405–416 (1977).

Greiner, J.W., Evans, C.H. and DiPaolo, J.A. Carcinogen-induced anchorage-independent growth and *in vivo* lethality of human MRC-5 cells. Carcinogenesis. **2**: 359–362 (1981).

Haber, D.A., Fox, D.A., Dynan, W.S. and Thilly, W.G. Cell density dependence of focus formation in the C3H 10T½ transformation assay. Cancer Res. **37**, 1644–1648 (1977).

Haber, D.A. and Thilly, W.G. Morphological transformation C3H 10T½ cells subcultured at low cell densities. Life Sciences **2**, 1663–1674 (1978).

Hayflick, L. and Moorehead, P.S. The serial cultivation of human diploid cell line. Exp. Cell Res. **25**, 585–621 (1961).

Heidelberger, C., Freeman, A.E., Pienta, R.J., Sivak, A., Bertran, J.A., Casto, B.C., Dunkel, V.C., Francis, M.C., Kakunaga, T., Little, J.B., and Schechtman, L.M. Cell transformation by chemical agents: A review and analysis of the literature. Mutation Research **114**, 283–385 (1983).

Hennings, H., Michael, D., Cheng, C., Steinert, P., Holbrook, K., and Yuspa, S.H. Calcium regulation of growth and differentiation of mouse epidermal cells in culture. Cell **19**, 245–254 (1980).

Hesterberg, T.W. and Barrett, J.C. Asbestos and mineral fiber induced cell transformation depends on fiber dimensions. Cancer Res. **44**, 2170–2180 (1984).

Hollstein, M., McCann, J., Angelosant, F.A., and Nichols, W.W. Short term tests for carcinogens and mutagens. Mutation Res. **65**, 289–356 (1979).

Huberman, E. and Sachs, L. Cell susceptibility to transformation and cytotoxicity by the carcinogenic hydrocarbon benzo(a)pyrene. Proc. Natl. Acad. Sci. U.S.A. **56**, 1123–1129 (1966).

Huberman, E., Magern, R., Sachs, L. Mutagenesis and transformation of normal cells by chemical carcinogens. Nature **264**, 360–361 (1976).

IARC Monograph on the Evaluation of Carcinogenic Risks of Chemical to Man. (1979), Lyon. Sex Hormones (II), Vol. 21.

IARC Monograph, Supplement 2, Long-term and short-term screening assays for carcinogen in a critical appraisal, 185–200 (1980).

Ishii, Y., Elliott, J.A., Mishra, N.K., and Lieberman, M.W. Quantitative studies of transformation by chemical carcinogen and ultraviolet radiation using a subclone BHK$_{21}$ clone 13 Syrian hamster cells. Cancer Res. **37**, 2023–2029 (1977).

Jacobs, L. and DeMars, R. Chemical mutagenesis with diploid human fibroblasts. In: *Handbook of Mutagenicity Test Procedures*, eds. Kilbey, *et al*, pp. 193–220 (1977). Elsevier, Amsterdam.

Kakunaga, T. A quantitative system for assay of malignant transformation by chemical carcinogens using a clone derived from Balb/3T3. Int. J. Cancer **12**, 463–463 (1973).

Kakunaga, T. Neoplastic transformation of human diploid fibroblasts cells by chemical carcinogens. Proc. Natl. Acad. Sci. U.S.A. **75**, 1334–1338 (1978).

Kakunaga, T., Lo, K., Leavitt, J. and Ikenaga, M. Relationship between transformation and mutation in mammalian cells. In: *Carcinogenesis: Fundamental Mechanisms and Environmental Effects*, eds. B. Pullman, P.O.P. Ts'o, and H. Gelboin, pp. 527–541 (1980) Reidel, Dordrecht.

Kennedy, A.R., Cairns, J., and Little, J.B. Timing of the steps in transformation of C3H 10T½ cells by X-irradiation. Nature **307**, 85–86 (1984).

Kennedy, A.R., Fox, M., Murphy, G., and Little, J.B. Relationship between X-ray exposure and malignant transformation in C3H 10T½. Cells. Proc. Natl. Acad. Sci. U.S.A. **77**, 7262–7266 (1980).

Kennedy, A.R. and Little, J.B. Investigation of the mechanism for the enhancement of radiation transformation *in vitro* by TPA. Carcinogenesis, **1**, 1039–1047 (1980).

Kopelovich, L., Bias, N.E., and Helson, L. Tumor promoter alone induces neoplastic transformation of fibroblasts from humans genetically predisposed to cancer. Nature **282**, 619–621 (1979a).

Kopelovich, L., Pfeffer, L.M. and Bian, N. Growth characteristics of human skin fibroblasts *in vitro*. Cancer **43**, 218–223 (1979b).

Kulesz-Martin, M., Koehler, B., Hennings, H., Yuspa, S.H. Quantitative assay for carcinogen altered differentiation in mouse epidermal cells. Carcinogenesis, **1**, 995–1006 (1980).

Landolph, J.R. and Heidelberger, C. Chemical carcinogens produce mutations to ouabain resistance in transformable C3H 10T½ C18 mouse fibroblasts. Proc. Natl. Acad. Sci. U.S.A. **76**, 930–934 (1979).

Lang, D.R. Measurement of the transformation mutation ratio in BALB/3T3 cells. In Vitro **15**, 223–224 (1979).

Luria, S.E., and Delbruck, M. Mutations of bacteria from virus sensitivity to virus resistance. Genetics **28**, 491–511 (1943).

Marquardt, H. Induction of mutation to ouabain resistance and of malignant transformation by chemicals in cloned mouse M2 fibroblasts. Carcinogenesis **1**, 215–218 (1980).

McCann, J. and Ames, B.N. Detection of carcinogens as mutagens in the Salmonella/microsome test assay of 300 chemicals. Discussion. Proc. Natl. Acad. Sci. U.S.A. **73**, 950–954 (1976).

McCann, J., Choi, E., Yamasaki, E., and Ames, B.N. Detection of carcinogens as mutagens in the Salmonella/microsome test: Assay of 300 chemicals. Proc. Natl. Acad. Sci. U.S.A. **72**, 5135–5139 (1975).

McCormick, J.J., Silinskas, K.C., and Maher, V.M. Transformation of diploid human fibroblasts by chemical carcinogens. In: *Carcinogenesis: Fundamental Mechanisms and Environmental Effects*, eds. B. Pullman, P.O.P. Ts'o, and H. Gelboin, pp. 491–498 (1980). D. Reidel Publishing Company, Holland, Vol. 13.

Metzler, M., Gottschlich, R., and McLachlan, J.A. In: *Estrogens in the Environment*, ed. J.A. McLachlan, p. 293 (1980). Elsevier North Holland, Inc., Amsterdam.

Milo, G.E., and DiPaolo, J.A. Presensitization of human cells with extrinsic signals to induced chemical carcinogenesis. Int. J. Cancer. **26**: 805–812 (1980).

Milo, G.E. Jr., and DiPaolo, J.A. Neoplastic transformation of human diploid cells *in vitro* after chemical carcinogen treatment. Nature **275**, 130–132 (1978).

Milo, G.E., Weisbrode, S.A., Zimmerman, R., and McCloskey, J.A. Ultraviolet radiation-induced neoplastic transformation of normal human cells *in vitro*. Chem. Biol. Interactions. **36**: 45–59 (1981).

Miyaki, M., Akamatsu, N., Hirono, U., Ono, T., Tonomura, A., and Utsunomiya, J. Transformation of fibroblasts from a patient with adenomatosis coli by treatment with a chemical carcinogen. Gann **71**, 741–742 (1980).

Miyaki, M., Akamatsu, N., Ono, T., Tonomura, A., and Utsunomiya, J. Morphological transformation and chromosomal changes induced by chemical carcinogens in skin fibroblasts from patients with familial adenomatosis coli. J. Nat'l Cancer Inst. **68**: 563–571 (1982).

Mondal, S. and Heidelberger, C. *In vitro* malignant transformation by methylcholanthrene of the progeny of single cells derived from C3H mouse prostate. Proc. Natl. Acad. Sci. U.S.A. **65**, 219–225 (1970).

Namba, M., Nishitani, K., and Kimoto, T. Carcinogenesis in tissue culture. 20:Neoplastic transformation of a normal human diploid cell strain, WI-38 with Co-60 gamma rays. Jap. J. Expt. Med. **48**, 308–311 (1978).

Nettesheim, P., and Barrett, J.C. Tracheal epithelial cell transformation: A model system for studies on neoplastic progression. In: Goldber, L. (ed.), *Critical Previews of Toxicology*, Vol. 12, CRC Press, Boca Raton, Fla. p. 215–239, (1984).

Nettesheim, P., Klein-Szanto, A.J.P., Marchok, A.C., Steele, V.E., Terzaghi, M., and Topping, D.C. Studies of neoplastic development in respiratory tract epithelium. Arch. Pathol. and Lab. Med. **105**, 1–10 (1981).

O'Neill, J.P. and Hsie, A.W. The CHO/HGPRT mutation assay: experimental procedure. In: *Banbury Report 2: Mammalian Cell Mutagenesis*, eds. A.W. Hsie, J.P. O'Neill, V.K. McElheny, pp. 55–69 (1979). Cold Spring Harbor Laboratory, New York.

Oshimura, M., Hesterberg, T.W., Tsutsui, T. and Barrett, J.C. Correlation of asbestos-induced cytogenetic effects with cell transformation of Syrian embryo cells in culture. Cancer Res. **44**, 5017–5022 (1984).

Parodi, S. and Brambilla, G. Relationships between mutation and transformation frequencies in mammalian cells treated *in vitro* with chemical carcinogens. Mutation Research **47**, 53–74 (1977).

Pienta, R.J., Poiley, J.A., and Lebherz, W.B. III. Further evaluation of a hamster embryo cell carcinogenesis bioassay. *Proc. of Third International Symposium on Detection and Prevention of Cancer*, Marcel Dekker, N.Y. (1977).

Pienta, R.J. Transformation of Syrian hamster embryo cells by diverse chemicals and correlations with their reported carcinogenic and mutagenic activities. In: *Chemical Mutagens*, eds. F.J. deSerres adn A. Hollaender, pp. 175–202 (1980).

Reznikoff, C.A., Bertran, J.S., Brankow, D.W. and Heidelberger, C. Quantitative and qualitative studies of chemical transformation of cloned C3H mouse embryo cells sensitive to postconfluence inhibition of cell division. Cancer Res. **33**, 3239–3249 (1973).

Reznikoff, C.A., Brankow, D.W. and Heidelberger, C. Establishment of characterization of a cloned line of C3H mouse embryo cells sensitive to postconfluence inhibition of cell division. Cancer Res. **33**, 3231–3238 (1973).

Rheinwald, J.G. and Green, H. Epidermal growth factor and the multiplication of cultured human epidermal keratinocytes. Nature **265**, 421–422 (1977).

Rheinwald, J.G. and Beckett, M.A. Detective terminal differentiation in culture as a consistent and selectable character of malignant human keratinocytes. Cell **22**, 629–632 (1980).

Rhim, J.S., Huebner, R.J., Arnstein, P., and Kopelovich, L. Chemical transformation of cultured human skin fibroblasts derived from individuals with hereditary adenomatosis of the colon and rectum. Int. J. Cancer **26**, 565–569 (1980).

Robbins, A.R. and Baker, R.M. (Na, K)ATPase activity in membrane preparations of ouabain-resistant HeLa cells. Biochem. **16**, 5163–5168 (1977).

Ronen, A. 2-Aminopurine. Mutation Res. **75**, 1–47 (1979).

Saxholm, H.J.K. and Digernes, V. Progressive loss of DNA and lowering of the chromosomal mode in chemically transformed C3H 10T½ cells during development of their oncogenic potential. Cancer Res. **40**, 4254–4260 (1980).

Sharkey, F.E., Fogh, J.M., Hajdu, S.E., Fitzgerald, P.J., and Fogh, J. Experience in surgical pathology with human tumor growth in the nude mouse. In: *The Nude Mouse in Experimental and Clinical Research*, eds. J. Fogh and B.C. Giovanella pp. 187–214 (1978). Academic Press, N.Y.

Shimada, H., Shibuta, H., and Yoshikawa, M. Transformation of tissue-cultured Xeroderma pigmentosum fibroblasts by treatment with N-methyl-N'-nitro-N-nitrosoguanidine. Nature**264**, 547–548 (1976).

Silinskas, K.C., Kateley, S.A., Tower, J.E., Maher, V.M., and McCormick, J.J. 1981. Induction of anchorage-independent growth in human fibroblasts by propane sultone. Cancer Res. **41**: 1620–1627.

Siminovitch, L. On the nature of heritable variation on cultured somatic cells. Cell **7**, 1–11 (1976).

Slaga, T.J., Viaje, A., Bracken, W.M., Buty, S.G., Miller, D.R., Fischer, S.M., Ritcher, C.K., and Dummont, J.N. *In Vitro* transformation of epidermal cells from newborn mice. Cancer Res. **38**, 2246–2252 (1978).

Spandidos, D.A. and Siminovitch, L. The relationship between transformation and somatic mutation in human and Chinese hamster cells. Cell **13**, 651–662 (1978).

Stoker, M. and MacPherson, I. Syrian hamster fibroblast cell line BHK$_{21}$ and its derivatives. Nature **203**, 1355–1357 (1964).

Styles, J.A. Studies on the detection of carcinogens using a mammalian cell transformation assay with liver homogenate activation. In: *Short term test systems for detecting carcinogens*, eds. K.H. Norpoth, and R.C. Gardner, pp. 226–238 (1980). Springer-Verlag, Berlin.

Sugiura, K., Teller, M.N., Parham, J.C., and Brown, G.B. A comparison of the oncogenicities of 3-hydroxyxanthine, guanine 3-N-oxide, and some related compounds. Cancer Res. **30**, 184–188 (1970).

Sutherland, B.M., Cimino, J.S., Delihas, N., Shih, A.G., and Oliver, R.P. Ultraviolet light-induced transformation of human cells to anchorage-independent growth. Cancer Res. **40**, 1934–1939 (1980).

Tejwani, R., Witiak, D.T., Inbasekaran, M.N., Cazer, F.D., and Milo, G.E. Characteristics of benzo(a)pyrene and A-ring reduced 7,12-dimethyl benz(a)anthracene induced neoplastic transformation of human cells *in vitro*. Cancer Lett. **13**: 119–127 (1981).

Terzaghi, M. and Little, J.B. X-irradiation-induced transformation in the C3H mouse embryo derived cell line. Cancer Res. **36**, 1367–1374 (1976).

Thomassen, D.G., Gray, T., Mass, M.J., and Barrett, J.C. High frequency of carcinogen-induced early, preneoplastic changes in rat tracheal epithelial cells in culture. Cancer Res. **43**, 5956–5963 (1983).

Todaro, G.J., and Green, H. Quantitative studies of the growth of mouse embryo cells in culture and their development into established lines. J. Cell Biol. **17**, 299–313 (1963).

Trainin, N., Kaye, A.M., and Berenblum, I. Influence of mutagens on the initiation of skin carcinogenesis. Biochem. Pharmacol. **13**, 262–267 (1964).

Tsutsui, T., Barrett, J.C., Ts'o, P.O.P. Morphological transformation, DNA damage, and chromosomal aberrations induced by a direct DNA perturbation of synchronized Syrian hamster embryo cells. Cancer Res. **39**, 2356–2365 (1979).

Tsutsui, T., Maizumi, H., McLachlan, J.A., and Barrett, J.C. Aneuploidy induction and cell transformation by diethylstilbestrol: a possible chromosome mechanism in carcinogenesis. Cancer Res. **43**, 3814–3821 (1983).

Tsutsui, T., Maizumi, H., and Barrett, J.C. Induction by modified purines (2-aminopurine and 6-N-hydroxyl-aminopurine) of chromosome aberrations and aneuploidy in Syrian hamster embryo cells. Mutation Res. in press (1984).

Yamamoto, T., Rabinowitz, A., and Sachs, L. Identification of the chromosomes that control malignancy. Nature New Bio. **243**, 247–250 (1973).

Zimmerman, R.J., and Little, J.B. Starvation for arginine and glutamine sensitizes human diploid cells to the transforming effect of N-acetoxy-2-AAF. Carcinogenesis. **2**: 1303–1310 (1981).

CHAPTER IX

A COMPARISON OF THE ANIMAL AND HUMAN CARCINOGENICITY OF ENVIRONMENTAL, OCCUPATIONAL AND THERAPEUTIC CHEMICALS

G.M. Williams, B. Reiss, J.H. Weisburger
Naylor Dana Institute for Disease Prevention
American Health Foundation
Valhalla, New York 10595

A. INTRODUCTION

I. Background

The chemical causation of cancer in humans was first recognized from the occurrence of cancer in occupational settings (see Weisburger and Williams, 1982a). Subsequently, a significant number of chemicals or combinations of chemicals has led to the development of cancer in exposed individuals (International Agency for Research on Cancer, 1983). These associations, arising primarily during occupational or therapeutic exposures, have firmly established the principle of chemical causation of some human cancers.

Virtually all of the chemicals that have been demonstrated to be causative agents of cancer in humans also produce cancer in a variety of animal models (International Agency for Research on Cancer, 1983). On the basis of this substantial background of evidence that human carcinogens can be revealed in animal models, it has been widely assumed that chemicals that are carcinogenic in animal models are likely to be potential cancer hazards to humans. This assumption has been reinforced by instances in which chemicals have been demonstrated to be carcinogenic in animals before subsequent identification of cancer causation in humans; examples of this are vinyl chloride (Haley, 1975; Maltoni and Lefemine, 1975; Maltoni, 1977) and bis-(chloromethyl) ether (Van Duuren *et al.*, 1972).

[a]This research was supported by Contract NO1-ES-6-2130 from the National Institute of Environmental Health Sciences.

The authors thank Dr. Hildegarde Marquardt and Mrs. Alena Leff for assistance with portions of the work.

Laboratory animal experiments are effective and efficient for the assessment of the safety of compounds with respect to their toxicity and carcinogenicity; however, mechanistic considerations are required for the correct evaluation and interpretation of animal data and the extrapolation of these data to humans (Kroes, 1979; Kolbye, 1980; Higginson, 1981; Munro and Krewski, 1981; Weisburger and Williams, 1981). This is especially important for chemicals that produce select neoplasms in one or more species at specific organ sites. For example, certain chemicals tested under a wide variety of conditions in several species have either exclusively or predominantly induced cancers of the liver in some mouse strains, or cancer of the kidneys or bladder in mice or rats, or both. Some of these results were achieved only at very high dose levels, with a relatively sharp cutoff, i.e., no neoplasms at all were produced at lower levels. Such observations indicate that it is necessary to understand species responses and acquire insight into the underlying relevant mechanisms of these responses in order to properly interpret the significance of such data obtained in tests for the determination of human cancer risk.

In the extrapolation of animal carcinogenicity data for the purpose of projecting human risk, both qualitative and quantitative considerations are involved. The qualitative, or at best semi-quantitative determination must address the issue of the reliability of the data obtained in animal bioassays and how such data can be meaningfully and realistically translated into a basis for hazard assessment in humans. Beyond this lies the component that is truly quantitative and deals with the delineation of the potency of the chemical under the conditions of the test and the relative sensitivity of animals and humans. Furthermore, the question of extrapolation from high dosage level animal testing in a limited number of experimental animals to the often prevailing low level human exposure, but with large numbers of individuals potentially at risk, needs to be addressed.

Technical papers and reviews describing the effects of chemical carcinogens in animal models usually have referred to a potential or actual effect in humans. However, even when data for both animals and humans were available on these chemicals, relatively few systematic evaluations of the available data base have been made to categorize and specify responses in animals compared to those in humans.

A continuing effort at correlation of animal bioassays with evidence of human effects has been made in the International Agency for Research on Cancer monograph series, which discusses the key literature on individual chemical carcinogens (Tomatis *et al.*, 1978). Each monograph includes an evaluation of all animal carcinogenicity data available for each agent, but the interpretation of species differences is not part of this undertaking. Moreover, although human effects are noted where available, no interpretation of discordances with animal data is attempted.

A number of papers have utilized the few truly adequate experimental data in dose-response studies in animals to delineate and extrapolate risk to humans on a quantitative basis. For example, several authors, particularly Mantel and Scheiderman (1975) and Cornfield (1977), have developed mathematical techniques for risk assessment from the classic experiment of Bryan and Shimkin (1943) in which subcutaneous sarcomas were induced by a range of doses of polycyclic aromatic hydrocarbons. Others, including Albert and Altschuler (1973), Hoel et al. (1975), Crump (1976), Guess et al. (1977), Peto (1977), and Preussman (1978) have made important contributions to these approaches. Although the experiment of Bryan and Shimkin was simple and the end point, subcutaneous sarcoma, readily visualized, most cancers in humans are of epithelial origin and thus do not correspond to the type of neoplasm produced in this study. Furthermore, most chemical carcinogens exhibit much steeper dose response curves (Shimkin et al., 1966; Druckrey, 1967; Shimkin et al., 1967; Littlefield et al., 1975; Schmähl et al., 1977) than was observed with the insoluble polycyclic aromatic hydrocarbons, which remain at an injection site for an unusually prolonged time interval. Thus, the existing mathematical formulations need to be reexamined, and the results from the Bryan and Shimkin experiment must be compared with the results from studies of other kinds of chemical carcinogens in models in which epithelial cancers are the measured end point. Druckrey, Schmähl and associates (1967; 1977) have published data on the induction of epithelial neoplasms that may be appropriate for this purpose. Also, in a major effort in this regard, the National Center for Toxicological Research performed a large scale study with 2-acetylaminofluorene in mice and has presented dose-response analyses of the results of these studies [Innovation in Cancer Risk Assessment (ED_{01}) Study, 1979]. This type of study is designed to reveal the shape of the dose-response curve at low doses.

A pertinent series of papers from an NIEHS Extrapolation Conference on risk assessment (Hoel and Rall, 1978) reports the views of several individuals on the applicability of specific tests to risk assessment in humans and discusses the feasibility of establishing thresholds for chemical responses. Likewise, mathematical modeling was discussed by several authors at a recent conference on risk analysis (Richmond et al., 1981).

Using a somewhat different approach, Meselson and Russell (1977) have reviewed the carcinogenic potency in laboratory rodents and mutagenic potency in Salmonella of several test compounds; they reported that these potencies were approximately equal except for the nitroso compounds which were considerably more potent as carcinogens. They suggested that the carcinogenic potency of a mutagenic compound in humans may be similar to that in rodents if its potency is expressed in terms of the average normal life-span of the respective species. Limitations in this approach stemming from the imbalances of subcellular metabolizing systems used in bacterial mutagenicity studies have been pointed out by Williams (1981).

The Consultative Panel on Health Hazards and Chemical Pesticides of the National Academy of Sciences published a useful document on comparative carcinogenicity (Meselson, 1975) In this report, the panel selected and tabulated studies on 13 chemical carcinogens of varied types and attempted a qualitative and quantitative comparison of the results of animal bioassays with human cancer occurrences. The relative sensitivity of humans was, therefore, evaluated by means of extrapolation.

Each of these reports dealing with dose-response relationships and extrapolation procedures has served a valuable purpose, but none represents a comprehensive attempt to identify and account for species differences in carcinogenicity through consideration of factors known to affect carcinogenicity (Weisburger and Williams, 1982a; 1983a).

To evaluate species differences in carcinogenicity, Williams *et al.* (1978) performed a data analysis in which the literature was searched for reports on six chemicals: aflatoxin B_1, benzidine, chlornaphazine, diethylstilbestrol, dimethylnitrosamine, and vinyl chloride. These chemicals were chosen becuase they had all been shown to be carcinogenic in animal models, and many studies of their effects in various animal species had been performed. Four of these chemicals, benzidine, chlornaphazine, diethylstilbestrol, and vinyl chloride, are accepted as carcinogenic in humans as well (International Agency for Research on Cancer, 1983); aflatoxin B_1 has been considered by many to be a probable human carcinogen (Linsell and Peers, 1977), and human exposure to dimethylnitrosamine has occurred although human carcinogenicity has not been documented. Only those studies that seemed appropriate to the question of species to species comparison and human extrapolation were selected for evaluation. The most important criteria for inclusion of a carcinogenicity study were the adequacy of the study (i.e. sufficient detail on dosages and sufficient numbers of animals) and the reliability of the diagnosis of the pathological lesions. The data were compared and the relative sensitivity of animal species was determined. Factors that might account for differences in response between species such as route of exposure, dose rate, age and sex of the animals, diet, metabolic activities, detoxification, etc. (Weisburger and Williams, 1982b) were researched and evaluated for the various compounds in order to provide insight into species differences and possible modes of action.

II. Mechanisms of Chemical Carcinogenesis

The molecular effects of chemical carcinogens have been intensively studied in a number of laboratories during the last fifteen years, culminating in the concept that many carcinogens operate as electrophilic reactants (Miller and Miller, 1981). The realization that certain chemical carcinogens ultimately had specific properties leading to interaction with tissue macromolecules, including DNA, has led to a strengthening of the relationship between mutagenesis and carcinogenesis. As a further extension, the term "genotoxicity" was introduced to cover the toxic, lethal and heritable effects of carcinogens on DNA (Ehrenberg *et al.*, 1973). The use of tests for genetic effects has confirmed the genotoxicity of most electrophilic compounds where appropriate metabolic pathways were provided. These short-term tests have been demonstrated to be reliable not only as preliminary tools for the detection of potential carcinogens but also as a method for determining whether specific carcinogens are DNA-reactive, i.e. genotoxic (Williams, 1978; 1979).

210

Considerable evidence of various types has been obtained that not all carcinogens react with DNA (Williams, 1979a; 1979b). Based on such information, Weisburger and Williams (1980) introduced the categorization of carcinogens into DNA-reactive or genotoxic substances that have the ability to damage DNA and epigenetic agents that lack DNA-damaging ability but produce another biologic effect that could be the basis for carcinogenicity. The nature of the risk from exposure to these two types of agents appears to be different (Weisburger and Williams, 1981). Thus, in the analysis, any relevant data pertaining to whether the agent is or is not reliably DNA-reactive was included in the qualitative risk evaluation for humans.

In the quantitative risk extrapolation, two parameters were considered: (1) the latent period of neoplasm development and (2) the total yield of neoplasms, i.e., the percentage of subjects with neoplasms, or actually, the percentage of subjects with neoplasms at a specific organ site. A further refinement in experimental studies was the evaluation of the number or multiplicity of neoplasms in affected organs, but little comparative data of this type were found.

In extensive dose response testing of a series of carcinogenic arylamines and nitrosamines, Druckrey and associates (1967) established several concepts for carcinogens of the type that are now considered to be DNA-reactive. One concept maintained that the total final yield of neoplasms in a given organ is a function of the total dose. Another concept was that the latent period until cancer appears in a specific organ is a function of the daily dose rate of a specific carcinogen. These concepts applied only to situations in which the exposure to the carcinogen was continuous for the entire duration of the test. For a limited exposure to a carcinogen followed by a carcinogen-free holding period, the final yield of neoplasms could still be proportional to the total dose. However, administration of many powerful carcinogens at lower dose rates for a longer time interval yielded a higher cancer incidence than the same total dose at higher dose rates for a shorter interval; the basis for this different outcome probably resided in effects on the operation of several processes, including the ratio of activation/detoxification reactions, DNA repair, cell replication rates, etc. Nevertheless, in the quantitative evaluation performed, data on cumulative doses and incidences were used since these provided the best means for quantitative comparison of species responses. However, whereas cumulative exposures to animals could usually be calculated from reported experimental protocols, determination of human exposures to agents such as benzidine necessitated a consideration of the length of service of an individual at a chemical plant and specific plant function in order to compute the cumulative exposure. For these calculations, knowledge of pertinent biochemical data on each agent was employed.

This review is a condensation and update of the interspecies carcinogenicity assessment of Williams et al. (1978). Four known human carcinogens from that study, benzidine, chlornaphazine, diethylstilbestrol and vinyl chloride, as well as the likely human carcinogen, aflatoxin B_1, are discussed here. Only selected data from the original report to support its main conclusions are presented in this review. The analysis of Williams et al. (1978) revealed that the chemicals that were carcinogenic in humans were carcinogenic in a number of animal species over a wide range of doses, including low doses. However, significant species differences in carcinogenic response were found for every chemical for which reliable data were available. In some cases, these could be accounted for by differences in parameters known to affect carcinogenicity. Nevertheless, the species closest to humans in sensitivity varied for each chemical and could not be predicted from any available collateral data.

B. COMPARISON OF ANIMAL AND HUMAN CARCINOGENICITY DATA

I. Environmental Carcinogens:

Among the carcinogens examined in the study of Williams *et al.* (1978), aflatoxin B_1 is a naturally-occurring carcinogen present in the human environment, specifically as a fungal derived contaminant in the diet. High levels occur in certain foods in Africa and Asia. In the United States levels of up to 20 parts per billion are permitted in human foods. For animal fodder, the action level has recently been raised to 200 parts per billion. Although this agent is a potent animal carcinogen, quantification of human carcinogenicity has been difficult. Indeed, working groups of the International Agency for Research on Cancer have considered the evidence for carcinogenicity in humans to be only limited (International Agency for Research on Cancer, 1983), mainly because of the concurrent presence of other potentially causative agents, including hepatitis B virus that could be an enhancing factor due to liver cell damage and replication alterations. Thus, the evaluation of aflatoxin B_1 illustrates the difficulty of ascertaining the human carcinogenicity of an environmental agent. This is exemplified by the broad experience of the International Agency for Research on Cancer (1983); in the ascertainment of human carcinogens, no useful evidence was derived from general environmental exposures.

1. Aflatoxin B_1 (AFB$_1$):

Aflatoxins are polyheterocyclic fungal toxins that occur in nature as heterogeneous mixtures contaminating certain foods. These mixtures always contain AFB_1 which has been found to be carcinogenic in a variety of species. AFB_1 is a genotoxic carcinogen which, in sensitive animal species, including the trout, rat, duck and monkey, has predominantly or exclusively caused liver neoplasms. Humans in certain geographic regions are exposed to AFB_1 in the diet, and suffer a high incidence of liver cancer.

Only a few dose-response animal studies have been conducted with AFB_1, but a comparison of animal species showed that rainbow trout was the most sensitive (Sinnhuber and Wales, 1968), followed by the rat (Wogan *et al.*, 1974), duckling (Carnaghan, 1965) and monkey (Lin *et al.*, 1974). The mouse was relatively resistant (Wogan, 1976).

Rats predominantly responded to AFB_1 by developing liver neoplasms (Wogan et al., 1974; Epstein et al., 1969), with total doses of 2-7 mg/kg producing an 80% or greater incidence of liver neoplasms (Table I); less typically and in lower incidence, cancers of the stomach (Butler and Barnes, 1966), colon (Ward et al., 1975), and kidney (Epstein et al., 1969) were produced. In mice, AFB_1 was only weakly oncogenic, increasing the incidence of pulmonary adenomas in strain A mice (Wieder et al., 1968) and lymphomas in Swiss mice (Louria et al., 1974). In the only long term study of oral administration, a total dose of 11.5 mg/kg failed to produce liver neoplasms in mice of the C57BL/6NB strain exposed and observed for 20 months (Table I). However, AFB_1 produced liver neoplasms in new-born mice (Vesselinovitch et al., 1972). Thus, the adult rat was clearly more sensitive to liver carcinogenesis by AFB_1 than the adult mouse.

AFB_1 undergoes biotransformation in mammals (Wogan, 1976) and metabolic activation is required to convert AFB_1 to the chemically reactive forms which presumably are responsible for its potent biological effects, including DNA damage and mutagenicity. The biotransformation is complex (Weisburger and Williams, 1982b), but sound evidence has shown the reactive electrophile, the 2,3 epoxide, to be the ultimate carcinogenic metabolite (Miller and Miller, 1981). Detoxified metabolites are conjugated with glutathione and excreted.

To elucidate species differences in the carcinogenicity of reactive carcinogens, direct determinations of the formation of the ultimate carcinogenic metabolites have not been possible because of their reactivity. Thus, indirect measurements have often been used. AFB_1 was found by Garner and Wright (1975) to bind to protein in rat and hamster liver and kidney in constant proportion, but binding of AFB_1 to nucleic acids was much higher than to protein, particularly in rat liver, the target organ of a susceptible species. The observation of binding to DNA indicated that AFB_1 is a DNA-reactive type of carcinogen, which is supported by studies using in vitro systems (McCann et al., 1975; Williams, 1977b). Indirect measurement of the formation of the activated metabolite as a mutagenic metabolite generated by liver enzyme preparations revealed rat liver preparations to be approximately four times as active as those from mouse liver (Hsieh, 1977), thus providing a further correlation with species sensitivity. Likewise, AFB_1 was found to be more genotoxic in rat than in mouse hepatocytes (McQueen et al., 1983a).

The work of Essigmann et al. (1982) further substantiated the species and organ selectivity of aflatoxin activation. They found the levels of aflatoxin-DNA adducts in the liver of the rat to be about 10 times those of the kidney, as indicated by the maximal concentration of AFB_1-N'-guanine, the major DNA adduct, as well as the concentrations of other minor adducts. In the Swiss mouse liver, however, despite the presence of a fully representative spectrum of adducts, the levels of all of the aflatoxin-DNA adducts were approximately 0.1% of those in the rat liver. These data indicate that the mouse liver activated AFB_1 through essentially the same pathways as rat liver but possessed some mechanisms leading to lower levels of critical interactions. Studies of the amounts of DNA repair in rat and mouse hepatocytes revealed a lower level in the mouse (McQueen et al., 1983a), suggesting that rapid removal of adducts in the mouse was probably not the basis for these low levels. Therefore, limited capacity for activation or greater detoxification appears to be responsible for the lower sensitivity of mice. Male rats were more sensitive to AFB_1 than female rats (Kamden et al., 1982). The higher incidence of lung neoplasms in male rats as compared to female rats was suggested by Kamden et al. to be a consequence of lower activity of AFB_1-inactivating liver enzymes in the male.

A relationship exists between human exposure to aflatoxins and liver cancer (Linsell and Peers, 1977; Linsell, 1982). The most important studies on the effects of aflatoxin ingestion in humans were several investigations performed in geographic areas with high incidences of liver cancer, i.e., certain African countries and Thailand. It was estimated that 40% of all neoplasias in Mozambique were primarily liver cancers. In these regions, contamination of agricultural products such as corn, peanuts and beans by mycotoxins was found to be relatively high. These reported levels of exposure suggested a reasonable quantitative relationship between aflatoxin ingestion and liver cancer.

Both Peers et al. (1976) and Shank (1977) calculated a linear dose response for aflatoxin consumption and liver cancer; males particularly have a very high incidence of this disease (Table II). The fact that liver cancer first presents itself in Africa and Asia at a very young age, compared to regions of low aflatoxin exposure, suggests that the causative factors in the two situations: (1) are different, (2) are present at higher levels in the environment of high risk regions, (3) exert their influence at a younger age, perhaps through the mother's milk or even while in utero in high risk regions, and (4) operate together in synergism with other elements (hepatitis B, for example) in high risk regions.

There are a number of considerations that enter into the evaluation of human studies:

1) Aflatoxin carcinogenesis was first described in 1960; thus, no data are available on levels prevailing in the human environment in various parts of the world prior to that time.

2) The aflatoxins present in the diet are a mixture which may be subject to seasonal variations.

3) Estimation of the human dose may be inaccurate because of variations in the type of aflatoxin and amount of diet. Nevertheless, the apparent range is not great (Table II), and therefore, the averages are probably representative. Also, the reported doses could probably be tolerated on a chronic basis since the acutely toxic dose is in the range of 2-6 mg/day (Krishnamachari et al., 1975).

4) All human studies were done in areas where epidemiology is difficult, and case ascertainment may thus be imprecise. Nevertheless, the similarity in rates among the countries (Table II) suggests that the figures may be reasonable.

5) All studies were conducted in regions where hepatitis-B-virus was suspected to contribute to liver cancer incidence (Blumberg et al., 1975) either through oncogenic activity, or by producing chronic hepatitis and cirrhosis. As far as is known, such interaction has not been demonstrated in rodents. In non-human primates, a small test (Lin et al., 1974) did not provide unambigu-

ous evidence of a viral-chemical interaction. Regardless, the possibility of hepatitis-B-virus determining the development of liver cancer independently or in conjunction with aflatoxin or other mycotoxins must be considered. The relevant interactions and mechanisms remain to be defined.

In spite of these limitations, AFB_1 is concluded to be causally involved in human liver cancer. Comparison of the animal dose-response data (Table I) and the human (Table II) reveal that humans are only slightly less sensitive than rats to AFB_1 carcinogenesis.

II. Occupational Carcinogens

The two chemicals from the study of Williams et al. (1978) which represent carcinogenic hazards in the work place are benzidine and vinyl chloride. With occupational agents, the ascertainment of effects on humans is considerably easier than with environmental carcinogens, primarily because exposed individuals can be definitely identified. However, as will be seen, the determination of exposure levels is still difficult and thus limits the precision of quantitative assessment. Moreover, other known risk factors for human cancer are generally present (Weisburger and Williams, 1982a) and can be confounding unless proper controls are used for comparison.

1. Vinyl Chloride (VC)

VC is a synthetic halogenated ethylenic hydrocarbon used in the production of polyvinyl chloride. VC is a DNA-reactive carcinogen active in several species, including mice, rats, rabbits and hamsters. Several organs, including the liver, kidney, ear duct, skin and forestomach have been affected by VC, depending on the species. VC exposure has led to the frequent production in mice of hepatic and extrahepatic angiosarcomas, rare forms of neoplasia. In occupationally exposed humans, VC has induced hepatic angiosarcomas and has been associated with the occurrence of brain, lung and other types of neoplasms (Selikoff and Hammond, 1975).

VC induced liver angiosarcomas in rats (Maltoni, 1977; Lee et al., 1978), mice (Holmberg et al., 1976; Maltoni, 1977), and hamsters (Maltoni, 1977). The maximum incidence in mice was 13-18% and in rats 15%. This occurred at a lower total dose in mice (Table III) and, thus, mice appear to be more sensitive. Hamsters were less sensitive than either mice or rats.

Due to various limitations in animal experimentation with VC, the current information on VC is not adequate for a complete assessment of species differences. One of the limitations arises from the fact that VC is a gas at room temperature and hence inhalation is the appropriate mode of administration in VC carcinogenicity studies. Intraperitoneal and subcutaneous injections were found to be highly ineffective; therefore, studies concerning VC usually contained descriptions of the dosage in terms of gaseous concentration and duration of exposure. However, no data have been developed on absorption by different species or the effective doses reaching target organs, such as the liver.

In particular, metabolic capacity in animals studied was saturated at 250 ppm and carcinogenic effects in the liver plateaued between 250 and 500 ppm. As shown in Table III, there is almost no increase in liver tumor incidences at exposure concentrations above 250 ppm.

VC is metabolized by liver subcellular preparations (Bartsch *et al.*, 1975) and liver cells (Shimada *et al.*, 1985) to a genotoxic moiety. The DNA-reactive metabolites stem from conversion of VC to chloroethylene oxide by cytochrome P-450-dependent monooxygenases and then rearrangement to 2-chloroacetaldehyde (Zajdela *et al.*, 1980; Anders, 1983). Enzyme preparations from mouse liver were reported to be at least 3 times more active than those from rat liver in generating mutagenic metabolites (Bartsch *et al.*, 1975). These findings suggested that the greater susceptibility of mice to VC carcinogenesis was due to a greater capability for metabolic activation.

In humans, angiosarcoma of the liver was first recognized as a VC-associated cancer in 1974 (Creech and Johnson, 1974). Studies have also suggested that individuals working and living near PVC-polymerization facilities had excess mortality from cancer of the brain and lung (Monson *et al.*, 1974; Tabershaw and Gaffey, 1974). There is some indication that the large-cell undifferentiated type of lung cancer is more prevalent than expected in VC-exposed populations. In these populations, excess mortality from "other respiratory disease" has also been found (Waxweiler *et al.*, 1976), and a slight but significant excess was noted for deaths from lymphomas.

Hepatic angiosarcoma is the best defined VC-induced cancer in humans. Most of the neoplasms have been observed in reactor cleaners. The published incidence in humans for angiosarcoma is 3 to 6%; cumulative exposures for these incidences were calculated to be of the order of 400 g/kg. However, since reactor cleaners are virtually the only exposed humans with recorded cases of angiosarcoma, previous calculations of incidence based on the total work force at a VC plant really combine populations with distinctly different levels of risk. Published data on cancer in reactor cleaners are inadequate, but can be interpreted to indicate that the incidence for this group is probably greater than 3% and may be as high as 20-25%.

Typically, occupational liver angiosarcoma was diagnosed in men ranging in age from 36 to 58 (mean 47 years) following 7 to 28 (mean 18) years of employment. In almost all cases, the latent period exceeded 10 years. However, in one documented case, exposure at a "high concentration" for 4 years led to the development of hepatic angiosarcoma and death eight years after the first exposure (Fox and Collier, 1977). Nevertheless, on the average, the latent period was closer to 20 years (Anonym., 1976), and a typical employment period in the reactor-cleaning job (usually followed by years in a lower exposure job) ranged from several months to several years. The general consensus (Nicholson *et al.*, 1975; Barnes, 1976) is that a polymerization plant operator was exposed to an average VC concentration of 1,000 ppm. Assuming that this was a reasonable estimate for a reactor cleaner, a year spent at this job corresponds to a total dose of 33 g/kg. This value was derived from multiplication of the concentration of VC in the air breathed by a reactor cleaner, i.e. 2.56 mg/L (= 1000 ppm; Hefner *et al.* 1975) by the volume of air inhaled (10 L/min; Guyton, 1947; Meselson *et al.*, 1975) and the length of time exposed per day (6 hrs/day), per week (5 days/week) and per year (50 weeks/year). Thus: (2.56 mg/L) (10 L/min) (6 hr/day) (5 days/wk) (50 wks/yr) = 2,304 g/yr or 33 g/kg/yr.

After 18 years (the average employment of known cases of VC-attributed cancer) the cumulative dose of 583 g/kg was inhaled. This value assumes complete absorption of inhaled compound and therefore the true value may have been somewhat smaller (Bolt *et al.*, 1976). Furthermore, the exposures reported probably did not represent effective doses because, in animal studies, metabolic capacity was saturated at 250 ppm and carcinogenic effects in the liver plateaued between 250 and 500 ppm. Thus, calculated effective cumulative liver carcinogenic exposures in humans for 18 years, with consideration of this limitation, may have been 150 g/kg instead of 600 g/kg. Using the lower estimate of the carcinogenic dose for humans, the sensitivity of humans is estimated to be within the same order of magnitude or at least no more than 10-fold less sensitive than animal models. However, extrahepatic neoplasms in animal models did not show a plateau and although human data so far have not given parallel indications, they should be monitored.

2. Benzidine (BZD)

BZD or 4,4'-diaminobiphenyl, is an organic chemical intermediate used in dyestuff manufacturing. It is also a reagent employed in clinical laboratories. BZD is a DNA-reactive carcinogen active in several species including: mice (Bonser *et al.*, 1956; Prokofjeva, 1971; Vesselinovitch, *et al.*, 1975; Nelson *et al.*, 1982), rats (Spitz *et al.*, 1950; Boyland *et al.*, 1954; Griswold *et al.*, 1968; Steinhoff, 1974), hamsters (Saffiotti *et al.*, 1977), rabbits (Bonser *et al.*, 1956) and dogs (Spitz *et al.*, 1950).

A significant species difference in response was that in the rabbit and dog, BZD produced urinary bladder cancer whereas in rodents, males usually developed liver neoplasms, and females developed mammary cancer. In humans, exposure to BZD induced urinary bladder cancer.

In mice, Bonser *et al.* (1956) and Prokofjeva (1971) obtained predominantly liver neoplasms. However, in those studies, high mortality due to infection (Bonser *et al.*, 1956) or toxicity (Prokofjeva, 1971) resulted in relatively low tumor incidences. Vesselinovitch et al. (1975) studied the carcinogenic effect of BZD dihydrochloride in B6C3F$_1$ mice under varying experimental conditions. Depending on the conditions, the mice developed liver neoplasms, lung adenomas, Harderian-gland cystadenomas and lymphoreticular neoplasms (Table IV). A positive dose response relationship was observed for liver neoplasms with three different dose levels (50, 100 and 150 ppm) administered daily in the diet for 84 weeks to male and female mice. A total dose of 5000 mg/kg body weight given to females produced a 64% incidence of liver tumors whereas 6250 mg/kg given to males yielded only a 22% incidence of liver tumors and a 36%

incidence of Harderian gland tumors (Table IV). No dose-response study was available for rats; however, in the extensive study by Spitz *et al.* (1950), a total dose of 2400 mg/kg injected into Sherman strain rats produced an 80% incidence of Zymbal gland tumors. Also, it induced an 11% incidence of hepatomas in males and 0.4% in females. Based on these studies in which rats displayed high susceptibility to Zymbal gland tumors, and others (Griswold *et al.*, 1968; Steinhoff, 1974) in which female rats were shown to be highly susceptible to mammary tumors, the rat appears to be more sensitive than the mouse. However, while male rats appear to be more sensitive to liver carcinogenesis by BZD than male mice, female rats were more sensitive than female mice.

In rabbits and dogs, BZD produced urinary bladder cancer (Table IV). A total dose of 1,800 mg/kg produced a 14% incidence in female rabbits at 3.5 years while 30,000 mg/kg produced a 16% incidence in dogs at 8 years.

BZD is an aromatic amine which undergoes biotransformation similar to other compounds of this class, including acetylation, ring and N-hydroxylation and conjugation reactions (Haley, 1975a). Several metabolic pathways were proposed from studies with *in vitro* liver preparations. In the first proposed pathway, BZD was converted to N-acetylBZD, then N,N'-diacetylBZD followed by N-hydroxy-N,N'-diacetylBZD which bound to DNA (Morton *et al.*, 1979). A study using isolated perfused liver identified the metabolites, monoacetylBZD and diacetylBZD, as well as BZD-N-glucuronide and acetylBZD-glucuronide (Lynn *et al.*, 1983). The rate of formation of diacetylBZD was consistent with the metabolic pathway proposed by Morton *et al.*, 1979. The second pathway proposed that N-acetylBZD was hydroxylated to N-hydroxy-N-acetylBZD which was then acetylated to N-hydroxy-N,N'-diacetylBZD and subsequently converted to N-hydroxy-N-acetylBZD (Martin *et al.*, 1982). N-(deoxyguanosin-8-yl)-N'-acetylBZD was identified as a DNA adduct (Morton *et al.*, 1979; Martin *et al.*, 1982). A third route of metabolism demonstrated in renal medullary microsomes involved co-oxidative metabolism (Zenser *et al.*, 1980).

Following activation, BZD was genotoxic in several of the rapid bioassay tests. McCann *et al.* (1975) found BZD to be active as a mutagen in the *Salmonella typhimurium* test in the presence of liver microsomes. Williams (1978) obtained a positive response in the rat hepatocyte primary culture/DNA repair test with BZD and other aminobiphenyl derivatives. BZD also induced DNA repair in rabbit hepatocytes (McQueen *et al.*, 1983b).

Species differences in the rate of formation of BZD metabolites were observed in *in vitro* studies (Morton *et al.*, 1979). The rates of acetylation of both BZD and N-acetylBZD were highest in the hamster, followed by the guinea pig, mouse and rat. These findings, however, do not account for species differences in carcinogenicity (Table IV).

The pharmacokinetics of BZD differ between rodents and larger animals. In rodents a greater proportion was excreted in the bile; the dog and monkey, however, excreted BZD primarily in the urine (Haley, 1982). This difference could account for the occurrence of neoplasms in the bladder of larger animals.

Occupational exposure to BZD was found to increase the risk of bladder

TABLE I
Carcinogenicity of Aflatoxin B_1 in Various Species

Species Strain Sex	Dose and Regimen	Total Dose (mg/kg)	Duration of Exposure	Observation Period	Latent Period	Type of Cancer	Incidence (%)	Reference
Rat								
Fisher Adult male Inbred	Control	0		109 weeks	—	liver	0	Wogan et al., 1974.
	50 ppb[a]	1.42–1.99	71–97 weeks	97 weeks	82 weeks		80	
	100 ppb[a]	2.16–3.51	54–88 weeks	88 weeks	54 weeks		100	
Wistar Adult male Outbred	Control	0		100 weeks	—	liver (kidney)	0 (0)	Epstein et al. 1969
	250 ppb[a]	1.84	21 weeks		106 weeks		67 (23)	
	500 ppb[a]	3.63	21 weeks	89 weeks	89 weeks		72 (28)	
	1000 ppb[a]	7.35	21 weeks	87 weeks	87 weeks		86 (57)	
Mouse C57 B1/6NB	150 ppm[a]	11.5	20 months	20 months	—	liver	0	Wogan, 1976

[a] Administered in diet.
[b] i.p.

TABLE II

Association of Aflatoxin Consumption with Liver Cancer in Humans

Region	Period	Dietary Alfa- ng/kgbw/day[a]	Accumulated dose μg/kg/yr	Hepatoma incidence[b] (Cases/10^5/year)			Reference
				M	F	Total	
Swaziland	1972-73						Peers et al 1976
Highland		7.7	2.8	7.0	1.4		
Midland		13.3	4.9	14.8	2.2		
Lowland		64.7	23.6	26.7	5.6		
Lembombo		23.1	8.4	18.7	0		
Tot. Popul'n		27.2	9.9	16.8	3.1	10.0	
Thailand	1972-73						Shank et al 1972
Singburi		51-55	19-20	5		14.0	
Ratburi		31-48	11-18	2	1	6-(7.6)	
Shongkhla		5-6?	2?			2.0	

[a]Calculated on an average weight of 70 kg.
[b] = crude rate.

cancer in humans and decrease the age of onset of this cancer (Table V). Zavon *et al.* (1973) reported an incidence of over 50% in a group of 25 men who worked in one U.S. BZD plant in 1958. However, this is probably an overestimate because workers with no cancer seemed under-represented. Furthermore, the hygiene in that particular plant may have been deficient, exposing most employees to high levels. The highest levels of contamination were located around filter presses and occurred during shoveling of the product into drums. If reports were accurate, the incidence would be extremely high; this suggested that estimates of exposure based on urine analysis of diazotizable or quinone-reactive material were unrealistic and far too low. A more reasonable estimate of incidence was obtained by Case *et al.* (1954) who analyzed data from 21 British factories for the years 1920 to 1950. It was noted that as many as 5-10% of all men engaged in manufacture (not use) of BZD in the period under study developed cancer or papilloma of the bladder.

On the average, bladder tumors (papillomas or carcinomas) could be diagnosed 16 ± 5 years after the first exposure, although cases appearing as early as two years and as late as 45 years after the first exposures were recorded (Case *et al.*, 1954). In terms of risk, heavy occupational exposure (such as was encountered in the manufacturing process prior to hygienic regulation) increased 20-fold the chance of dying from bladder cancer (10 certified deaths among workers against the 0.54 expected).

The carcinogenic effect of BZD seems to have been dose-related, although absolute doses actually inhaled, absorbed through the skin and/or ingested in chemical plants could only be estimated. For example, a dose response relationship between exposure to BZD and the incidence of bladder tumors was derived from the observation that significantly fewer cases were found in plants with low-risk exposure than in those with heavier exposure (Case *et al.*, 1954). A drop in the occurrence of new cases occurred following semiautomation of an old process which decreased human contact with the carcinogen (Vigilani and Barsotti, 1961). This decreased incidence further suggests a dose-response relationship for BZD.

A factor complicating the analysis of the human carcinogenicity of BZD is the fact that humans display a genetically-determined polymorphism in the rate of acetylation of arylamines including BZD (Glowinski *et al.*, 1978). Metabolism studies with innocuous substrates for acetylation have shown that individuals can be classified as rapid or slow acetylators, with rapid acetylation being the dominant trait (Knight *et al.*, 1959; Evans *et al.*, 1960). A similar polymorphism exists in rabbits (Gordon *et al.*, 1973). It has been proposed that acetylator phenotype could affect susceptibility to the carcinogenicity of aromatic amines (Lower and Bryan, 1976; Lower *et al.*, 1979). In fact, a recent study observed an excess of slow acetylators among bladder cancer patients who were occupationally exposed to aromatic amines (Cartwright *et al.*, 1982). It is noteworthy that the species that mimics the human response, i.e., cancer of the bladder, is the rabbit, which also displays a polymorphism in BZD activation (McQueen *et al.*, 1983b).

Based on the assumption that urinary excretion multiplied by a recovery

TABLE III
Carcinogenicity of Vinyl Chloride in Various Species

Species Strain Sex	Dose and Regimen	Total Dose (mg/kg)	Duration of Exposure	Observation period (week)	Latent Period (week)	Type of Cancer	Incidence (%)	Reference
Rat:								
Sprague-Dawley, both sexes	Control	0	12 months	for life	135 weeks	—	0	Maltoni, 1977
	250 ppm[a]	7,500[b]	12 months	for life	135 weeks	Nephroblastoma; Liver angio-sarcoma; Zymbal gland;	10 / 7 / 26	
	10,000 ppm[a]	320,000	12 months	for life	135 weeks	Liver angio-sarcoma; Brain neuro-blastoma Nephroblastoma	15 / 11 / 8	
Mouse:								
Swiss, both sexes	Control	0	30 months	for life	81 weeks	Lung	5	Maltoni 1977
	250 ppm[a]	48,800	30 months	for life	81 weeks	Lung Mammary Liver angio-sarcoma	55 / 37 / 18	
	2,500 ppm[a]	479,600	30 months	for life	81 weeks	Lung Mammary Liver angio-sarcoma	50 / 30 / 18	
	10,000 ppm[a]	1,920,000	30 months	for life	81 weeks	Lung Mammary Liver angio-sarcoma	58 / 43 / 13	

222

TABLE III (cont.)
Carcinogenicity of Vinyl Chloride in Various Species

Species Strain Sex	Dose and Regimen	Total Dose (mg/kg)	Duration of Exposure	Observation period (week)	Latent Period (week)	Type of Cancer	Incidence (%)	Reference
Golden Hamster:	Control	0	30 w	for life	—	Forestomach	3	Maltoni, 1977
						Skin	3	
	6,000 ppm[a]	305,000	30 w	for life	—	Forestomach	22	
						Skin	6	
						Liver angio-sarcoma	3	
	10,000 ppm[a]	507,000	30 w	for life	—	Forestomach	26	
						Skin	17	

[a]By inhalation
[b]calculated by Barnes, 1976.

factor of 70 equals exposure, the carcinogenic dose for humans has been calculated to be 50 to 200 mg/kg (Vigilani and Barsotti, 1961; Zavon *et al.*, 1973; Meselson *et al.* 1975). However, this estimate has been shown to be unrealistically low since it depends upon the analysis of urinary BZD in workmen. It is now known that only a very small part of the ingested BZD is excreted as such but is present in the urine as diverse metabolites. Because the methods used for measuring exposure to BZD did not consider the fact that BZD can be biotransformed *in vivo* to a variety of metabolites (Lynn *et al.*, 1983) with unknown properties, an estimation of exposure without determination of the presence of most of these metabolites would underestimate exposure. Also, because exposure to low levels of BZD requires a long latent period for cancer development, it was difficult to document the resulting tumor development in relation to an antecedent BZD exposure. Lastly, cigarette smoking, which is also a risk factor for bladder cancer (Wynder and Goldsmith, 1977), may also be additive or even synergistic, but this has not been recorded.

We conclude that the dose of BZD which effectively led to urinary bladder cancer in humans with a latent period of 5-15 years was at least 200 gms. Hygienic conditions in BZD chemical plants prevailing at the time that the surveys were conducted are consistent with this estimate. It is not known whether lower exposures would also lead to cancer in humans after a longer latent period.

Using these figures, humans are calculated to be about as sensitive to BZD as the rabbit, which also displays acetylation polymorphism, and more sensitive than the dog. Rodents are more sensitive than any of these species, but develop liver rather than bladder tumors.

III. Therapeutic Carcinogens

In the study of Williams *et al.* (1978), two carcinogenic drugs, chlornaphazine and diethylstilbestrol were evaluated. In principle, carcinogenic drugs should offer the best possibility for developing data on human dose response effects because of well-defined therapeutic regimens. Even here, however, the evalution was limited because of a lack of information on actual dosages administered. In addition, for certain carcinogenic drugs, the underlying disease condition that necessitated therapy and the use of several drugs further complicated evaluation.

1. Chlornaphazine (CNZ)

CNZ is a nitrogen mustard derivative of 2-naphthylamine. CNZ was originally synthesized at the Chester Beatty Institute in London for use in cancer chemotherapy and was used as a therapeutic agent in Denmark. It is a DNA-reactive carcinogen that has produced cancer in mice in several organs (Boyland *et al.*, 1961, 1964; Shimkin *et al.*, 1966), but studies in other animal species were not available for adequate species comparisons. Its therapeutic use was found to

TABLE IV
Carcinogenicity of Benzidine in Various Species

Species Strain Sex	Dose and Regimen	Total Dose (mg/kg)	Duration of Exposure	Observation period (week)	Latent Period (week)	Type of Cancer	Incidence (%)	Reference
Rat: Sherman, Male	15 mg/wk[a]	2,400	64 weeks	—	—	Heptatoma Zymbal gland Colon adenocacinoma	11 80 6	Spitz et al., 1950
Female	15 mg/wk[b]	2,400	64 weeks	—	—	Hepatoma Zymbal gland Colon adenocarcinoma	0.4 80 0	
Mouse: C57BL/6J X C3Heb/FeJ F$_1$ Male	50 ppm[c]	3,150	84 weeks	84	84 weeks	Liver Harderian gland Lung;	6 18 4	Vesselino-vitch, et al., 1975
	100 ppm[c]	6,250	84 weeks	84	84 weeks	Liver Harderian gland	22 36	
	150 ppm[c]	5,900	39 weeks	84	84 weeks	Liver	70	
Female	50 ppm[c]	5,000	84 weeks	84	84 weeks	Liver Harderian gland Lung	64 6 4	
	150 ppm[c]	7,500	84 weeks	84	84 weeks	Liver	94	
Rabbit: Female	75-150[d] mg/wk[d]	375-3,400	—	44	—	—	0	Spitz et al., 1950
Female	20 mg/wk[b]	1,800	3.5 years	—	3.5 years	Invasive bladder carcinoma	14	Bonser, 1959
Dog: Mixed breed Male	200-300 mg[e] 6 times/week	30,000	5 years	—	8 years	—	0	Spitz et al., 1950
Female	200-300 mg[e] 6 times/wk	30,000	5 years	—	8 years	Bladder carcinoma	16	Spitz et al., 1950

[a] p.o. in oil; [b] p.o. in diet; [c] p.o. daily in diet; [d] s.c. in oil; [e] p.o. capsule.

TABLE V
Urinary Bladder Neoplasms in Men Exposed to Benzidine

Type of Exposure	Duration of Exposure (yrs)	Latent Period Years	Incidence[a]		Reference
			Number	%	
Manufacture	4 to 32 (X = 16)	8 to 32 (X = 15.9)	23/198[a]	12[b]	Scott, 1952
Handling	15 to 27 (X = 27)	15 to 27 (X = 27)	7/86[a]	8[b]	
Manufacture		2 to 45 (16 ± 5)	38/496	5–10	Case et al., 1954
Manufacture 1912 to 1962		4 to 31 (X = 16.6)	17/76[b]	21[c]	Goldwater et al., 1965
Manufacture 1929 to 1960	6 to 28 (X = 13.6)	4 to 31 (X = 16.6)	13/25[c]	50[d]	Zavon et al., 1973

[a]Includes both papillomas and carcinomas.
[b]Incidence not corrected for latent period, hence underestimated.
[c]Incidence not corrected for latent period, date probably incomplete.
[d]Data on tumor-free workers probably incomplete (hence incidence probably overestimated).

TABLE VI

Carcinogenicity of Chlornaphazine in Mice

Species Strain Sex	Dose and Regimen	Total Dose (mg/kg)	Duration of Exposure	Observation period	Type of Cancer	Incidence (%)	Reference
A/J both sexes	0.1ml[a] of 2% polyethylene glycol sol'n 2 × weekly	780	1 year	18 months	Vaginal and cervical carcinoma	46	Boyland et al., 1961
A/J both sexes	0.2ml[b] in 0.5% acacia 3 × weekly	0	4 weeks	39 weeks	lung tumor nodules	0.5	Shimkin et al., 1966
		75				0.5	
		300				0.9	
		1200				2.0	
		4800				3.6	

[a]intravaginal.
[b]i.p.

TABLE VII
Bladder Tumor Distribution Among Three Dose Groups of
Patients Treated with Chlornaphazine[a]

Total Dose			Incidence
g	mg/kg	Number of Tumors	%
< 100	200	3/41	7.3
> 100	1,900	2/12	16.7
> 175	3,500	5/8	62.5

[a]Adapted from Thiede and Christensen (1969).

be associated with a high risk for bladder cancer, which in fact should have been expected since 2-naphthylamine was known at the time to be a bladder carcinogen in animals and humans.

In the mouse, CNZ implanted in the bladder increased the frequency of bladder neoplasms, and intravaginal application induced vaginal and cervical carcinoma (Boyland et al., 1961, 1964). The nature of the exposure made it impossible to estimate the available doses in these experiments. CNZ also considerably increased the incidence and multiplicity of lung tumors in strain A mice (Shimkin et al., 1966). A dose-response effect was observed (Table VI).

CNZ is a nitrogen mustard in which the alkyl group has been replaced by the 2-naphthyl group and therefore it probably functions as a direct acting alkylating agent which does not require metabolism for its carcinogenicity. This may account for the vaginocervical (Boyland et al., 1961) and bladder (Boyland et al., 1964) carcinogenicity of CNZ following direct application. Furthermore, since many other nitrogen mustard derivatives were found to induce pulmonary adenomas in mice (Shimkin et al., 1966), the induction of such neoplasms in mice by CNZ may have resulted from the presence of the alkylating group (Shimkin et al., 1966). The lack of a requirement for metabolism is also supported by the observation that CNZ was directly mutagenic to Salmonella (McCann et al., 1975).

For human exposure, detailed information on the doses of CNZ given therapeutically was readily available. The recorded data revealed that people treated with total doses of more than 200 gms had a high risk for developing urinary bladder cancer within 5-15 years; however, cases of bladder cancer were seen by 5 years and even after as short a latent period as 2 years (Thiede and Christensen, 1969) (Table VII).

Men and women seemed equally sensitive to the carcinogenic effects of CNZ treatment (Videbaek, 1964; Thiede and Christensen, 1969; Laursen, 1970). The age of the individual did not appear to influence the response; however, most of the patients studied were 50 years and older. There were no data on younger individuals.

A number of patients given lower doses failed to develop bladder cancer within the time period of 15 years, but further follow-up histories of these patients were not documented. Therefore, no reliable information on the incidence of cancer following low pharmacological exposure levels was in the literature. Although no conclusion could be drawn from data on low dose administration, it was clear that at the higher dose levels or duration of administration, this drug induced cancer in humans proportional to dose and duration.

The bladder carcinogenicity of CNZ in humans was more likely due to a 2-naphthylamine derivative since 2-naphthylamine but not nitrogen mustard type compounds are known to act as bladder carcinogens in rats, hamster, dogs, monkeys and humans (Arcos and Argus, 1974). The exact mechanism of bladder cancer induction of the 2-naphthylamine derivative is still unclear but as with most carcinogenic arylamines, the N-hydroxylated derivative, 2-naphthylhydroxylamine, was mutagenic without metabolic activation (Belman *et al.*, 1968; McCann *et al.*, 1975).

The sensitivity of humans to CNZ appears to be comparable to that of mice. The reliability of this comparison, however, is tenuous, since in the only relevant animal study (Shimkin *et al.*, 1966), lung neoplasms rather than bladder cancer as in humans were induced. Thus, the mechanisms of tumor induction in humans and the mouse were probably different, and the existing data could not be considered adequate for sound extrapolation. Since the mouse strain used was not sensitive to bladder cancer induction by 2-naphthylamine, this species was not a good model for the relevant human cancer. Thus, although the cumulative carcinogenic dose in mg/kg in the mouse and human were comparable, the probable differences in mechanism suggest that this similarity may have been a coincidental consequence of comparable sensitivity of different organs to different carcinogenic moieties.

2. Diethylstilbestrol (DES)

DES is a synthetic stilbene with an estrogenic potency about ten-fold higher than that of the natural steroid estrogen, estradiol. It was used in agriculture for increasing the feed efficiency of animals for meat production and was also utilized in medicine for various indications requiring estrogen supplementation, including pharmacological use in short courses to suppress lactation and more prolonged treatment to support pregnancies; it was also administered in chemotherapy of prostate cancer. DES produced cancer in several animal species and, in two clinical applications, associated cancers were reported, including vaginal cancer in the female offspring of pregnant women treated with sizable amounts of DES to maintain pregnancy.

DES produced cancer in the mouse (Hall and Moore, 1966; Gass *et al.*, 1974; Highman *et al.*, 1977), rat (Geschickter and Byrnes, 1942), male Syrian golden hamster (Kirkman and Bacon, 1952a; Rustia and Shubik, 1979), dog (Jabara, 1959, 1962) and squirrel monkey (McClure and Graham, 1973). Species differed from one another with respect to the tissues (organs) affected, but most, if not all, tumors involved endocrine glands or hormone-responsive tissues.

DES was carcinogenic in several distinct animal models and, therefore, the animal studies were divided into two groups: (a) chronic exposures and (b) *in utero* and neonatal exposures. Different mechanisms appear to be involved in producing the effects observed under these two sets of conditions.

a) Chronic Exposure: DES induced mammary tumors in the mouse, rat and hamster following long-term exposure (Table VIII). In the mouse, the presence of a mammary tumor virus was required or otherwise mammary tumors were not induced up to a total dose of 774 mg/kg (Highman *et al.*, 1977). Thus, in this situation, the mammary tumor virus may have acted as the "initiating" agent with DES producing a "promoting" effect. Interestingly, the presence of the mammary tumor virus factor also increased the frequency of vaginal adenoses and cervical and endometrial carcinoma (Highman *et al.*, 1977).

Testicular tumors in males and hyperplasia with keratosis of the vaginal mucosa in females were induced in adult mice of specific strains, such as BALB/c, with subcutaneous pellets of 20% DES in cholesterol, but the doses could not be calculated. Certain strains of mice, such as C3H, were resistant, for as yet unknown reasons. The resistant strains exhibited atrophy of the gonads, whereas sensitive strains exhibited hyperactive gonads (Shimkin *et al.*, 1941; Andervont *et al.*, 1960).

Male Syrian golden hamsters typically responded to DES treatment with renal carcinoma in a dose-related fashion (Kirkman and Bacon, 1952a,b). The mechanism of carcinogenesis in this case is unknown, but presumably a hormonal effect induced by DES played a role; the hamster kidney tumor is known to have estrogen receptors (Li *et al.*, 1976) and to be prolactin-sensitive (Hamilton *et al.*, 1975). Hence the mechanism in this excretory organ may be akin to that in the usual endocrine-responsive organs.

In a study designed specifically to compare two species with respect to DES carcinogenicity, a suspension of DES inserted into the vagina induced folliculomas of the ovary in mice and chromophobe adenomas of the pituitary in rats (Volfson, 1974). In other rat studies, mammary neoplasms were induced in animals of both sexes (Geschickter and Byrnes, 1942; Dunning *et al.*, 1947) with subcutaneous injections, or with pellets containing DES in cholesterol.

b) "*In Utero*" and Neonatal Exposures: A single treatment of ICR/JCL mice on day 15 or day 17 of gestation led to significant ovarian cancer development after birth (Nomura and Kanzaki, 1977; Table IX). McLaughlan (1977) administered DES to both sexes of mice transplacentally; following birth, uterine adenocarcinomas developed in the female and noncancerous genital-tract lesions occurred in the males. Exposure of NMRI female mice to DES at 10 days of age produced lesions presumed to be precancerous in the epithelium of the vagina and uterine cervix (Forsberg, 1975).

In hamsters, transplacental DES-treatment led to neoplasms and abnormalities of the genital tissues in both sexes (Rustia and Shubik, 1979). Not only the uterus and cervix were affected in the female hamster offspring but also the ovaries were cystic and lacked corpora lutea. Some evidence of a dose effect was seen in this study, although not enough information was presented to formulate a definitive interpretation of the data.

Napalkov and Anisimov (1979) demonstrated a tumor incidence in the

TABLE VIII

Carcinogenicity of Diethylstilbestrol in Adults of Various Species

Species Strain Sex	Dose and Regimen	Total Dose (mg/kg)	Duration of Exposure	Observation period	Latent Period	Type of Cancer	Incidence (%)	Reference
Rat: Adult albino	Control	0	—	92–222 days	—		0	Geschickter and Byrnes, 1942
both sexes	10μg/day[a]	36.8–88.8	104–222 days	92–222 days	92–222 days		50 (M) 88 (F)	
Mouse: Adult female	Control	0	—	52–102 weeks	—		0	Highman, Norvell and Shellenbergee, 1977
C3H/HeJ[b]	100 ppb[c]	7.58–14.88	52–102 weeks		52–102 weeks to sacrifice	Mammary Uterus, cervix	8 1	
	500 ppb[c]	37.92–74.38				Mammary Cervix	7 2	
C3Heb/FeJ[d]	Control	0		52–93 weeks			0	
	100 ppb[c]	7.58–13.50	52–93 weeks		52–93 weeks to sacrifice	Cervix, vagina	1	
	500 ppb[c]	37.92–67.81				Cervix	1	
Syrian Golden Hamster; adult male	0.6mg[e] on alternate days	45–60	150–199 days		—	Kidney	10	Kirkman and Bacon, 1952
		60–75	200–249 days		—		66	
		75–180	250–599 days		—		95–100	

[a] By injection in oil
[b] High-titer to mouse mammary tumor virus (MTV) factor
[c] Dissolved in corn oil and added to diet.
[d] Low-titer to MTV factor.
[e] By s.c. injection in oil or s.c. pellet.

TABLE IX

Carcinogenicity of Diethylstilbestrol in the Fetuses of Various Species

Species Strain Sex	Dose and Regimen	Total Dose (mg/kg)	Duration of Exposure	Observation period	Latent Period (week)	Type of Cancer	Incidence (%)	Reference
Hamster: Syrian Golden 1 × 20 mg/kg[a]		20	1–2 days	for life	—	—	0	Rustia and Shubik, 1979
Fetus, female	1 × 40 mg/kg	40			22–61 weeks	Cervix, vagina	28	
	2 × 40 mg/kg	80			26–55 weeks	Cervix, vagina, uterus	50	
Mouse: ICR/JCL Fetus, both sexes	d15 of gest.[b] or d17 of gest.	10 to mother	single treatment	12 mo. after birth	—	Ovarian (24% lung)	18	Nomura and Kanzaki, 1977
						Ovarian (17% lung)	40	
	control					Ovarian (9% lung)	1.3	
CD-1 Fetus both sexes	0.01 μg/kg/day[c] on d9–16 of gestation.	0.00008 to mother	8 days	6–15 mo. after birth		Uterine adenocarcinoma, epidermoid tumors of cervix and vagina.	10	McLachlan, 1977

[a] By gavage during 14th or 15th day of gestation.
[b] By s.c. injection in water.
[c] By s.c. in corn oil.

offspring of rats treated with DES during gestation that was 3 times higher than in controls. Tumors of the ovary and the corpus uteri were found only in the experimental group; this increase in tumor incidence in the female offspring might depend on hormone-metabolic changes induced by alteration of the hypothalamus-directed sexual differentiation during the perinatal period.

In studies of *in utero* and neonatal exposure, the mouse appeared to be more sensitive than the hamster (Table IX), but the mouse data were not complete.

The mode of action of DES as a carcinogen is controversial. Metzler (1981) suggested that DES could be activated to a reactive species. However, evidence of genotoxicity of DES has not been clear (Upton *et al.*, 1983). Thus at present, it seems likely that the hormonal action of DES is the main factor in its oncogenicity, both in chronic studies and *in utero*.

In the chronic studies, DES, through its estrogenic effects, or interactions with the endocrine system, including the pituitary gland, probably created a hormonal stimulus that enhanced or promoted tumor development by pre-existing neoplastic cells, such as those transformed by the mammary tumor virus. This concept was supported by the finding that natural estrogens, including estradiol, exerted a similar effect (Highman *et al.*, 1977). Chronic exposure studies have demonstrated tumor production in other endocrine-sensitive organs as well, indicating that in these organs hormonal imbalance plays an important role in DES carcinogenesis. Restriction of DES carcinogenicity to endocrine-sensitive tissues supports the concept of action through the potent hormonal effects of DES rather than DNA-reactive which could have affected other sites.

The carcinogenic effects of *in utero* and neonatal exposure to DES also appeared to be related to its hormonal action. Under these conditions the production of urogenital anomalies was a consistent occurrence. Altered development of the vaginal and cervical epithelium was particularly prevalent following DES exposure, and sequential studies of the fate of this abnormal epithelium in mice suggested that it was the site of origin of cancers. Thus, one aspect of the carcinogenicity of DES under these conditions appeared to include a teratogenic action. Furthermore, the presence of DES *in utero* may have produced another kind of developmental effect known as imprinting (Einarsson, 1973, Lucier, 1978). Agents that affect the hypothalamo-pituitary axis can produce a permanent alteration in the function of this system. With sexual development, excessive estrogen production can occur at puberty resulting in stimulation of target organs (Forsberg, 1976). Rustia and Shubik (1979) demonstrated that neonatal DES sensitizes hamsters to mammary cancer induction by 7,12-dimethylbenz(a)anthracene in this manner. If the production of developmental abnormalities is contributory to transplacental carcinogenesis by DES, then species differences in response must be related to the state of differentiation of the urogenital and endocrine systems at the time of exposure.

In the human, DES has been associated with an increased risk of clear cell adenocarcinoma of the vagina and/or cervix at puberty in daughters of women treated during pregnancy with DES or the related dienestrol during the first 17 weeks of gestation (Herbst *et al.*, 1971; Greenwald *et al.*, 1971; Vooijs *et al.*, 1973). There is some indication that later in the lives of transplacentally-exposed persons, invasive squamous carcinoma of the cervix may occur with increased incidence. Vaginal adenosis, found in the majority of women with intrauterine exposure and in all cancer cases, has been suspected to be a precursor of the clear-cell adenocarcinoma (Herbst *et al.*, 1975). Males born from estrogen-supported pregnancies have been reported to have lowered semen quality, epididymal cysts, and hypotrophic testes, but an increased cancer incidence has not been found thus far (McMartin *et al.*, 1978). Cancer and anomalies have been associated with other estrogens (MacMahon, 1973), again pointing to a hormonal rather than genotoxic action for DES.

Whereas in laboratory animals, chronic feeding of large doses of DES increased the incidence of tumors in hormone-responsive organs, neoplasms as a result of chronic exposure were not definitively demonstrated in humans (McMartin *et al.*, 1978).

The finding of vaginal adenosis in females exposed to DES or other estrogens *in utero* together with the observation that clear-cell adenocarcinomas of the vagina and/or uterus were almost always accompanied by adenosis (Herbst *et al.*, 1975) indicates that the carcinogenic process in humans may be related, at least in part, to DES teratogenicity, as in the animal studies. Moreover, the appearance of the neoplasms at puberty suggested a role for a developmental alteration of the endocrine system.

The available data on dose response in humans are inadequate for the demonstration of dose dependence, and the effective dose of DES leading to cancer in humans is unknown (Table X). Nonetheless, in offspring of patients treated in the midwest of the United States, especially at the Mayo Clinic in Rochester, Minnesota, where lower daily doses of DES were prescribed, four cases of squamous-cell carcinoma *in situ* of the cervix were recorded among a total of 404 girls, aged 13 to 29 (average 22 years) whose mothers were treated during the first trimester; however, no cases of vaginal or cervical cancer were found (Lanier *et al.*, 1973). On the other hand, in the Atlantic states, doses were progressively increased to as much as 125 mg DES per day and cancer was produced (Table X). It is clear that a critical review of the Mayo Clinic data compared to those of Herbst, Greenweld, and of Vooijs indicate a much higher risk of vaginal cancer with high doses of DES, with a hint, but not proof, of a threshold dose. These limited data suggest that animals are more sensitive than humans.

The most likely explanation for the production of cancer in female offspring is that transplacental application of substantial amounts of DES caused abnormal differentiation and development of the female genital tract tissue, resulting in tissue that was more susceptible to cancer development (Mattingly and Stafl, 1976). Robboy *et al.* (1982) recently described an *in vivo* model for the study of human uterovaginal development that permits study of DES effects. Intact reproductive tracts from human embryos and fetuses 5.0 to 17.7 weeks of age obtained after dilation and curettage were grown for four weeks in athymic mice, both untreated and implanted with a DES pellet. Specimens exposed to DES exhibited anomalies, many of which mimicked those observed clinically in young women exposed prenatally to DES. Since most DES-associated clear-

TABLE X

Maternal Dose and Age of Daughter at Diagnosis in 27 Clear-Cell Adenocarcinoma Patients with Confirmed Prenatal Exposure to DES or other Nonsteroidal Synthetic Estrogens

| Total Dose Before 18 Weeks | | Age of Diagnosis | Status | | References |
mg	mg/kg (maternal)		At Diagnosis	Last Known	
375	6.3	18			Hill, 1973
630–735	10.5–12.3	15			Noller et al., 1974
750	12.5	17			Hill, 1973
700–1,400	11.7–23.3	?			Gilson et al., 1973
1,125	18.8	18			Greenwald et al., 1973
1,225	20.4	?			Sherman et al., 1974
1,225	20.4	?			Sherman et al., 1974
1,260	21.0	19			Bivens and Zimmerman, 1974
1,350	22.5	18			Greenwald et al., 1971
1,225–1,750	20.4–29.2	7			Noller et al., 1974
875–2,100	14.6–35.0	19			Fetherston et al., 1972
1,750	29.2	16			Kantor et al., 1973
875–2,600	14.6–43.3	20			Herbst et al., 1971
875–2,600	14.6–43.3	16			Herbst et al., 1971
875–2,600	14.6–43.3	18			Herbst et al., 1971
875–2,600	14.6–43.3	16	s	1	Herbst et al., 1971
875–2,600	14.6–43.3	16	s	1	Herbst et al., 1971
875–2,600	14.6–43.3	19	s	1	Herbst et al., 1971
875–2,600	14.6–43.3	22	s	1	Herbst et al., 1971
2,600	43.3	16	a	1	Hill, 1973
2,900	48.3	17	s	1	Greenwald et al., 1971
3,200	53.3	15	s	d	Greenwald et al., 1971
3,200	53.3	15	s	d	Greenwald et al., 1971
6,300	105.0	14	s		Kantor et al., 1973
7,900	131.7	11	a	d	Voojis et al., 1973
10,500	175.0	18	s	d	Voojis et al., 1973
12,000	200.0	18	s	1	Williams and Schweitzer, 1971

[a] Doses were obtained by subtracting from total reported dose the amount received after week 18 of gestation.

s = Symptomatic; a = Asymptomatic; d = Dead; 1 = Living; ? = Information not given.

TABLE XI
Species to Species Comparison of Carcinogenicity

| Carcinogen | Species Comparison | | Associated Neoplasms in Humans | Animal Response comparable to Human |
	Sensitive	Resistant		
Aflatoxin B₁	Rat	Mouse	Liver	Rat
Vinyl Chloride	Mouse	Hamster	Liver	Mouse
				also Brain and Lung
Dimethylnitrosamine	All	None	—	—
Chlornaphazine	Mouse	Unknown[a]	Bladder	None
Benzidine	Rat	Unknown[a]	Bladder	Rabbit
Diethylstilbestrol	Neonatal Mouse	None	Vagina and Cervix	Neonatal Mouse

[a]For mechanistic reasons, we suggest that the guinea pig would be resistant, but it has not been tested.

cell adenocarcinomas in humans were diagnosed at puberty, hormones were suspected to trigger the growth of the abnormal tissue; however, it is not known what caused the malignant transformation. Studies in mice suggested that a virus, such as the *herpes simplex* virus, might be an analog for the mammary tumor virus virus in mice and could be necessary for the development of cervical and vaginal cancer in humans (Highman *et al.*, 1977); however, there are no data on the incidence of this virus in pubescent girls exposed to DES *in utero* who developed vaginal lesions.

Thus, it is difficult to compare the sensitivity of the human and mouse fetuses on the basis of existing studies because of differences in experimental design and exposure conditions. Furthermore, it must be emphasized that reliable dose response data were not available for humans even though numerous case reports exist. Therefore, any attempt at quantitative extrapolation of the animal data to the human would not be appropriate.

In consideration of the postulated difference in mechanism for tumor development between chronic and *in utero*/neonatal exposures, only the latter could be considered to be appropriate models for transplacental human carcinogenicity. Recent data in mice and hamsters appear promising for human extrapolation, but because of a paucity of retrospective, accurate data on dosages used, the degree of human sensitivity is still not known. It may be calculated that the 27 cases in humans with documented dosages received an average total of about 46 mg/kg by week 17. In order to properly establish human sensitivity, precise knowledge of how many female offspring had mothers who received doses of that order is required. With this information (i.e. the denominator) the percentage of cases treated identically that developed cancer could be established; however, such information was not available and therefore we used the apparent minimum effective dose (6.3 mg/kg) and the average incidence (0.14%) for our comparison. With such data, mice and hamsters exposed *in utero* appeared to be more sensitive than humans, but since the human data are inadequate, the apparent degree of difference cannot be specified.

C. CONCLUSIONS

Comparison of the carcinogenicity of five chemicals in several species revealed distinct differences in responses (Table XI). For example, the environmental carcinogen aflatoxin B_1 produced liver cancer in several species, probably including humans. However, although a dietary level of parts per million was sufficient for neoplasm development in rats, mice were resistant to even the highest doses. In contrast, with an occupational carcinogen, the mouse was slightly more sensitive than the rat to vinyl chloride in the induction of hepatic angiosarcomas, the same neoplasm associated with exposure to the carcinogen in humans.

With benzidine, another occupational carcinogen, bladder cancer was produced in dogs, rabbits and humans. Benzidine induced mainly liver cancer in mice, rats and hamsters; it was also a potent mammary carcinogen in female rats. Thus, rodents were an inappropriate model for the human carcinogenicity of this agent, in respect to target organ affected. Moreover, the human genetic polymorphism of acetylation, a reaction critical to the activation of benzidine, is inherent only in the rabbit.

The drug chlornaphazine produced pulmonary adenomas in mice, but adequate data were not available for other animal species. Treatment of humans with chlornaphazine produced urinary bladder cancer, demonstrating a difference between the rodent and human response, which may, however, be due to insufficient testing in other laboratory animal species such as rats or hamsters.

The synthetic estrogenic drug diethylstilbestrol was the only carcinogen studied that was not clearly DNA-reactive. In humans, diethylstilbestrol caused the development of reproductive organ cancers in the female children of mothers treated with large doses during pregnancy. Many animal models developed similar tumors not only as a result of intra-uterine exposure but also, unlike humans, following chronic treatment. Animals appeared to be more sensitive to diethylstilbestrol than humans, but factors such as developmental status in the case of transplacental exposure and the presence of mammary tumor virus in mice used for chronic studies complicated comparisons. Of course, the role of any virus in human cancer causation is unknown at this time.

In some, but not all cases, species differences in carcinogenicity could be accounted for in terms of known factors and mechanisms affecting tumor production. For example, metabolic activation and detoxification of aflatoxin B_1 were found to differ between sensitive and resistant species. In humans, however, another factor, endemic hepatitis B, may have augmented the development of neoplasms and had to be considered in the assessment of hepatocarcinogenicity of aflatoxin B_1. For the quantification of vinyl chloride carcinogenicity, it was found that the saturation levels of absorption and metabolism of the chemical had to be taken into account.

In comparing animal responses to human carcinogenicity data, for aflatoxin B_1, vinyl chloride, benzidine and diethylstilbestrol, at least one animal system (although different in each case) was found to be as responsive as or more responsive than the most sensitive human groups (Table XI). For chlornaphazine, there was also a more responsive animal, but the nature of the carcinogenic effect was different from that seen in humans, and therefore, the reliability of comparison was uncertain. Thus, from multispecies animal testing, the most sensitive species can be taken as the upper limit of human sensitivity. An important qualification, however, is that with the exception of diethylstilbestrol, all of the carcinogens evaluated were DNA-reactive. For genotoxic carcinogens, the finding of comparable sensitivity between at least one animal species and humans supports the suggestion that such carcinogens represent definite hazards to humans (Weisburger and Williams, 1981).

As an example of a carcinogen that does not damage DNA but rather operates by another mechanism, (Weisburger and Williams, 1980), the findings with diethylstilbestrol clearly show that such agents can cause cancer in humans. However, this study does not permit general conclusions regarding extrapolation to humans of effects in animal models. The nature of the hazard posed by these agents may be qualitatively different from DNA-reactive carcinogens (Weisburger and Williams, 1981; 1983b). At present, only a few epigenetic carcinogens, including diethylstilbestrol, have been associated with cancer in humans (International Agency for Research on Cancer, 1983). This situation has often been attributed to the difficulty of identifying carcinogenicity in humans because of a long latent period. However, this study, it was possible to identify the minimum latent period in humans for several carcinogens, these were as follows: chlornaphazine, 2 years; vinyl chloride, 4 years; and benzidine, 2 years. These observations show that in situations where significant exposures have occured, cancer is manifested within a sufficiently short time to incriminate the causative agent. The same seems to be true for liver tumors associated with the use of oral contraceptives (International Agency for Research on Cancer, 1982). Therefore, the absence of human carcinogenicity in situations of intense exposure to epigenetic carcinogens such as phenobarbital and saccharin seems to represent a qualitatively different response of humans. At present, limitations in the human data on diethylstilbestrol do not permit quantitative extrapolation of animal data to humans.

This analysis leads to some definite recommendations on the process of risk extrapolation. There is, apparently, no single animal species that reliably predicts cancer risk for humans. Furthermore, each type or class of chemicals, due to its pathways of biotransformation or reactivity, displays a selectively of specificity in its effects. Thus, in order to formulate a picture of any potential cancer risks in humans, it is necessary to acquire fundamental information in several animal species. In the light of current knowledge of the mechanisms of carcinogenesis, it is also evident that data derived from biochemical studies and a battery of rapid *in vitro* tests for genotoxicity which reflect the presence or absence of DNA reactivity are essential for risk assessment and extrapolation (Williams and Weisburger, 1981; Weisburger and Williams, 1983a).

The species *homo sapiens* is not uniform and each individual probably differs in sensitivity as a result of genetic and developmental factors which are further modified by environmental agents such as diet and smoking (Williams *et al.*, 1982). For example, given equal exposure to cigarette smoke, not all individuals develop lung cancer. For exposure to an occupational carcinogen, a Japanese workman on his typical dietary regimen may not be at the same risk as his U.S. or British counterpart on a different diet. Specifically, it is known that asbestos is considerably more dangerous as a lung carcinogen to a smoker than to a nonsmoker (Selikoff *et al.*, 1968; Saracci, 1977). These factors make estimations of human risk imprecise and support the suggestion that DNA-reactive carcinogens should be treated as qualitative hazards (Weisburger and Williams, 1981).

The process of risk analysis is clearly complex, but with systematic acquisition of data utilizing contemporary knowledge of the relevant mechanisms, it should be possible to provide protection for the public from real hazards and thereby contribute to the prevention of cancer.

REFERENCES

Albert, R.E. and Altshuler, B. Considerations relating to the formulation of limits for unavoidable population exposures to environmental carcinogens. In: Radionuclide

Carcinogenesis. C.L. Sander, R.H. Busch, and J.R. Ballou (eds.), pp. 233–253. U.S. Atomic Energy Commission, CONF-720505, NTIS, Springfield, Va. (1973).

Anders, M.W. Mechanisms of haloalkene and haloalkene biotransformation. In: Drug Metabolism and Distribution (Laruble, J.W., ed.), pp. 95–98. Elsevier Biomedical Press, Amsterdam (1983).

Andervont, H.B., Shimkin, M.B. and Canter, H.Y. Susceptibility of seven inbred strains of the F_1 hybrids to estrogen-induced testicular tumors and occurrence of spontaneous testicular tumors in strain BALB/c mice. J. Natl. Cancer Inst. **25**, 1069–1081 (1960).

Arcos, J.C. and Argus, M.F. Chemical Induction of Cancer, Vol. II-B, Academic Press, New York (1974).

Barnes, A.W. Vinyl chloride and the production of PVC. Proc. R. Soc. Med. **69**, 277–281 (1976).

Bartsch, H., Malaveille, C. and Montesano, R. Tissue mediated mutagenicity of vinylidene chloride and 2-chlorobutadiene in Salmonella 1 typhimurium. Nature **255**, 641–643 (1975).

Belman, S., Troll, W., Teebor, G., Werner, B., Hesser, J.E., Millman, I., Saimot, G., and Payet, M. The carcinogenic and mutagenic properties of N-hydroxy-aminonaphthalines. Cancer Res. **28**, 535 (1968).

Bivens, M.D. and Zimmerman, E.A. Clear-cell adenoma of the vagina. Rocky Mountain Med. J. **71**, 512 (1974).

Blumberg, B.S., Larouze, B., London, W.T. et al. The relation of infection with the hepatitis B agent to primary hepatic carcinoma. Am. J. Pathol. **81**, 669–682 (1975).

Bolt, H.M., Kappus, H., Buchter, A., and Bolt, W. Disposition of (1,2-14C) vinyl chloride in the rat. Arch. Toxicol. **35**, 153–162 (1976).

Bonser, G.M., Clayson, D.B. and Jull, J.W. The induction of tumors in the subcutaneous tissues liver and intestine in the mouse and certain dye stuffs and their intermediates. Brit. J. Cancer **10**, 653–667 (1956).

Boyland, E., Busby, E.R., Dukes, C.E., Grover, P.L. and Manson, D. Further experiment on implantation of materials into the urinary bladder of mice. Brit. J. of Cancer **18**, 575–581 (1964).

Boyland, E., Charles, R.T. and Gowing, N.F.C. The induction of tumors in mice by intravaginal application of chemical compounds. Brit. J. Cancer **15**, 252–256 (1961).

Boyland, E., Harris, J. and Horning, E.J. The induction of carcinoma of the bladder in rats with acetamidofluorene. Brit. J. Cancer **8**, 647 (1954).

Bryan, W.R. and Shimkin, M.B. Quantitative analysis of dose-response data obtained with three carcinogenic hydrocarbons in strain C3H male mice. J. Natl. Cancer Inst. **3**, 503 (1943).

Butler, W.H. and Barnes, J.M. Carcinoma of the glandular stomach in rats given diets containing aflatoxin. Nature (Lond.) **209**, 90 (1966).

Carnaghan, R.B.A. Hepatic tumors in ducks fed a low level of toxic ground nut meal. Nature (Lond.) **208**, 308 (1965).

Cartwright, R.A., Glasnan, R.W., Rogers, H.J., Ahmad, R.A. Barham-Hall, D., Higgins, E., Kahn, M.A. Role of N-acetyltransferase phenotypes in bladder carcinogenesis: a pharmacogenetic epidemiological approach to bladder cancer. Lancet **2**: 842–845 (1982).

Case, R.A.M., Hosker, M.E., McDonald, D.B. and Pearson, J.T. Tumors of the urinary bladder in workmen engaged in the manufacture and use of certain dyestuff intermediates in the British chemical industry. Brit. J. Indust. Med. **11**, 75–104 (1954).

Cornfield, J.: Carcinogenic risk assessment. Science **198**, 693 (1977).

Creech, J.L. and Johnson, M.N. Angiosarcoma of the liver in the manufacture of polyvinyl chloride. J. Occup. Med. **16**, 150 (1974).

Crump, K.S., Hoel, D.G., Langley, C. and Peto, R. Fundamental carcinogenic processes and their implications for low dose risk assessment. Cancer Res. **36**, 2973–2979 (1976).

Druckrey, H. Quantitative aspects in chemical carcinogenesis. In: Potential Carcinogenic Hazards from Drugs, Evaluation of Risks. R. Truhaut (ed.), pp. 60– . UICC Monograph Series, No. 7. Springer Verlag, Berlin (1967). Dunning, W.F., Curtis, M.R. and Segaloff, A. Strain differences in response to diethylstilbestrol and the induction of mammary gland and bladder cancer in the rat. Cancer Res. **7**, 511–521 (1947).

Ehrenberg, L., Brookes, P., Druckrey, H., Lagerlof, B., Litwin, J. and Williams, G.M. The relation of cancer induction and genetic damage. In: Evaluation of Genetic Risks of Environmental Chemicals. C. Ramel (ed.). Ambio Special Report No. 3, pp. 15–16 (1973).

Einarsson, K., Gustafsson, J., Stenberg, A. Neonatal imprinting of liver microsomal hydroxylation and reduction of steroids. J. Biol. Chem. **248**: 4978–4997 (1973).

Epstein, S.M., Bartus, B. and Farber, C.M. Renal epithelial neoplasms induced in male Wistar rats by oral aflatoxin B_1. Cancer Res. **29**, 1045–1050 (1969).

Essigmann, J.M., Croy, R.G., Bennett, R.A. and Wogan, G.N. Metabolic activation of Aflatoxin B_1: Patterns of DNA adduct formation removal and excretion in relation to carcinogenesis. Drug Metabolism Reviews **13**, 581–602 (1982).

Evans, D.A.P., Manley, K.A. and McKusick, V.A. Genetic control of isoniazid metabolism in man. Brit. Med. J. **2**, 486–491 (1960).

Fetherston, W.C., Meyers, A. and Speckhard, M.E. Adenocarcinoma of the vagina in young women: The stilbestrol-adenosis adenocarcinoma of the vagina syndrome. Wis. Med. J. **71**, 87 (1972).

Forsberg, J.G. Late effects in the vaginal and cervical epithelia after injections of diethylstilbestrol into neonatal mice. Am. J. Obstet. Gynecol. **121**, 101–104 (1975).

Forsberg, J.G. Animal model: Estrogen-induced adenosis of vagina and cervix in mice. Am. J. Path. **84**, 669 (1976).

Fox, A.J. and Collier, P.F. Mortality experience of workers exposed to vinyl chloride monomer in the manufacture of polyvinylchloride in Great Britain. Brit. J. Ind. Med. **34**, 1–10 (1977).

Garner, R.C. and Wright, C.M. Binding of ^{14}C-aflatoxin B_1 to cellular macromolecules in the rat and hamster. Chem. Biol. Interactions **11**, 123–131 (1975).

Gass, G.H., Brown, J. and Okey, A.B. Carcinogenic effects of oral diethylstilbestrol on C3H male mice with and without the mammary tumor virus. J. Natl. Cancer Inst. **53**, 1369–1370 (1974).

Geschickter, C.F. and Byrnes, E.W. Factors influencing the development and time of appearance of mammary cancer in the rat in response to estrogen. Arch. Pathol. **33**, 334–356 (1942).

Gilson, M.D., Dibona, D.D. and Korab, D.R. Clear-cell adenocarcinoma in young females. Obstret. Gynecol. **41**, 494 (1973).

Glowinski, I.B., Radtke, H.E. and Weber, W.W. Genetic Variation in N-acetylation of carcinogenic arylamines by human and rat liver. Mol. Pharmacol. **14**, 940–949 (1978).

Goldwater, L.S., Rosso, A.J. and Kleinfeld, M. Bladder tumors in a coal tar dye plant. Arch. Environ. Health **11**, 814 (1965).

Gordon, G.R., Sharizadeh, A.G. and Peters, J.H. Polymorphic acetylation of drugs in rabbits. Xenobiotica **3**, 133–150 (1973).

241

Greenwald, P., Barlow, J.J., Nasca, P.C. and Burnett, W.S. Vaginal cancer after maternal treatment with synthetic estrogens. N. Eng. J. Med. **285**, 390–392 (1971).

Greenwald, P., Nasca, P.C., Burnett, W.S. Prenatal stilbestrol experience of mothers of young cancer patients. Cancer **31**, 568 (1973).

Griswold, D.P., Casey, A.E., Weisburger, E.K. and Weisburger, J.H. The carcinogenicity of multiple intra-gastric doses of aromatic and heterocyclic nitro or amino derivatives in young female Sprague-Dawley rats. Cancer Res. **28**, 924–933 (1968).

Guess, H., Crump, K. and Peto, R. Uncertainty estimated for low-dose-rate extrapolations of animal carcinogenicity data. Cancer Res. **37**, 3475–3483 (1977).

Guyton, A.C. Measurement of the respiratory volumes of laboratory animals. Am. J. Physiol. **150**, 70–77 (1947).

Haley, T.J. Benzidine revisited: A review of the literature and problems associated with the use of benzidine and its congers. Clin. Toxicol. **8**, 13–42 (1975a).

Haley, T.J. Vinyl Chloride: How Many Unknown Problems. J. Toxicol. Env. Health. **1**, 47–73 (1975b).

Hall, W.T. and Moore, D.H. Effects of estrogenic hormones on the mammary tissue of agent-free and agent-bearing male mice. J. Natl. Cancer Inst. **36**, 184–185 (1966).

Hamilton, J.M., Flaks, A., Saliya, P.G. et al. Hormonally induced renal neoplasia in the male Syrian hamster and the inhibitory effect of 2-bromo-^{a}-ergocryptine methane sulfonate. J. Natl. Cancer Inst. **54**, 1385 (1975).

Hefner, R.E., Watanata, P.G., Gehrings, P.J. Preliminary studies of the fate of inhaled vinyl chloride monomer in rats. Ann. N.Y. Acad. Sci. **246**, 135–148 (1975).

Herbst, A.L., Poskanzer, D.C., Robboy, S.J., Friedlander, L. and Scully, R.E. Prenatal exposure to stilbestrol. A prospective comparison of exposed female offspring with unexposed controls. N. Eng. J. Med. **292**, 334–339 (1975).

Herbst, A.L., Ulfelder, H. and Poskanzer, D.C. Adenocarcinoma of the vagina: Association of maternal stilbestrol therapy with tumor appearance in young women. N. Eng. J. Med. **28**, 878–881 (1971).

Higginson, J. Rethinking the environmental causation of human cancer. Fd. Cosmet. Toxicol. **19**, 533–538 (1981).

Highman, B., Norvell, M.J. and Shellenberger, T.E. Pathologic changes in female C3H mice continuously fed diets containing diethylstilbestrol or 17^b-estradiol. J. Environ. Path. Toxicol. **1**, 1–30 (1977).

Hill, E.C. Clear-cell carcinoma of the cervix and vagina in young women: A report of six cases with association of maternal stilbestrol therapy and adenosis of the vagina. Am. J. Obstet. Gynecol. **116**, 470 (1973).

Hoel, D.G. and Rall, D.P. (eds.) Conference in Pinehurst, North Carolina, on the extrapolation of carcinogenesis data. Environ. Health Perspect. **22**: 127 (1978).

Hoel, D.G., Rall, D.P., Gaylor, D.W., Kirschstein, R.L., Saffiotti, U., Schneiderman, M.A. Estimation of risks of irreversible delayed toxicity. J. Toxicol. Environ. Health Perspect. **1**, 133–151 (1975).

Holmberg, B., Kronevi, T. and Wineill, M. The pathology of vinylchloride exposed mice. Acta. Vet. Scand. **17**, 328–342 (1976).

Hsieh, D.P.H.G.., Wong, J.J., Wong, Z.A., Michas, C. and B.H. Ruebner. Hepatic transformation of aflatoxin and its carcinogenicity. Cold Spring Harbor Conferences on Cell Proliferation. Origins of Human Cancer, Book B: Mechanisms of Carcinogenesis. (H.H. Hiatt, J.D. Watson, J.A. Winsten, eds.) Cold Spring Harbor Laboratory, pp. 697–708 (1977).

International Agency for Research on Cancer Monograph program on the evaluation of the carcinogenic risk of chemicals to humans, Chemicals, industrial processes and industries associated with cancer in humans, Vols. 1–29, International Agency for Research on Cancer, Lyon (1983).

Innovation in Cancer Risk Assessment (ED_{01} Study). Proceedings of a symposium sponsored by National Center for Toxicological Research, U.S. Food and Drug Administration and the American College of Toxicology. J.A. Staffa and M.A. Mehlman (eds.), Pathotox. Publishers Inc., Park Forest South, Il (1979).

Jabara, A.G. Canine ovarian tumors following stilbestrol administration. Austral. J. Exp. Biol. **37**, 549–565 (1959).

Jabara, A.G. Induction of canine ovarian tumors by diethylstilbestrol and progesterone. Austral. J. Exp. Biol. **40**, 139–152 (1962).

Kamden, L., Siest, G. and Magdalon, J. Differential toxicity of Aflatoxin B_1 in male and female rats: relationship with hepatic drug-metabolizing enzymes. Biochem. Pharm. **31**, 3057–3062 (1982).

Kirkman, H. and Bacon, R.L. Estrogen-induced tumors of the kidney. 1. Incidence of renal tumors in intact and gonadectomized male golden hamsters treated with diethylstilbestrol. J. Natl. Cancer Inst. **13**, 745–756 (1952a).

Kirkman, H. and Bacon, R.L. Estrogen induced tumors of the kidney. II. Effect of dose, administration, type of estrogenic and age on the induction of renal tumors in intact male golden hamster. J. Natl. Cancer Inst. **13**, 757–765 (1952b).

Knight, R.A., Selin, M.J. and Harris, H.W. Genetic factors influencing isoniazid blood levels in humans. Trans. Conf. Chemother. Tuberac. **18**, 52–60 (1959).

Kolbye, A.C. Jr. Impact on short-term screening tests on regulatory action. In: The Predictive Value of short-term Screening Tests in Carcinogenicity Evaluation. (G.M. Williams, R. Kroes, H.W. Waaijers, K.W. van de Poll, eds.). Elsevier/North Holland and Biomedical Press, Amsterdam, pp. 311–326 (1980).

Kroes, R. Animal data, interpretation, and consequences. In Environmental Carcinogenesis: Occurrence, Risk Evaluation, and Mechanisms. Eds. Emmelot, P., and Kriek, E. Elsevier/North Holland Biomedical Press, Amsterdam, pp. 287–301 (1979).

Lanier, A.P., Noller, K.L., and Decker, D.G. Cancer and stilbesterol. A follow-up of 179 persons exposed to estrogens *in vitro* from 1943–1959. Mayo Clin. Proc. **48**, 793 (1973).

Laursen, B. Cancer of the bladder in patients treated with chlornaphazine. Brit. Med. J. **3**, 684 (1970).

Lee, C.C., Bhandari, J.C., Winston, J.M. et al. Carcinogenicity of vinyl chloride and vinylidene chloride. J. Toxicol. Environ. Health **4**, 15–30 (1978).

Li, J.J., Talby, D.S., Li, S.A. Reception characteristics of specific estrogen binding in the renal adenocarcinoma of the golden hamster. Cancer Res. **36**, 1127–1132 (1976).

Lin, J.J., Lin, C., and Svoboda, D.J. Long-term effects of aflatoxin B_1 and viral hepatitis on marmoset liver. A primary report. Lab. Invest. **30**, 267–278 (1974).

Linsell, A. Carcinogenicity of mycotoxins. In: Environmental Carcinogens: Selected Methods of Analysis, Vol. 5 (Egan, R., Stoloff, L., Scott, P., Castegnaro, M., O'Neill, I.K., Bartsch, H., eds.) International Agency for Research on Cancer, pp. 3–14 (1982).

Linsell, A. and Peers, F.G. Field studies on liver cell cancer. In: Origins of Human Cancer, Book A. (H.H. Hiatt, J.D. Watson, J.A. Winston, eds.) Cold Spring Harbor Lab., p. 549–556. (1977).

Littlefield, N.A., Cueto, C., Davis, A.K. and Medlock, K. Chronic dose-response studies in mice fed 2-AAF. J. Toxicol. Env. Health **1**, 25–37 (1975).

Louria, D.B., Finkel, G., Smith, J.K. and Buse, M. Aflatoxin-induced tumors in mice. Sabouraudia **12**, 371–375 (1974).

Lower, G.M., Hilsoon, T., Nelson, G.E., Wolf, H., Ganskey, T.E. and Bryan, G.T. N-acetyltransferase phenotype and risk in urinary bladder cancer: Approaches in molecular epidemiology. Environ. Health Perspect. **29**, 71–79 (1979).

Lower, G.M. and Bryan, G.T. Enzymatic deacetylation of carcinogenic arylacetamides by tissue microsomes of the dog and other species. J. Toxicol. Environ. Health **1**, 421–432 (1976).

Lucier, G. Differences in metabolic deactivation during development. Delivered at Toxicology Forum in Washington, D.C. February 19, 1978.

Lynn, R.K., Garvie-Gould, C., Milam, D.F., Scott, K.F., Eastman, C.L. and Rodgers, R.M. Metabolism of the human carcinogen benzidine in the isolated perfused rat liver. Drug. Metab. Disposition **11**, 109–114 (1983).

MacMahon, B., Cole, P. and Brown, J. Etiology of human breast cancer. A review. J. Natl. Cancer Inst. **50**, 21–42 (1973).

Maltoni, C. Vinyl chloride carcinogenicity: An experimental model for carcinogenesis studies. In: Origins of Human Cancer. (H.H. Hiatt, J.D. Watson, J.A. Winsten, eds.) Cold Spring Harbor Laboratory. 119–146 (1977).

Maltoni, C., and Lefemine, G. Carcinogenicity bioassays of vinyl chloride: current results. Ann. N.Y. Acad. Sci. **246**, 195–219 (1975).

Mantel, N. and Schneidermann, M.A. Estimating "safe" levels, a hazardous undertaking. Cancer Res. **35**, 1379 (1975).

Martin, C.N., Beland, F.A., Roth, R.W. and Kadlubar, F.F. Covalent binding of benzidine and N-acetylbenzidine to DNA at the C-8 atom of deoxyguanosine *in vivo* and *in vitro*. Cancer Res. **42**, 2678–2696 (1982).

Mattingly, R.F. and Stafl, A. Cancer risk in diethylstilbestrol-exposed offspring. Am. J. Ob. Gyn. **126**, 543–548 (1976).

McCann, J., Choi, E., Yamasaki, E. and Ames, B. Detection of carcinogens as mutagens in the Salmonella/microsome test: Assay of 300 chemicals. Proc. Natl. Acad. Sci. USA, **72**, 5135–5139 (1975).

McClure, H.M. and Graham, C.E. Malignant uterine mesotheliomas in squirrel monkeys following diethylstilbestrol administration. Lab. Animal Sci. **23**, 493–498 (1973).

McLachlan, J.A. Prenatal exposure to diethylstilbestrol in mice: Toxicological studies. J. Toxicol. Environ. Health **2**, 527–537 (1977).

McMartin, K.E., Kennedy, K.A., Greenspan, P., Alam, S.N., Greiner, P. and Yam, J. Diethylstilbestrol: A review of its toxicity and use as a growth promotant in food-producing animals. J. Environ. Path. Toxicol. **1**, 279–313 (1978).

McQueen, C.A., Kreiser, D.M. and Williams, G.M. The hepatocyte primary culture/DNA repair assay using mouse or hamster hepatocytes. Environ. Mutagenesis. **5**, 1–8 (1983a).

McQueen, C.A., Maslansky, C.J. and Williams, G.M. The role of acetylation polymorphism in determining susceptibility of cultured rabbit hepatocytes to DNA damage by aromatic amines. Cancer Res. **43**, 3120–3123 (1983b).

Meselson, M.S. Contemporary Pest Control Practices and Prospects: The Report of the Executive Committee, Vol. 1: National Academy of Sciences. Washington, D.C. (1975).

Meselson, M. and Russel, K. Comparisons of carcinogenic and mutagenic potency. In: Origins of Human Cancer, Book C, Human Risk Assessment (eds. Hiah, H.H., Watson, J.D., Winsten, J.A.) Cold Spring Harbor Laboratory, Cold Spring Harbor, N.Y., p. 1473–1482 (1977).

Metzler, M. Studies on the mechanism of carcinogenicity of diethylstilbestrol: Role of metabolic activation. Fd. Cosmet. Toxicol. **19**, 611–615 (1981).

Miller, E.C. and Miller, J.A. Mechanisms of chemical carcinogenesis. Cancer **47**, 1055–1064 (1981).

Monson, R.R., Peters, J.M. and Hansen, M.N. Proportional mortality among vinyl-chloride workers. Lancet **1**, 397–398 (1974).

Morton, K.C., King, C.M. and Baetcke, K.P. Metabolism of Benzidine to N-hydroxy-N,N'-diacetylbenzidine and subsequent nucleic acid binding and mutagenicity. Cancer Res. **39**, 3107–3113 (1979).

Munro, I.C. and Krewski, D.R. The role of risk assessment in regulatory decision making. In: Health Risk Analysis (eds. Richmond, C.R., Walsh, P.J., Copenhaver, E.D.) The Franklin Institute Press, Philadelphia, PA, p. 443–460 (1981).

Napalkov, N.P. and Anisimov, U.N. Transplacental effect of diethylstilbestrol in female rats. Cancer Letters **6**, 107–114 (1979).

Nelson, C.J., Baetcke, K.P., Frith, C.H., Kodell, R.L. and Schieferstein, G. The influence of sex, dose, time and cross on neoplasia in mice given benzidine dihydrochloride. Toxicol. Appl. Pharmacol. **64**, 171–186 (1982).

Nicholson, W.J., Hammond, E.C., Seidman, H. and Selikoff, I.J. Mortality experience of a cohort of vinyl chloride-polyvinyl chloride workers. Ann. N.Y. Acad. Sci. **246**, 225–230 (1975).

Noller, K.L., Decker, D.G., Dockerty, M.B. Mesohephric clear cell carcinoma of the vagina and cervix. A retrospective analysis. Obstet. Gynecol. **43**, 640 (1974).

Nomura, T. and Kanzaki, T. Induction of urogenital anomalies and some tumors in the progeny of mice receiving diethylstilbestrol during pregnancy. Cancer Res. **37**: 1099–1102 (1977).

Peers, F.G., Gilman, G.A., and Linsell, C.A. Dietary aflatoxins and human liver cancer. A study in Swaziland. Int. J. Cancer **17**, 167–176 (1976).

Peto, R. Epidemiology, multistage models and short-term mutagenicity tests. In: Origins of Human Cancer (H.H. Hiatt, J.D. Watson, and J.A. Winsten, eds.) Cold Spring Harbor Laboratory, 1403–1428 (1977).

Preussmann, R. Toxicological aspects of food safety—carcinogenicity and mutagenicity. Arch. Toxicol. Suppl. **1**, 69–84 (1978).

Prokofjeva, O.G. Induction of hepatic tumors in mice by benzidine. Vop. Onkol. **17**, 61–64 (1971).

Richmond, C.R., Walsh, P.J., Copenhaver, E.D. Health Risk Analysis. The Franklin Institute Press. Philadelphia (1981).

Robboy, S.J., Taguchi, O., and Cunha, G.R. Normal development of the human female reproductive tract and alterations resulting from experimental exposure to diethylstilbestrol. Human Pathol. **13**: 190–198 (1982).

Rustia, M. and Shubik, P. Effects of transplacental exposure to diethylstilbestrol on carcinogenic susceptibility during postnatal life in hamster progeny. Cancer Res. **39**, 4636–4644 (1979).

Saffiotti, U. Identifying and defining chemical carcinogens. In: Origins of Human Cancer. (H.H. Hiatt, J.D. Watson and J.A. Winsten, eds.) Cold Spring Harbor Laboratory. 1311–1326 (1977).

Saracci, R. Asbestos and lung cancer: An analysis of epidemiological evidence on the asbestos-smoking interaction. Int. J. Cancer **20**, 323–331 (1977).

Schmahl, D., Thomas, C., and Auer, R. Iatrogenic Carcinogenesis. Springer-Verlag. Berlin. (1977).

Scott, T.S. Carcinogenic and Chronic Toxic Hazards of Aromatic Amines. Elsevier Press. New York. (1962).

Selikoff, I.J. and Hammond, E.C. Health Hazards of Asbestos Exposure, Vol. 330. Ann. N.Y. Acad. Sci.: NY Acad Sci., New York (1979).

Selikoff, I.J. and Hammond, E.C. Toxicity of Vinyl Chloride-Polyvinyl Chloride, Vol. 246. Ann. N.Y. Acad. Sci.: NY Acad Sci., New York (1975).

Selikoff, I.J., Hammond, E.C. and Chung, J. Asbestos exposure, smoking and neoplasia. J. Amer. Med. Assoc. **204**, 106–112 (1968).

Shank, R.C., Bhamarapravati, N., Gordon, J.E. and Wogan, G.N. Dietary aflatoxins and human liver cancer. IV. Incidence of primary liver cancer in two municipal populations in Thailand. Fd. Cosmet. Toxicol. **10**, 171–179 (1972).

Shank, R.C. Epidemiology of aflatoxin carcinogenesis. In: Environmental Cancer, Vol. 3. Kraybill, H.F.S. and Mehlman, M.A., eds., Halstead Press, New York, 1977, p. 291.

Sherman, A.I., Goldrath, M., Berlin, A. Cervical-vaginal adenosis after *in utero* exposure to synthetic estrogens. Obstet. Gynecol. **44**, 531 (1974).

Shimada, T., Swanson, A., Leber, P., and Williams, G.M. Activities of chlorinated ethane and ethylene compounds in the salmonella/microsome mutagenesis and hepatocyte DNA repair assays under vapor phase exposure conditions. Cell Biol Toxicol 1000–000 (1985).

Shimkin, M.B., Grady, H.G. and Andervont, H.B. Induction of testicular tumors and other effects of stilbestrol-cholesterol pellets in strain C mice. J. Natl. Cancer Inst. **2**: 65 (1941).

Shimkin, M.B., Weisburger, J.H., Weisburger, E.K., Gubareft, N., and Suntzeff, V. Bioassay of 29 alkylating chemicals by the pulmonary-tumor response in strain A mice. J. Natl. Cancer Inst. **36**: 915–935 (1966).

Shimkin, M.B., Wieder, R., Marzi, D., Gubareff, N., and Suntzeff, V. Lung tumors in mice receiving different schedules of urethane. In: Proceedings of the Fifth Berkeley Symposium on Mathematical Statistics and Probability. University of California Press. Vol. IV, 707 (1967).

Sinnhuber, R.O., Wales, J.H., Ayers, J.L. et al. Dietary factors and hepatoma in rainbow trout (Salmogairdneri) I. Aflatoxins in vegetable protein feedstuffs. J. Natl. Cancer Inst. **41**, 711–718 (1968).

Spitz, S., Maguigan, W.H. and Dobriner, K. The carcinogenic action of benzidine. Cancer **3**, 789–804 (1950).

Steinhoff, D. Cancerogenic effects of benzidine in female Sprague-Dawley rats. Naturwissenschaften **61**, 276–277 (1974).

Tabershaw, I.R. and Gaffey, W.R. Mortality study of workers in the manufacture of vinyl chloride and its polymers. J. Occup. Med. **16**, 509 (1974).

Thiede, T. and Christensen, B.C. Bladder tumors induced by chlornaphazine. A five year follow up study of chlornaphazine-treated patients with polycythemia. Acta Med. Scand. **185**, 133–137 (1969).

Tomatis, L., Agthe, C., Bartsch, H., Huff, J., Montesano, R., Saracci, R., Walker, E., and Wilbourn, J. Evaluation of the carcinogenicity of chemicals: A review of the monograph program of the international agency for research on cancer (1971 to 1977). Cancer Res. **38**, 877–885 (1978).

Upton, A.C., Clayson, D.G., Jansen, J.D., Rosenkrantz, H. and Williams, G. Report of ICPEMC task group on the differentiation between genotoxic and nongenotoxic carcinogens. In preparation (1983).

Van Duuren, B.L., Katz, C., Goldschmidt, B.M., Frenkel, R. and Sivak, A. Carcinogenicity of halo-ethers. II. Structure-activity relationship of analogs of bis(chloromethyl)ether, J. Natl. Cancer Inst. **48**, 1431–1439 (1972).

Vesselinovitch, S.D., Rao, K.V.N. and Milhailovich, N. Factors modulating benzidine carcinogenicity bioassay. Cancer Res. **35**: 2814 (1975).

246

Vesselinovitch, S.D., Milhailovich, N., Wogan, G.N., Lombard, L.S. and Rao, K.V.N. Aflatoxin B_1, a hepatocarcinogen in the infant mouse. Cancer Res. **32**, 2289–2291 (1972).

Videbaek, A. Chlornaphazine (Erysan) may induce cancer of the urinary bladder. Acta Med. Scand. **176**, 45–50 (1964).

Vigliani, E.C. and Barsotti, M. Environmental tumors of the bladder in some Italian dye-stuff factories. Med. Lavoro **52**, 241–250 (1961).

Volfson, I.I. The blastomogenic action of sinestrol during intravaginal insertions. Neoplasma **21**, 569–576 (1974).

Vooijs, P.G., Ng, A.B.P. and Wentz, W.B. The detection of, vaginal adenosis and clear cell carcinoma. Acta Cytol. **17**, 59–63 (1973).

Ward, J.M., Sontag, J.M., Weisburger, E.K. and Brown, C.A. Effect of lifetime exposure to aflatoxin B_1 in rats. J. Natl. Cancer Inst. **55**, 107–113 (1975).

Waxweiler, R.J., Stringer, W., Wagoner, J.K. and Jones, J. Neoplastic risk among workers exposed to vinyl chloride. Ann. N.Y. Acad. Sci. **271**, 40–48 (1976).

Weisburger, J.H. and Williams, G.M. Chemical carcinogens. In: Toxicology: The Basic Science of Poisons, 2nd Edition (Eds. Doull, J., Klaassen, C.D. and Amkdur, M.O.) pp. 84–138, Macmillan, NY (1980).

Weisburger, J.H. and Williams, G.M. Basic requirements for health risk analysis: the decision point approach for systematic carcinogen testing. In: Proceedings of the Third Life Sciences Symposium on Health Risk Analysis, Franklin Press, pp. 249–271 (1981).

Weisburger, J.H. and Williams, G.M. Chemical Carcinogenesis. In: Cancer Medicine, 2nd Edition, Eds. J.F. Holland and E. Frei III, Lea and Febiger, Philadelphia, pp. 42–95 (1982a).

Weisburger, J.H. and Williams, G.M. Metabolism of chemical carcinogens. In: Cancer: A Comprehensive Treatise, 2nd Edition, Ed. F.F. Becker, Plenum Press, N.Y., p. 241–333 (1982b).

Weisburger, J.H. and Williams, G.M. Bioassay of Carcinogens: *In Vitro* and *In Vivo* Tests. In: Chemical Carcinogens, Chapter 2, Ed. C.E. Searle, in press (1983a).

Weisburger, J.H. and Williams, G.M. The distinct health risk analysis required for genotoxic carcinogens and promoting agents. Environ. Health Perspect. **50**, 233–245 (1983b).

Wieder, R., Wogan, G.N. and Shimkin, M.B. Pulmonary tumors in strain A mice given injections of aflatoxin B_1. J. Natl. Cancer Inst. **40**, 1195 (1968).

Williams, G.M. Further improvements in the hepatocyte primary culture DNA repair test for carcinogens. Detection of carcinogenic biphenyl derivatives. Cancer Letters, **4**, 69 (1977).

Williams, G.M. The detection of chemical carcinogens by unscheduled DNA synthesis in rat liver primary cell cultures. Cancer Res. **37**, 1845 (1977b).

Williams, G.M. Further improvements in the hepatocyte primary culture DNA repair test for carcinogens: Detection of carcinogenic biphenyl derivatives. Cancer Letts. **4**, 69 (1978).

Williams, G.M. A comparison of *in vivo* and *in vitro* metabolic activation systems, In: Critical Reviews in Toxicology—Strategies for Short-term Testing for Mutagens/Carcinogens, (Butterworth, B. ed.) C.R.C. Press, West Palm Beach, FL; p. 96 (1979a).

Williams, G.M. The status of *in vitro* test systems utilizing DNA damage and repair for the screening of chemical carcinogens. Journal Association of Official Analytical Chemists, **62**, 857 (1979b).

Williams, G.M. Classification of genotoxic and epigenetic hepatocarcinogens using liver culture assays. Annals New York Academy of Sciences, **349**: 273–282, 1980.

Williams, G.M. Mammalian culture systems for the study of genetic effects of N-substituted aryl compounds. In: Carcinogenic and Mutagenic N-Substituted Aryl Compounds, Eds. S. Thorgeirsson and E.K. Weisburger, National Cancer Institute Monograph, **58**: 237–242, 1981.

Williams, G.M., Lerr, A. and Weisburger, J.H. A species to species comparison of carcinogenicity data with human extrapolation. Final Report NIEHS Contract NO 1-ES-6-2130 (1978).

Williams, G.M. and Weisburger, J.H. Systematic carcinogen testing through the decision point approach. Annual Review of Pharmacology and Toxicology, **21**: 393–416 (1981).

Williams, G.M., Weisburger, J.H. and Wynder, E.L. Lifestyle and cancer etiology. In: Carcinogens and Mutagens in the Environment, Food Products, (H.F. Stich, eds.) CRC Press, Boca Raton, FL, pp. 53 (1982).

Williams, R.R. and Schweitzer, R.J. Clear cell carcinoma of the vagina in a girl whose mother had taken diethylstilbestrol. Calif. Med. **118**, 53 (1973).

Wogan, G.N. In: Hepatocellular carcioma: Aflatoxins and the irrelationship to hepatocellular carcinoma. 25–41 (1976).

Wogan, G.M., Paglialunga, S., and Newberne, P.M. Carcinogenic effects of low dietary levels of aflatoxin B_1 in rats. Fd. Cosmet. Toxicol. **12**, 681–685 (1974).

Wynder, E.L. and Goldsmith, R. The epidemiology of bladder cancer: a second look. Cancer **40**, 1246–1268 (1977).

Zajdela, F., Croisy, A., Barbin, A., Malaveille, C., Tomatis, L. and Bartsch, H. Carcinogenicity of chloromethylene oxide, an ultimate reactive metabolite of vinyl chloride and bis(chloromethyl)ether after subcutaneous administration and in initiation-promotion experiments in mice. Cancer Res. **40**, 352–356 (1980).

Zavon, M.R., Hoegg, U. and Bingham, E. Benzidine exposure as a cause of bladder tumors. Arch. Environ. Health **27**, 1–7 (1973).

Zensen, T.V., Mattammal, M.B., Armbrecht, H.J., and Davis, B.B. Benzidine binding to nucleic acids mediated by the peroxidative activity of prostaglandin endoperoxide synthetase. Cancer Res. **40**: 2839–2845 (1980).

CHAPTER X

THE QUESTION OF THE EXISTENCE OF THRESHOLDS: EXTRAPOLATION FROM HIGH TO LOW DOSE

David W. Gaylor
National Center for Toxicological Research

A. INTRODUCTION

The discussion here is directed toward assessing disease risk in animal populations from exposure to chemicals. In order to detect potential adverse health effects due to exposure to a chemical with a reasonable number of animals, it generally is necessary to use experimental dosage levels well above expected human exposure. The problem is to predict adverse health effects in a laboratory animal species at extremely low dosage levels from experiments in which dosage levels may be many times higher.

B. THRESHOLDS

Some toxicologists postulate the existence of a threshold dose below which no adverse effect occurs. If such thresholds exist, absolute safety could be assured by determining the threshold dose and regulating the use of the chemical so that the threshold dose is never exceeded. Some toxicologists postulate that there do not appear to be threshold doses for direct acting carcinogens and mutagens (see e.g., Druckrey, 1967). Even if threshold doses do exist, they can not be accurately estimated from animal bioassay data.

We must distinguish between two types of thresholds: individual and population. An individual threshold applies to a particular animal under a given set of conditions. A population threshold applies to a large group of animals such that a dose is found at which no animals develop an adverse effect, that is the minimum of the individual animal threshold dosages in the group.

It might appear that animal bioassays have proven the existence of individual thresholds since some of the animals administered a given dose of a carcinogen produce tumors while others do not. One might argue for those animals not possessing tumors that the dose was below a threshold. However, carcinogenesis is a process that involves time. It may be that environmental and genetic differences among animals alter the rate at which the carcinogenic process proceeds. Thus, at the termination of a chronic animal bioassay, not all animals are at the same stage of the carcinogenic process. Those in the advanced stages possess a tumor and those in the early stages do not. Considering only the proportion of animals with tumors may incorrectly lead one to conclude that the threshold dose had been surpassed only for the tumor bearing animals. In fact, carcinogenesis may have been induced in all animals but not have progressed to tumors in all animals before the termination of a study or before their death due to other causes. Also, the detection of internal microscopic tumors is subject to sampling variation. Typically, one microscopic slide per animal tissue is examined. Thus, internal microscopic tumors may be detected in some animals and missed in other animals according to their location. Also, if carcinogenesis is a stochastic process such that the development of a tumor is a chance event resulting when certain conditions exist with a small probability, then these conditions may occur by chance earlier in some animals than in others. Thus, the existence of tumors at some point in time in some animals and not in others does not necessarily mean that the threshold dose was surpassed for some animals and not for others. Mathematical distribution functions such as the logit (Berkson, 1944) and the probit (Mantel and Bryan, 1961) often are used to describe a mathematical relationship between the proportion of animals with tumors and dose. This should not be interpreted as providing a distribution of individual animal thresholds. Even if individual thresholds exist, many factors may influence the induction and progression of the carcinogenic process such as to make the determination of a population threshold value a nearly impossible task.

The existence of dose response relationships for tumors might also lead one to incorrectly assume the existence of thresholds. As dosage is decreased the prevalence of an observable biological effect (e.g., the proportion of animals with tumors) diminishes to zero. Eventually, a dosage is reached below which the experiment has essentially no resolving power to distinguish between the spontaneous background rate and small induced biological effects. The observance of no tumors in a group of animals exposed to a given dosage of a chemical does not mean that a subthreshold dosage has been found. It only means that the true prevalence rate of tumors is low. For example, if no tumors are observed in 100 animals, the upper 99% confidence limit on the true proportion of animals with tumors is 0.045. We can only be relatively certain that the true tumor rate is less than 4.5%.

If no toxic effects were observed at a dosage, this dosage often is called the "no effect" or more correctly the "no observable effect" dosage. Because of the limitations of any given experiment, it is realized that the "no observable effect" dosage is not a precise estimate of a true no effect level. As an added precaution the "no observable effect" level is divided by an arbitrary safety factor, often 100, to establish allowable dosages. How much protection does this procedure provide? If the true tumor rate is zero, there is no problem. On the other hand, even though no animals out of 100 animals were observed to have tumors, the tumor rate at the experimental dosage level might be as high as 4.5%. If the tumor rate is proportional to dosage (arguments for low dose linearity will be presented later), dividing the "no observable effect" level by a safety factor of 100 would also divide the tumor rate by a factor of 100 resulting in a "maximum" risk of 0.00045 (450 per million). This may be an unacceptable risk in many circumstances.

Thresholds can not be established statistically. Increasing the number of animals will provide a more precise estimate of the tumor rate, but can never guarantee absolute safety. Suppose, no animals in 10,000 exhibit a particular type of tumor. Again, this does not mean a subthreshold dose has been found. The upper 99% confidence limit on the true tumor rate is 0.00045. Observing no tumors with increasing sample sizes reduces the upper limit on the potential tumor rate, but can never reach zero.

If a chemical acts through the same mechanism to produce tumors as for spontaneous tumors, then an addition of the chemical will simply increase the tumor incidence no matter how low the exposure to the additional chemical (Peto, 1978). This can be demonstrated graphically (Figure 1). Suppose the true

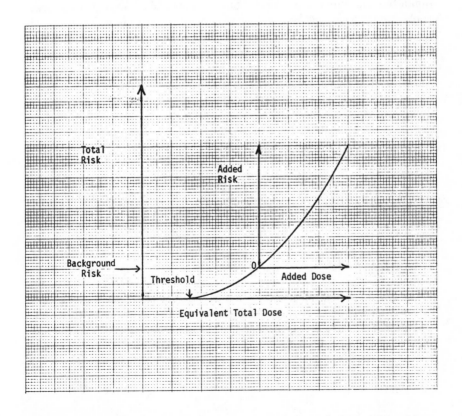

FIGURE 1. Additivity of response above background from equivalent additional dose.

dose response is represented by the curve with a threshold dose. The occurrence of tumors in control animals indicates that one or more factors are already operating to produce tumors. Consider a chemical which acts through one or more of the same factors to produce the same kind of tumors already occurring in control animals. With the addition of a chemical, the starting point 0 is actually at the equivalent total dose of those factors producing the background tumor rate (Figure 1). Since this point is beyond the threshold dose, the addition of the chemical simply adds to the carcinogenic burden resulting in added risk without any threshold effect for the chemical. The only conceivable way in which a chemical could have a threshold dose is for it to act through a unique mechanism to produce tumors in a manner not already in progress.

Cornfield (1977) proposed a kinetic model for describing dose response relationships which included the potential for a threshold dose. However, this kinetic model in a way, argues against thresholds in that threshold doses in this system could only be achieved with immediate and complete deactivation.

With the issue of thresholds unresolvable by dose response animal bioassays, we must turn to other approaches to provide safety with exposure to chemicals. Unfortunately, the use of fixed safety factors applied to "no observable effect" levels benefit the poorer experiments. The fewer animals used the less likely a tumor bearing animal will appear. Thus, with fewer animals higher "no observable effects" levels will be obtained resulting in higher allowable levels. The fixed safety factor procedure works in exactly a manner opposite to what is desired. As the number of animals is decreased, higher dosages are required in order to detect toxic effects, resulting in higher "no observable effect" levels and subsequently higher allowable dosages. Procedures for extrapolating from high to low doses which circumvent the fixed safety factor paradox are discussed in the next section.

C. MATHEMATICAL MODELS

Some of the mathematical models that have been proposed to describe dose response relationships in carcinogenesis for low dose extrapolation will be presented. None of these models have a population threshold. However, some of these models allow for the possibility of individual animal thresholds.

I. One-Hit Model

The one-hit model is a stochastic model based on the concept that a tumor can be induced when a single susceptible receptor is exposed to a single quantum of a chemical. The probability of tumor induction by exposure to a chemical at a dose of $d \geq 0$ is

$$P(d) = 1 - \exp(-\gamma d)$$

where γ is an unknown parameter that represents the slope of the dose response curve at $d = 0$. In rare cases the dose may be the dose delivered to a target tissue, but more often it is the dose administered to the whole animal expressed in dose per body weight, per surface area, or as concentration in the diet.

II. Multi-Hit (k-Hit) Model

The k-hit model is a stochastic model for which k hits of a susceptible receptor are requried to induce cancer. The probability of a tumor resulting from an exposure of dose, d, is

$$P(d) = 1 - \sum_{i=0}^{k-1} (\lambda d)^i e^{-\lambda d} / i!$$

For small values of λd, the k-hit model may be approximated by $P(d) = (\lambda d)^k$ which plots as a straight line on log-log graph paper with a slope of k.

III. Multistage Model

A generalization of the multi-hit model is the multistage stochastic model proposed by Armitage and Doll (1961).

$$P(d) = 1 - \exp\left[- \prod_{i=1}^{k} (\alpha_i + \beta_i d)\right]$$

where $\alpha_i \geq 0$, $\beta_i \geq 0$, and k is the number of stages for the carcinogenic process. The α's represent the spontaneous background occurrence and the β's are the proportionality constants induced by the dose for each stage. The multistage model can be written in a simpler form

$$P(d) = 1 - \exp[-(\gamma_0 + \gamma_1 d + \gamma_2 d^2 + ... + \gamma_k d^k)]$$

where $\gamma_1 \geq 0$, $i = 1, 2 ... , k$.

IV. Extreme Value Model

Chand and Hoel (1974) show that if the time-to-tumor distribution is a Weibull distribution the dose response is described by an extreme value model

$$P(d) = 1 - \exp[- \exp(\alpha + \beta \log d)].$$

V. Probit Log-Dose Model

The probit log-dose model has been used extensively in bioassay (see e.g. Finney, 1952). This model assumes that the distribution of log-doses that result in tumors is Gaussian (Normal). For the probit log-dose model the probability of a tumor is

$$P(d) = \Phi (\alpha + \beta \log d)$$

where Φ denotes the standard cumulative Gaussian (Normal) distribution. Chand and Hoel (1974) show that the probit log-dose response is obtained when the time-to-tumor distribution is log-normal.

VI. Logistic Model

Berkson (1944) proposed the logistic model for bioassay data

$$P(d) = [1 + \exp(\alpha + \beta \log d)]^{-1}$$

The logistic model closely approximates the probit log-dose model.

D. CHOICE OF MODEL

None of the mathematical models proposed can be validated on the basis of biological arguments. Unfortunately, most of these mathematical models fit the experimental data about equally well in the experimental dose range, but they may give substantially different estimates when extrapolated to low dose levels (FDA Advisory Committee on Protocols for Safety Evaluation, 1971). Since the shape of the dose response curve is unknown below the experimental data range, it is impossible to obtain point estimates of risk at low doses. Animal bioassay data can not resolve the true mathematical nature of dose response curves below the experimental dose range.

Recognizing that actual point estimates of risk or "safe" doses can not be obtained without knowing the true form of the dose response curve at low doses, Mantel and Bryan (1961) proposed a technique for "virtual safety." Their procedure is based on the observation that a large body of tumor bioassay data can be described by probit lines plotted as the logarithm of dosage with slopes greater than one. Since there is no guarantee that these slopes would apply at lower doses, Mantel and Bryan (1961) adopted a supposedly conservative convention by extrapolating to low doses with a slope of one. Thus, they chose to extrapolate to lower doses along a line for which the tumor rate does not decrease as rapidly with decreasing dose as was observed experimentally. Mantel and Bryan do not suggest that the true slope is one nor do they imply that the true dose response is probit log-dose at low doses. Their only assumption is that the dose response curve lies below this extrapolation line, thereby predicting a conservatively higher proportion of tumors than actually occur at low doses. Thus, the Mantel-Bryan procedure does not provide an actual estimate of tumor risk or "safe" dose, but hopefully provides a conservative upper limit on tumor risk at low doses.

The slope of the probit log-dose model approaches zero at low doses. If low dose linearity is the true state of nature, the Mantel-Bryan method will not be conservative. It has been shown by Guess *et al* (1977) that for risks on the order of 10^{-8} to 10^{-6}, the Mantel-Bryan procedure may overestimate the true "safe" dose by factors approaching 100-fold if the true dose response curve is linear at low dose. For the Mantel-Bryan procedure to be conservative, it is necessary to rule out low dose linearity. In view of the plausible arguments for low dose linearity by Crump *et al* (1976), Guess *et al* (1977), and Peto (1978), it appears that the Mantel-Bryan procedure may not provide the assumed conservatism. Also, the argument for low dose linearity is illustrated by Figure 1. Any segment of a continuous monotonic curve can be approximated within a specified small error by a sufficiently small straight line segment beginning at point 0.

A procedure does exist for making conservative low dose risk assessments which does not depend on any mathematical model for extrapolation. This is appealing since none of the proposed mathematical models can be verified biologically or by tumor bioassay data. By making one simple plausible assumption of a sigmoid shape for a dose response curve, which frequently is verifiable experimentally, it is possible to obtain an estimate of an upper limit on the risk at low doses using linear interpolation without adopting any particular mathematical model outside of the data range. This is particularly appealing because it does not depend on any theory of carcinogenesis. The only requirement for conservatism is that the dose response is curving upward at low doses, a condition that generally prevails in a wide variety of bioassays including mutagenesis and teratogenesis. This linear interpolation procedure is described in the next section.

E. LINEAR INTERPOLATION

Gaylor and Kodell (1980) provide an algorithm for performing linear interpolation. Linear interpolation does not consist of fitting a straight line through experimental bioassay data. In fact, most dose response data for carcinogens are nonlinear. Linear interpolation does not attempt to provide an estimate of risk in the low dose region. This can only be accomplished if the true form of the mathematical dose response model is known. Rather, linear interpolation only attempts to place an upper limit on the potential risk at low dosages. This can be accomplished under the simple condition that the dose response is curving upward (convex) for low dosages. In the low dose range where the response is convex, a line from a point in this range of the curve connected to the spontaneous background response at zero dose will always lie above the true dose response curve providing an overestimate of the true risk.

Due to inherent experimental variation, the true mathematical dose response relationship can not be determined exactly even in the experimental dose region. Because of this uncertainty interpolation proceeds from an upper confidence limit on the estimated tumor rate. Since the quantity of interest is the excess tumor rate above the spontaneous background rate, linear interpolation proceeds along a line from the upper confidence limits in the experimental region on the excess tumor rate to zero excess tumors at zero dose. Since the procedure is attempting to predict an intermediate response using the straight line connecting two points, the procedure is actually *linear interpolation.*

Linear interpolation over the low unobserved dose range is described by

$$P = Ud/d_e,$$

where P is the upper bound on the potential proportion of animals with excess tumors caused by the administration of a dosage, d, of a chemical and U is the upper confidence limit at a dosage, d_e, in the experimental dose range, as illustrated in Figure 2. Linear interpolation is used between zero and the upper confidence limit on the excess tumor rate estimated at the lowest experimental dosage. Any mathematical model can be used which adequately fits the data in the experimental dose range. The only purpose of this model is to obtain an upper confidence line in the experimental region. The fitted line is not extended below the experimental region.

The following steps constitute the procedure suggested by Gaylor and Kodell (1980) for linear interpolation:

1. Use any mathematical model which gives zero excess tumors at zero dose that adequately fits the data in the experimental data range.
2. Obtain the upper confidence limits on the excess tumor rate above the spontaneous background rate in the experimental dosage range.
3. Connect a straight line from the origin to the point on the upper confidence limit at the lowest experimental dosage.
4. Obtain upper limits of risk for low dosages or, conversely, dosages corresponding to low upper limits of risk from the interpolation line in Step 3.

The estimated risk at the lowest nonzero experimental dose may be quite low. Such estimates are likely to be highly dependent on the model fitted to the data. Since we are attempting to minimize the effect of the choice of the model, we would not recommend using a fitted model below an excess risk level of 1% and therefore we would start the linear low dose interpolation at that point.

In the special case where only one dosage level of a chemical is administered to animals, obviously no mathematical model can be obtained. The experimental range is confined to a single point so that interpolation proceeds along the line connecting the upper confidence limit for the excess tumor rate at the experimental dosage to the origin. With only one dosage point caution must be exercised because it is not possible to determine if the dose response is curving upward. This generally is not a serious problem for tumor rates below 50%.

Linear interpolation is not ultraconservative and gives "safe" doses comparable to those obtained from the multistage model (Gaylor and Kodell, 1980).

Both linear interpolation and multistage extrapolation may predict "safe" doses so low that they are not attainable. This is not a fault of the extrapolation procedures used but is simply a limitation of the animal bioassay. It is not possible to provide a high degree of safety from a bioassay on a small number of animals, particularly if tumors are obtained in animals at dose levels close to human exposure levels. Bioassays, at best, may resolve mathematical models in the experimental dose range, but can not be expected to determine precisely the nature of the true dose response relationship below the experimental region. For this reason, the linear interpolation limits the use of a parametric dose response model to obtaining an upper confidence limit at the lowest nonzero experimental dose, from which a linear interpolation is made over the unobserved dose region. Since linear interpolation does not extrapolate to doses below the experimental range by using a mathematical model fitted to the data, the unresolved issue of selecting a valid mathematical model for extrapolation is circumvented and the technique is applicable to bioassay data other than carcinogenesis.

F. EXAMPLE

To illustrate the use of linear interpolation, consider urinary bladder carcinoma dose response data obtained in a large study conducted at the National Center for Toxicological Research in which 2-acetylaminofluorene (2-AAF)

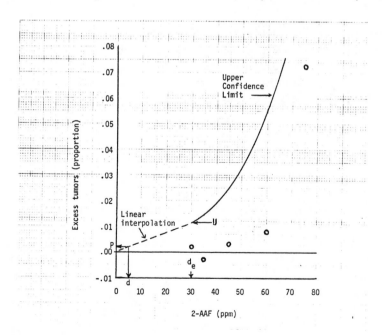

FIGURE 2. Potential lifetime incidence of bladder carcinoma for female BALB/c mice fed 2-AAF.

was fed to BALB/c female mice as described by Littlefield *et al* (1980). The proportion of animals dying with bladder carcinoma is given in Table 1. In spite of the large numbers of animals used, it is impossible to determine the shape of the dose response curve below the experimental data range (i.e., below 30 ppm). Linear interpolation was applied to these data to estimate the dosage of 2-AAF for which the lifetime tumor rate in these mice is less than one in a million with at least 97.5% confidence. The effect of the choice of the level of confidence from 95% to 99% is relatively unimportant.

In order to estimate the upper confidence limit at the lowest experimental dosage, 30 ppm, the multi-stage model

$$P = 1 - \exp[-(\beta_0 + \beta_1 d + \beta_2 d^2 + ... + \beta_k d^k)]$$

where P is the proportion of animals with bladder carcinoma and d is the dosage level of 2-AAF, was fit in the experimental dose range according to the procedure given by Crump *et al* (1977). The upper 97.5% confidence limit on the excess bladder carcinoma rate at 30 ppm is U = 0.0113. Linear interpolation over the unobserved low dose region below 30 ppm for the excess bladder carcinoma rate is given by

$$P = Ud/d_e = 0.0113d/30 = 3.77 \times 10^{-4} \times d.$$

Solving for d gives the dosage for which we are at least 97.5% confident that the excess bladder carcinoma rate does not exceed P. For example, the dosage of 2-AAF for which we are at least 97.5% confident that the excess bladder carcinoma rate does not exceed one in a million for BALB/c female mice under these experimental conditions is

$$d = 10^{-6}/3.77 \times 10^{-4} = 0.0027 \text{ ppm} = 2.7 \text{ ppb}.$$

For purposes of comparison, the corresponding dosage estimated by the proce-

TABLE 1. Proportion of mice with bladder carcinoma in the NCTR chronic feeding study of 2-AAF.

Dosage (ppm)	Bladder Carcinoma
0	3/360
30	15/1432
35	4/707
45	4/347
60	4/242
75	20/248
100	39/124
150	88/119

dure given by Crump *et al* (1977) using the multistage model is more conservative giving 0.08 ppb.

The experimental data for the lowest dosages, upper confidence limit in the experimental data range, and linear interpolation between 0 and 30 ppm are illustrated graphically in Figure 2.

It is of interest to compare the above approach using linear interpolation with the safety factor approach with these data. Ignoring the low dose trend and comparing the tumor rates at each dose with the controls results in the largest no observed effect level (NOEL) at 60 ppm. Since 2-AAF is an animal carcinogen, a relatively large safety factor should be employed. Suppose a safety factor of 1000 is used. This would result in an allowable dosage of 60 ppm $\div$ 1000 = 60 ppb. The question is how much safety does this level afford? The maximum upper 97.5% confidence limit on the excess proportion of animals with bladder carcinomas at 60 ppm is 0.039. Since the dose response is curving upward, reducing the dosage by a factor of 1000 will reduce the risk of bladder carcinoma by at least a factor of 1000. Hence, the risk at 60 ppb is less than 0.039 $\div$ 1000 = 39 $\times$ 10^{-6}. In order to reduce the upper limit on the potential risk to one in a million a safety factor of 39,000 would be required thus limiting the dosage to 60 ppm $\div$ 39,000 = 1.5 ppb. The method of linear interpolation gave a maximum dosage of 2.7 ppb. By utilizing all the experimental data and following the curvature of the dose response curve down to the lowest experimental dosage of 30 ppm, the linear interpolation method was less stringent than the safety factor approach.

G. SUMMARY

The existence of threshold doses for carcinogens can not be proved by the use of animal bioassays because it is impossible to observe and measure with absolute precision small increases in tumor rates above background. Thus, a set of experimental data may be equally compatible with either a threshold or nonthreshold model. Even if we knew that a threshold dose existed, this information is of no value since estimates of threshold doses can not be obtained. The question is not whether thresholds exist, but rather to what extent can risk be reduced at lower doses. The validity of various mathematical models for describing carcinogenic or mutagenic dose response relationships can not be established by animal bioassays below the measurable data range. However, linear interpolation can be used between zero and the lowest experimental data point for predicting potential low dose risk in animal populations. Linear interpolation does not depend on any theoretical development and hence can be applied to toxic effects other than carcinogenesis. The only condition required for conservatism is that the dose response is curving upward at low doses. Estimates of potential risk obtained by linear interpolation are widely applicable and often are not as high as those obtained from extending the multistage model to low doses (Gaylor and Kodell, 1980) or by the use of adequate safety factors.

REFERENCES

Armitage, P. and Doll, R. (1961). Stochastic models for carcinogenesis. *Proceedings of the Fourth Berkeley Symposium on Mathematical Statistics and Probability*, eds. L.M. LeCam and J. Neyman, pp. 19–38. Berkelely: Univ. of Calif. Press.

Berkson, J. (1944). Application of the logistic function to bio-assay. *J. Am. Stat. Assoc.* **39**: 357–365.

Chand, N. and Hoel, D.G. (1974). A comparison of models for determining safe levels of environmental agents. In *Reliability and Biometry: Statistical Analysis of Lifelength*, eds. F. Proschan and R.J. Serfling. Philadelphia: Soc. for Industrial and Applied Math.

Cornfield, J. (1977). Carcinogenic risk assessment. *Science* **198**: 693–699.

Crump, K.S., Guess, H.A., and Deal, K.L. (1977). Confidence intervals and test of hypotheses concerning dose response relations inferred from animal carcinogenicity data. *Biometrics* **33**: 437–451.

Crump, K.S., Hoel, D.G., Langley, C.H., and Peto, R. (1976). Fundamental carcinogenic processes and their implications for low dose risk assessment. *Cancer Res.* **36**: 2973–2979.

Druckrey, H. (1967). Quantitative aspects of chemical carcinogenesis. *Potential Carcinogenic Hazards from Drugs (Evaluation of Risks)*, ed. René Truhart, U.I.C.C. Monograph Series, Vol. 7, 60–78. New York: Springer-Verlag.

FDA Advisory Committee on Protocols for Safety Evaluation (1971). Panel on carcinogenesis report on cancer testing in the safety evaluation of food additives and pesticides. *Toxicol. Appl. Pharm.* **20**: 419–438.

Gaylor, D.W. and Kodell, R.L. (1980). Linear interpolating algorithm for low dose risk assessment of toxic substances. *J. Environ. path. and Toxicol.* **4**:305–312.

Guess, H.A., Crump, K.S., and Peto, R. (1977). Uncertainty estimates for low-dose-rate extrapolations of animal carcinogenicity data. *Cancer Res.* **37**:3475–3483.

Littlefield, N.A., Farmer, J.H., Sheldon, W.G. and Gaylor, D.W. (1980). Effects of dose and time in a long-term, low-dose carcinogenic study. *J. Environ. Path. and Toxicol.* **3**: 17–34.

Mantel, N. and Bryan, W.R. (1961). Safety testing of carcinogenic agents. *J. Natl. Cancer Instit.* **27**: 455–470.

Peto, R. (1978). Carcinogenic effects of chronic exposure to very low levels of toxic substances. *Environ. Health Perspectives* **22**: 155–159.

Watson, G.S. (1977). Age incidence curves for cancer. *Proc. Natl. Acad. Sci.* **74**: 1341–1342.

SUBJECT INDEX

acetaminophen, 93
2-acetylaminofluorene, 62
activation of products, 81
acute transforming retroviruses, 29
aflatoxins, 10, 89, 212–15
alkylating agents, 101–102
alkaline elution, 106, 131
alkaline sucrose gradient centrafugation, 131, 133
alkaline sucrose sedimentation, 106
alkaline unwinding of DNA, 107
alkyl benzanthracenes, 8
allyl isothiocyanate, 62
Ames test, 21, 64
anaplasia, 45
aneuploidy, 18, 36–40, 189–198
aniridia, 20
antimetabolites, 41
arginine deprivation, 66
aromatic amines, 2, 8, 91
aryl hydrocarbon hydroxylase, 86
asbestos, 69
assay systems, 64–67
ataxia telangiectasia, 18
autosomally linked recessive syndromes, 18
5-azacytidine, 43
azo dyes, 8, 61, 83

base excision, 130
base substitutions, 64
benzacridines, 4
benzanthracene, 3, 4
benzidine, 217–224
benzo(a)pyrene, 2, 3
benzphenanthrenes, 4
3,4-benzpyrene, 2
biotransformation processes, 81–83, 129
blastocysts, 17
Bloom's syndrome, 18
Burkitt's lymphoma, 38

carbon tetrachloride, 94
carcinogenesis,
clinical perspectives, 17–20
mechanisms of, 4–6
and mutagenesis of mammalian cells, 171–206
relation to toxicology, 7
somatic mutation model, 13–59
carcinogenic hydrocarbons, 1, 63
carcinogens,
as mutagens, 21–22
species and organ/tissue differences, 6
carcinomatoid tumors, 5
catalytically cracked petroleum residues, 4
cell death, 104
cell fusion, 24–28
cell mutagenesis systems, 153–170
cellular homologs, 28
cellular oncogenes, 28
chemical carcinogenesis,
historical perspective, 1–12
mechanisms of, 210–212
chemical carcinogens,
as mutagens, 61–78
chimney sweeps, 1
Chinese hamster ovary (CHO) cell assay, 65, 154–155, 158–61
chlornaphazine (CNZ), 224–229
chromosomal
aberrations, 65
abnormalities, 16
changes, 37–40
disorders, 36–40
imbalances, 37
instability, 18–19
protein binding, 97
variability, 39–40
chronic irritation theory, 2, 4
chronic toxicity test, 7
cigarette smoke, 4
clonal evolution hypothesis, 15
clonal hybrid strains, 27
coal tar, 1, 2, 4, 6, 7, 61
cocarcinogenesis, 5
codominant expression, 24

262

hydroxy derivatives, 3
hydroxyurea suppression, 66
hyperchromatic mitoses, 44
hyperdiploidy, 39
hypochromatic mitoses, 44
hypoxanthine-guanine phosphori-
    bosyl transferase (HGPRT),
    154–57

inplantation of plastics, 9
inactivation of drugs, 81
indirect acting agents, 79
individual thresholds, 249
initiation, 4
insertional mutagenesis, 35–36
insertions, 64
intercalation, 99, 104
isoenzyme patterns, 17

karyotypic changes, 37–40
keratoacanthomas, 5

L5178Y mouse lymphoma assay, 65,
    155, 163–66
large deletions, 64
linear interpolation, 255–257
liquid chromatography, 3
liquid scintillation counting, 133
logistic model, 254
long-term carcinogenicity bioassays,
    69–72

mammalian cell systems, 153–170
mammalian mutational assay sys-
    tems, 153–170
mass spectroscopy, 105, 132
metabolic activation, 63, 79–97
metabolic stress, 40
methyl carbamate, 10
methylcholanthrene, 3, 9, 63
methyl derivatives, 3
methylguanine, 10
microbial systems, 153
micronuclei, 66
micronutrients, 6
mitogenic hormones, 41
mitotic aneuploidy, 39

mitotic recombination, 36, 39
molecular cloning experiments, 31–32
monooxygenase activity, 85
mouse cell lines, 176–179
multi-hit model, 253
multiple loci assay, 154–55
multistage model, 253
multistep model, 35–36
mustard gas, 5, 62
mutagenic lesions in DNA, 19
mutation,
    induction, 64
    and transformation, compared,
        15–16
mutational etiology for tumors, 17
mutational markers, 184

Na/K ATPase, 158
β-naphthoflavone, 86
National Cancer Institute, 9
NCI/NTP protocol, 68
neoplastic
    phenotype, 24
    progression, 14–15
    transformation, 14–15, 173–83
Neurospora crassa, 64
neutral filter elution, 106
NIH3T3 cell transformation assay,
    30, 33
nitrosamines, 10, 92–93
nondisjunction, 36, 45
no observable effect dosage, 250
nuclear magnetic resonance, 105, 113
nucleoid sedimentation, 108
nucleotide excision, 130
nutrition and cancer, 6

occupational chemicals, carcinogeni-
    city of, 207–248
oncogene activation, 35
oncogenic viruses, 28
one-hit model, 252–253

paramecia, 9
parental DNA, 134
particulate-bound enzymes, 81–83
peripheral blood lymphocytes, 66

VOLUME VI
Applied Toxicology of Petroleum Hydrocarbons

Edited by H.N. MACFARLAND, Gulf Oil Corporation
C.E. HOLDSWORTH, American Petroleum Institute
J.A. MACGREGOR, Standard Oil of California
and M.L. KANE, American Petroleum Institute